The Lymphoid Leukaemias

The Lymphoid Leukaemias

Daniel Catovsky, MD, DSc (Med), FRCPath, MRCP
Professor of Haematology, Academic Department of Haematology and Cytogenetics,
Institute of Cancer Research, Royal Marsden Hospital, London

Robert Foa, MD
Associate Professor of Medicine, Dipartimento di Scienze Biomediche e Oncologia Umana,
Clinica Medica I, University of Turin, Turin, Italy

Butterworths
London   Boston   Singapore   Sydney   Toronto   Wellington

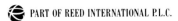
First published 1990

© Butterworth & Co. (Publishers) Ltd, 1990

British Library Cataloguing in Publication Data

Catovsky, Daniel
   The lymphoid leukaemias.
   1. Man. Blood. Leukaemia
   I. Title
   616.99419

ISBN 0-407-00259-6

Library of Congress Cataloging in Publication Data

Catovsky, D. (Daniel)
   The lymphoid leukaemias/Daniel Catovsky, R. Foa.
     p.   cm.
   Includes bibliographical references.
   ISBN 0-407-00259-6
   1. Lymphocytic leukemia. I. Foa, R. II. Title.
   [DNLM: 1. Leukemia. Lymphocytic.
WH 250 C366L]
RC643.C38   1990
616.99′419—dc20
DNLM/DLC
for Library of Congress   89-71252
                                 CIP

Composition by Genesis Typesetting, Borough Green, Kent
Printed in Great Britain at the University Press, Cambridge

Foreword

The lymphoproliferative diseases are unrivalled in the rich variety of their clinical presentations, natural history and pathological manifestations. Their devotees, infected with a passionate and life-long enthusiasm, have been called 'lymphomaniacs' by Alastair Robb-Smith, himself a distinguished pioneer. The authors of this book are outstanding members of the company and they are fortunate in having joined it at the most exciting stage in the development of their subject. Before the mid-1960s, work on the lymphoproliferative diseases had been largely based on the traditional methods of clinical observation and descriptive pathology. The discovery that most lymphocytes were either 'thymus-derived' or of 'bursa-equivalent' origin was soon followed by the invention of the hybridoma technique and the capacity to produce monoclonal antibodies. A torrent of research activity of unparalleled productivity poured out in all fields of biological enquiry including the lymphoid system and its pathology. Professor Catovsky and, a little later, Dr Foa, were among the first to apply the new technique to the study of the lymphoid leukaemias, and soon made original contributions of lasting value. The special merit of their research programme is its clinical orientation. They are skilled clinical haematologists with a wide experience in the management of all forms of lymphoproliferative disease, and between them they are equally skilled in cytomorphology, electron microscopy and cytogenetics. They are thus particularly well placed to explore the uncharted territory opened up by the new technology, and to interpret new discoveries whose message is often obscure if they are considered in isolation, but becomes apparent when methodically correlated with the findings of the traditional clinicopathological disciplines. This integrative approach is the secret of clinical research at its best, and explains the success of the authors' own research and of this book.

It is difficult for general haematologists to keep pace with the recent advances and to know how far their diagnostic and therapeutic strategies should be influenced by them. General physicians feel even more out of touch. The increasingly complex jargon of immunophenotyping means little to those who do not handle the reagents constantly. The authors have wisely introduced their readers to the basic methodology in their first chapter. Their lucid descriptions of clinical matters will also help non-clinical scientists to understand the clinical relevance of their work.

The authors have rendered outstanding service in bringing together the accumulated knowledge of the last decade, in the hope that their account will serve as a scaffold on which the new generation of molecular biologists will build for the practitioners of the next.

It is my privilege to have been associated with the authors for many years and I am delighted that the rich harvest I watched growing, and which they have now reaped, will be shared by so many others.

D. A. G. Galton
Formerly Honorary Director, MRC Leukaemia Unit and
Emeritus Professor of Haematological Oncology,
University of London, Royal Postgraduate Medical School

Preface

Major advances in diagnostic techniques in the last decade have made it necessary to revise and update our knowledge on the leukaemias arising from lymphoid cells. The application, world wide, of the current comprehensive system of immunophenotyping lymphocytes, led to the recognition of numerous subsets in each of the two known major B and T categories. The enormous heterogeneity thus revealed had to be incorporated rapidly into clinical practice. In this book we illustrate the advances which have resulted not only from the advent of monoclonal antibodies but also from the combined use of immunological studies with detailed morphological, ultrastructural, cytochemical and, more recently, molecular analyses. There are already many examples of how this approach has led to the recognition of discrete disease entities that differ in their natural history and prognosis and respond differently to certain treatments. Examples are hairy cell leukaemia and its variant form, prolymphocytic leukaemia (B and T types), splenic lymphoma with circulating villous lymphocytes and adult T-cell leukaemia/ lymphoma. The last named is also one of the best examples of the power of the combined and integrated clinical, morphological and phenotypic approach which, in this case, contributed to the epidemiology of the first human retrovirus, HTLV-I.

We hope that this book will be used as a multidisciplinary framework of the lymphoid leukaemias, constructed from the knowledge accumulated in the 1980s, onto which the discoveries in molecular mechanisms that are likely to emerge in the 1990s will be added. The non-random chromosome translocations with very specific breakpoints in most of the disorders described here are now being gradually interpreted at the molecular level and the new insight resulting from this should ultimately be clinically beneficial. The new methods include Southern blotting for the demonstration of immunoglobulin or T-cell receptor gene rearrangements to define B- and T-cell clonality and the polymerase chain reaction for the study of the Philadelphia chromosome in acute lymphoblastic leukaemia and the translocation t(14;18) in follicular lymphoma. We feel it is essential that the new advances should have direct clinical application and already the potential role of these techniques in the monitoring of minimal residual disease is beginning to be appreciated. These will also, directly or indirectly, reinforce the value of the traditional methods for the study of lymphoid malignancies because they acquire new significance and increased power when supported by the more precise information on underlying pathogenesis provided by the new methods.

We have written this book as haematologists, who are a unique breed working in the interface of pathology, oncology and clinical medicine. In some countries haematologists are only concerned with diagnosis (haematopathologists), in others only with treatment (haemato-oncologists) and perhaps, in most, with all aspects of clinical haematology, including advancing the frontiers of research. We hope that this book will be of interest to haematologists of all kinds, as well as to general physicians, oncologists, immunologists and scientists concerned with a better understanding of the mechanisms of lymphoid malignancies.

This book would not have been possible without the encouragement and the clinical laboratory contributions of many of our colleagues in London and Turin. We wish, first of all, to thank Professor Felice Gavosto who gave us the impetus to pursue this effort. We are particularly grateful for the elegant ultrastructural studies of Estela Matutes and Daniele Robinson who provided all the electron micrographs that illustrate the many morphological facets of the lymphoid leukaemias. The secretarial work initiated by Catherine Chmaj and completed by Wanda Malinowski has been extremely valuable.

Daniel Catovsky
Robert Foa
January 1990

Contents

Foreword   v

Preface   vii

List of abbreviations   xiii

1 Immunological markers   **1**
Introduction   1
Methodology   3
Immunological classification of lymphoid leukaemias   16
Lymphocyte functional assays   19

2 Acute lymphoblastic leukaemia   **32**
Introduction   32
Clinical features   32
Cytochemistry   36
Immunological classification   39
Prognostic factors   45
Special features of some ALL subtypes   47
Treatment   50
Pattern of relapse   54
Infectious complications   56
Bone marrow transplantation   57
Chromosome abnormalities   58
Epidemiology   64

3 B-cell chronic lymphocytic leukaemia   **73**
Introduction   73
Familial incidence   74
Clinical findings   75
Laboratory investigations   75
Prognostic factors   82
Staging systems   85
Complications   86
Transformation of B-CLL   90
Treatment   94
T-cell phenotype and function in B-cell leukaemias   100

Chromosome abnormalities in B-CLL   104
Tumour necrosis factor alpha (TNF) in B-CLL   106

4 T-cell chronic lymphocytic leukaemia/T-cell lymphocytosis   113
Introduction   113
Clinical and laboratory features   113
Diagnostic criteria   115
Differential diagnosis   118
Natural history and prognosis   120
Management   121
T-cell functional studies   123
Cytogenetic studies   126
Reactive or neoplastic nature of the T-cell proliferation   127

5 Prolymphocytic leukaemia   132
Introduction   132
Clinical and laboratory features   132
Diagnosis   133
Cytochemistry of B- and T-cell leukaemias   144
Prognosis and treatment   147
Chromosome abnormalities   150

6 Hairy cell leukaemia   156
Introduction   156
Clinical and laboratory features   156
Diagnostic features   157
Differential diagnosis   164
Prognostic features   165
Treatment   166
Complications and unusual associations   171
The origin of hairy cells   174
Special studies   177

7 The leukaemic phase of non-Hodgkin's lymphoma   182
Introduction   182
The classification of non-Hodgkin's lymphomas   182
Laboratory investigations for the study of NHLs in leukaemic phase 184
Incidence of a leukaemic phase   189
Prognostic significance   189
The leukaemic phase of follicular lymphoma   190
Intermediate or mantle zone (or centrocytic) NHL   195
Lymphoplasmacytic lymphoma   198
Splenic lymphoma with villous lymphocytes   199
Burkitt's lymphoma   205
Large cell NHL in leukaemic phase   207
Treatment of NHLs   209
Chromosome abnormalities in NHLs   212

8 Adult T-cell leukaemia/lymphoma   218
Introduction   218
Clinical features   218
Laboratory investigations   221

Histopathology of ATLL   228
The association of HTLV-I with ATLL   231
Epidemiology of ATLL   238
Prognosis and treatment   240
T-cell antigen receptor   243

9 Cutaneous T-cell lymphomas   **253**
Introduction   253
Clinical features   253
Diagnosis   256
Differential diagnosis   261
Natural history and prognosis   262
Treatment   264
Special studies   268
Chromosome abnormalities in CTCLs   269

10 Plasma cell neoplasias   **277**
Myelomatosis   277
Plasma cell leukaemia   294
Heavy chain disease   296
Waldenström's macroglobulinaemia   297
Special studies in plasma cell dyscrasias   299
T-cell abnormalities in multiple myeloma   300
Chromosome abnormalities   301

Index   **309**

List of abbreviations

ADA	adenosine deaminase
ALL	acute lymphoblastic leukaemia
AML	acute myeloid leukaemia
AMM	anterior mediastinal mass
ANAE	α-naphthylacetate esterase
Ara-C	cytosine arabinoside
ATLL	adult T-cell leukaemia/lymphoma
BACOD	bleomycin, doxorubicin (Adriamycin), cyclophosphamide, oncovin and dexamethasone
B-CLL	B-cell CLL
bcr	breakpoint cluster region
BMT	bone marrow transplantation
cALL	common-ALL
CD	cluster of differentiation
CGL	chronic granulocytic leukaemia
CHOP	COP + hydroxydaunorubicin
CLA	common leucocyte antigen
CLL	chronic lymphocytic leukaemia
CLL/PL	CLL with 11–55% prolymphocytes
CNS	central nervous system
COP	cyclophosphamide, oncovin and prednisolone
CR	complete remission
CTCL	cutaneous T-cell lymphoma
CyIg	cytoplasmic immunoglobulin
DAP	dipeptidylaminopeptidase
DCF	2′-deoxycoformycin
EBNA	EBV nuclear antigen
EBV	Epstein–Barr virus
E-rosettes	sheep RBC rosettes
ELISA	enzyme-linked immunosorbent assay
FAB	French–American–British
FL	follicular lymphoma
fl	femtolitres
HCL	hairy cell leukaemia
Ig	immunoglobulin
IHA	immune haemolytic anaemia

ITP	immune thrombocytopenic purpura
IL	interleukin
K cell	killer cell
LGL	large granular lymphocyte
LPL	lymphoplasmacytic lymphoma
M-BACOD	methotrexate plus BACOD
McAb	monoclonal antibody
MM	mulitple myeloma
M-rosettes	mouse RBC rosettes
NEP	neutral endopeptidase
NHL	non-Hodgkin's lymphoma
NK	natural killer
PB	peripheral blood
PCR	polymerase chain reaction
Ph	Philadelphia chromosome
PHA	phytohaemagglutinin
PTAs	parallel tubular arrays
PWM	pokeweed mitogen
RBCs	red blood cells
SLVL	splenic lymphoma with circulating villous lymphocytes
SmIg	surface (membrane) immunoglobulin
T-ALL	T-cell ALL
T-CLL	T-cell CLL
TCR	T-cell receptor
TdT	terminal deoxynucleotidyl transferase
T-LbLy	T-lymphoblastic lymphoma
TNF	tumour necrosis factor alpha
TPA	12-*O*-tetradecanoylphorbol-13-acetate
VAD	vincristine, Adriamycin (doxorubicin) and dexamethasone
VAMP	as VAD but methylprednisolone instead of dexamethasone
WBC	white blood cell

Chapter 1

Immunological markers

Introduction

Lymphoid leukaemias include, in a broad sense, all neoplasias arising from cells of the lymphoid lineage, from early lymphoblasts to mature plasma cells. As the term 'leukaemia' denotes blood and/or bone marrow involvement we will include in this account some of the non-Hodgkin's lymphomas, such as follicular lymphoma, in which leukaemic manifestations are common.

The characterization of haemopoietic cells has made remarkable progress in the last decade, particularly since the development of the hybridoma technology which has resulted in the production of a large number of monoclonal antibodies (McAbs) against previously unknown membrane antigens. Before this development the only tools available for studying the heterogeneity of lymphoid cells were rosetting methods and heteroantibodies to human immunoglobulins (Ig). The rapid expansion of this new technology and the wider use of monoclonal antibodies has

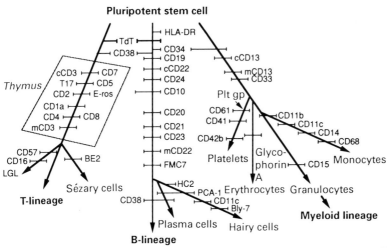

Figure 1.1 Scheme of haemopoietic differentiation from a common pluripotent stem cell into three major lineages: T-lymphoid, B-lymphoid and myeloid. The bars indicate the point at which specific antigens, recognized by monoclonal antibodies, appear on the maturing cells. Only the changes concerning the lymphoid lineage are discussed in this chapter

1

lead to a more precise knowledge of the antigenic changes during lymphoid differentiation. The numerous types of lymphoid malignancy which are now recognized reflect the heterogeneity of the lymphoid system and represent disorders arising from the various stages of B- and T-cell differentiation. The emerging picture, illustrated in Figure 1.1, based on information obtained using a number of monoclonal antibodies, is far from complete. Nevertheless, the prospect of a more precise characterization of the lymphoid cells involved in human neoplasias based on their membrane phenotype is becoming a reality today.

In parallel with advances in cellular immunology, other methods are also necessary for the analysis of leukaemic cell populations. All of them are important for a more accurate description of disease entities. One of them, the immunogold method[23], permits the simultaneous analysis of morphological features of single cells with immunological findings[85]. Ultrastructural morphology now plays a greater role in the cell characterization of lymphoid and myeloid malignancies[73].

The methodology currently available for the study of leukaemic cells with relevance to their cell origin, diagnosis and classification is outlined in Table 1.1.

Table 1.1 Methods for the study of leukaemic cells

Light microscopy	{	Morphology Cytochemistry
Electron microscopy	{	Cytochemistry Immunogold method
Lymphocyte markers	{	Rosetting methods Monoclonal antibodies SmIg and CyIg Terminal deoxynucleotidyl transferase Functional tests
Cytogenetics	{	Short-term cultures B- and T-cell mitogens Banding techniques
Molecular biology	{	Southern blot analysis for Ig and T-cell receptor gene rearrangement[a]

Abbreviations: Ig: immunoglobulin; SmIg: membrane Ig; CyIg: cytoplasmic Ig.
[a] See Chapters 2 and 8 respectively.

The description of the lymphoid markers will refer to them as applied by the authors and others to the study of individual patients. The advances in cytogenetics and molecular genetics have made it necessary to refer to these techniques in the account. Chromosome abnormalities are known to be specific to particular leukaemias and have also been shown to provide important clues about disease pathogenesis. The molecular analysis of DNA rearrangements of Ig genes and of T-cell receptor genes has improved our ability to detect the early signs of B- and T-cell differentiation. Such studies, now in active progress, have already yielded important information for the analysis of immature lymphoid cells[47] which are characteristic of acute lymphoblastic leukaemia (ALL) (see Chapter 2 for Ig genes and Chapter 8 for T-cell receptor genes). The possibility of defining monoclonality in T-cell chronic lymphocytic leukaemia (T-CLL) (see Chapter 4) and of clarifying the cell nature of hairy cell leukaemia, whose origin was disputed for many years (see Chapter 6), has also been advanced by the application of molecular biology techniques.

Methodology

There are many ways by which antigens or receptors can be demonstrated on the cell membrane and/or its cytoplasm. Rosetting methods are still used to demonstrate receptors for sheep red blood cells (RBCs) (E-rosettes), mouse RBCs (M-rosettes), the Fc portion of IgG (Fcγ) or IgM (Fcμ) (EA-rosettes) and for the third component of complement (EAC-rosettes). Most studies are carried out on cell suspensions from peripheral blood or bone marrow, usually mononuclear cell layers isolated by density gradient centrifugation, by direct or indirect immunofluorescence with fluorescein-conjugated antibodies. Reading of these preparations is carried out by means of fluorescence microscopy or by flow cytometry.

There is a growing tendency to utilize fixed cell preparations on cytocentrifuge-prepared slides or on blood or bone marrow films which can then be stained by the appropriate antibodies which are labelled with enzymes – peroxidase or alkaline phosphatase – which in turn can be demonstrated by appropriate cytochemical reactions. There are several advantages to such methods although they are, on the whole, more time consuming: (1) the slides can be examined with ordinary microscopes; (2) the preparations are permanent; (3) they permit better correlations with cell morphology; (4) they may require fewer cells for a particular test; (5) they may be more sensitive than a similar test performed on cell suspensions, for example the demonstration of Ig on B-cell chronic lymphocytic leukaemia (B-CLL) cells. Some antigens demonstrated by monoclonal antibodies

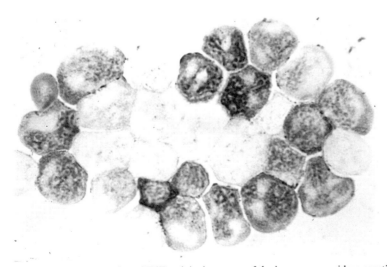

Figure 1.2 Demonstration of TdT activity by means of the immunoperoxidase reaction. The sample corresponds to a lymphoid–blast crisis of chronic granulocytic leukaemia (CGL). The TdT+ lymphoblasts have a dark stained nucleus and are smaller than the myeloid cells which are TdT− and are seen mainly in the centre of the preparation

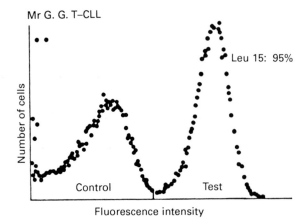

Mr G. G. T–CLL

Number of cells

Leu 15: 95%

Control   Test

Fluorescence intensity

Figure 1.3 Measurement of the immunofluorescence reaction in a sample from a case of T-CLL by means of an FACS analyser. The control cells represent the staining with the second layer without the monoclonal antibodies. The majority of cells in this sample reacted with the monoclonal antibody Leu15 (CD11b)

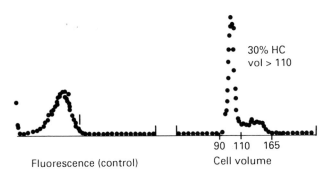

30% HC
vol > 110

Fluorescence (control)

90 110   165
Cell volume

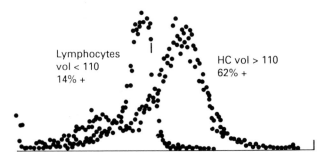

Lymphocytes
vol < 110
14% +

HC vol > 110
62% +

Fluorescence with McAb HC2

Figure 1.4 Example of the use of an FACS analyser in a sample of hairy cell leukaemia containing 30% hairy cells (HC) which can be recognized by their larger cell volume (>110). When the sample was stained with the monoclonal antibody HC2 25% of the mononuclear cells were positive. However, when the cells were gated according to their volume, 62% of the larger HC cells were shown to be positive whilst only a minority (14%) of those with a smaller volume were HC2+

do not react on fixed slides and others may not give the same result on slides as when studied in suspension. It is important to gain experience with particular reagents in order to ascertain when it is advantageous to use slides or suspensions. The enzyme terminal deoxynucleotidyl transferase (TdT) present in the nucleus of lymphoblasts is always investigated on slides[15] by immunofluorescence or immunoperoxidase (Figure 1.2). The use of fluorescence-activated cell sorters (FACS) offers the possibility of assessing accurately large numbers of cells in a short time (Figure 1.3). In some circumstances, for example in the study of hairy cell leukaemia cells, which can be identified by their large cell volume, the assessment of the reactivity with a particular monoclonal antibody by an FACS analyser has distinct advantages if the larger cells are 'gated' and the reactivity examined in that particular population (Figure 1.4).

The analysis of cell markers by immunological methods is not restricted to cell suspensions. The study of haemopoietic tissues (bone marrow, lymph nodes and spleen) may be carried out by immunohistochemical methods which often require the freezing of the initial biopsy specimen. Studies on tissue sections permit the examination of cells in their normal or pathological structural arrangement and, for the study of non-Hodgkin's lymphoma, this may have clear advantages.

Conventional B-cell markers

The presence of Ig on the membrane of B-cells (SmIg) is the chief distinguishing feature of these cells. It is also the best indicator of clonality in the B-cell disorders when the neoplastic cells are shown to have a single light chain[20]. The expression of SmIg assessed by the intensity of immunofluorescence (IF) staining increases with B-cell maturation and this is reflected in the B-cell leukaemias. B-CLL lymphocytes have weak expression of SmIg whilst cells of B-prolymphocytic leukaemia (B-PLL), B-cell non-Hodgkin's lymphoma and hairy cell leukaemia have strong SmIg staining.

The demonstration of Ig in the cytoplasm of fixed cells (CyIg) by immunofluorescence is used as a marker of B-cell differentiation[93]. Pre-B-cells lack SmIg but have a rim of cytoplasmic μ chain; plasma cells are also SmIg negative but have heavy and light chains (κ or λ) in the cytoplasm. When testing fixed cells, the immunoperoxidase method detects both SmIg and CyIg and is also more sensitive for the demonstration of SmIg, as demonstrated with B-CLL cells[59]. This advantage, however, should be weighed against the possibility of not being able to distinguish between SmIg and CyIg staining.

The binding of mouse RBCs (M-rosettes) is a specific B-cell feature and is a characteristic property of B-CLL lymphocytes. The binding to B-CLL cells is enhanced by pre-treatment of the lymphocytes with neuraminidase. The circulating cells in one-third of hairy cell leukaemia and follicular lymphoma cases also bind mouse RBCs although, as a rule, with lower percentages of M-rosettes than in B-CLL. Typical B-PLL cells only rarely form M-rosettes; the test is negative in the B-lineage blasts of ALL. The receptor for M-rosettes appears to be a distinct feature of B-CLL lymphocytes and of B-cells of intermediate maturation stages.

Conventional T-cell markers

The demonstration that sheep erythrocytes can bind to human leucocytes and form E-rosettes opened the way for the identification of T-lymphocytes. E-rosettes are best demonstrated by using AET-treated sheep erythrocytes[63] and this may be important when investigating immature T-lymphoblasts. In neoplastic T-cells with a mature membrane phenotype, notably Sézary cells, it is often necessary to treat also the lymphocytes with neuraminidase in order to increase the sensitivity of the E-rosette test. Sheep erythrocytes can be preserved adequately for at least 1 week and are available commercially in formalized preparations. E-rosettes are usually counted in suspension on chambers used for white blood cell (WBC) counts. E-positive cells can be examined in greater detail on cytocentrifuge made slides stained with Romanovsky stains. This permits the morphological identification of the E-positive cells which may be important when low proportions of abnormal T-cells or T-blasts are present in a sample which also contains normal T-lymphocytes.

The receptor for E-rosettes, which can now be recognized by a monoclonal antibody OKT11/Leu5 (CD2), is expressed on thymic cells at a later stage than the p40 antigen which characterizes early thymic or pre-thymic cells and is recognized by a monoclonal antibody of the CD7 cluster of differentiation (see Figure 1.1). E-rosettes are still a reliable, specific and easy to perform marker for normal and leukaemia T-cells. With the exception of pre-T-ALL, which by definition is E-rosette negative, 80% of T-cell disorders can be diagnosed by this test. There is a trend, however, to use monoclonal antibodies against T-cell antigens (see below) and these may have practical advantages and a greater reproducibility.

Monoclonal antibodies to B-cell antigens

There is now a wide range of reagents that recognize antigens present on the membrane of B-lymphocytes (Table 1.2). These antigens appear, and later disappear, at different stages during the process of differentiation from a B-cell precursor to a mature plasma cell. The characteristic constellation of antigens on a cell constitutes its membrane phenotype and this can be defined by the reactivity with several monoclonal antibodies. Because B-cell neoplasias arise from lymphocytes 'frozen' at different stages of B maturation, knowledge of the membrane phenotype not only permits a more objective characterization of these disorders but also helps to establish their cell of origin[4–6].

As shown in Table 1.2, many monoclonal antibodies are B-cell specific whilst others react also with cells of other lineages, e.g. anti-Ia and FMC8 (CD9). Of the B-cell-specific reagents, some react with most B-cells except for plasma cells, and are designated pan-B-markers, e.g. B4 (CD19), BA1 (CD24) and B1 (CD20), whilst others are restricted to particular maturation stages, e.g. B2 (CD21) in resting cells, FMC7 in mature B-cells, R1-3, PC-1 and PCA-1 in plasma cells. Several antigens are expressed on B-cells from very early stages before the expression of SmIg or CyIg. These cells have already rearranged their Ig genes, which is the first event during B-cell differentiation[47]. The pan-B monoclonal antibodies B4, BA1, B1 and J5 (CD10), which react with these early cells, are useful for the characterization of B-lineage ALL (see also Chapter 2). The value of a given monoclonal antibody will depend upon its specificity, the range of cells it reacts to (mature and/or immature), and the particular B-cell it helps to define, e.g. HC2 in activated B-cells and hairy cells.

Most antigens demonstrated by pan-B monoclonal antibodies can be equally demonstrated on the membrane and inside the cytoplasm of B-cells. Few others are expressed first in the cytoplasm and later on the cell membrane. One important

Table 1.2 Monoclonal antibodies against B-cell antigens[45a, 65a]

Monoclonal antibody[a]	Specificity	Mol.wt (kdal)	References
Anti-HLA-DR (OKIa[b])	Class II MHC ag; all B-cells except plasma cells; haemopoietic precursors; monocytes	29/34 (complex)	[33, 34, 56]
CD19 (B4[c]/Leu12[d])	Pan-B; all B-cells including precursors, except plasma cells	95	[67]
CD22 (Leu4[d], TO15)	Pan-B; early cytoplasmic expression (pre-B-cells) and late on the membrane (mature B-cells)	135	[21a, 60a, 77a, 94]
CD24 (BA1/L30)	Pan-B; as B4 but expressed slightly later in maturation	41/38	[3]
CD9 (FMC8[e]/BA2)	Not B-specific; early B-cells; PB B-cells; platelets; monocytes	24	[19, 44, 113]
CD10 (J5[c])[f]	Common ALL ag; pre-B-cells and follicular centre cells	100	[30, 45, 52, 84]
CD20 (B1[c]/Leu16[d])	Pan-B; mature B-cells except plasma cells	37/32	[68, 70, 98]
CD21 (B2[c])	B-restricted (resting B-cells); linked to EBV and C3d receptor CR2	140	[26, 69]
CD23 (MHM6)	Activated B-cells; Fce receptor	45–50	[23a, 29a, 112b]
Y29/55	PB and tissue B-cells; SmIg positive cells	Unknown	[28]
FMC7[e]	50% of PB B-cells; maturation linked ag	Unknown	[18, 22, 114]
HC1	Hairy cells; endothelial and epidermal basal cells	Unknown	[74, 75]
HC2	Hairy cells; activated B-cells	52–63	[74, 76]
R1-3	Late B-cells; plasma cells	Unknown	[87]
PC-1[c]	Plasma cells	28	[4]
PCA-1	Plasma cells; weakly expressed on monocytes and granulocytes	24	[6]
CD38 (OKT10[b])	B-precursors, germinal centre cells and plasma cells	45	[40, 83, 108]

Abbreviations: ag: antigens; CD: cluster of differentiation; EBV: Epstein–Barr virus; FMC: Flinders Medical Center; MHC: major histocompatibility complex; Mol. wt.: molecular weight; PB: peripheral blood.

[a] Listed according to the order in which they appear during B-cell differentiation.
[b] OKT series (Orthoclone).
[c] Coulterclone.
[d] Leu series (Becton Dickinson).
[e] Sera-Lab.
[f] Other monoclonal antibodies reactive with the same gp100: BA3, VIL-A1, AL2, anti-CALLA[d] and OKB-cALLA[b].

example is the monoclonal antibodies of the CD22 group (Table 1.2) which detect a cytoplasmic antigen on pre-B-cells and which only during the later stages of B-cell maturation are expressed on the membrane. Thus, in immature B-blasts (e.g. B-lineage ALL) and in B-CLL lymphocytes, CD22 will be only positive by immunocytochemical methods on fixed cells whilst on more mature B-lymphocytes (e.g. B-PLL cells and hairy cells) it will also be demonstrated by immunofluorescence on cell suspensions. Therefore the significance of a positivity with CD22 may be interpreted differently according to the method used.

For many years anti-Ia reagents were used for the characterization of B-cell disorders because most B-lymphocytes are positive and T-lymphocytes, except during activation, are negative. Nevertheless, HLA-DR determinants are not B-cell specific as they are also present in early haemopoietic cells and in monocytes. As more specific anti-B-cell monoclonal antibodies are now available, it is likely that they will replace the anti-Ia reagents for the typing of normal and leukaemic B-cells. The term 'HLA-DR' is commonly used to describe class II major histocompatibility complex (MHC) antigens. However, this designation may not be entirely adequate as there are at least three pairs of loci encoding for antigens in the HLA-D region: DP(SB), DR and DQ(DC)[34]. The majority of monoclonal antibodies used recognize common core determinants of products of these three different genes. Class II antigens are normally involved in antigen 'presentation' and are expressed differentially on the surface of certain cell types, including mononuclear phagocytes which ingest and process foreign antigens. Differences in the expression of these antigens are known to exist in some neoplastic B-cells. For example normal B-lymphocytes and follicular lymphoma cells are DP+, DR+, DQ+, whilst B-CLL cells, as well as non-T-ALL cells are DP+, DR+ but express DQ weakly or not at all[33, 34]. It is not clear whether these differences relate to the order in which these antigens are expressed during B-cell maturation, the suggested sequence being DP→DR→DQ, which parallels the order of the genes on chromosome 6[34], or to changes due to the leukaemic state.

The monoclonal antibodies of the CD10 cluster (e.g. J5), directed against the common-ALL (cALL) antigen, have similar reactivity to the rabbit anti-ALL-serum reported originally by Greaves; they all precipitate the same 100-kilodalton glycoprotein[30]. These reagents have been used for many years to define a distinct form of childhood ALL, cALL associated with good prognostic features. In recent years, partly as a result of studies on tissue sections, the cALL antigen has been found to be more widely expressed than previously recognized. For example, follicular centre cells, granulocytes and cultured tissue fibroblasts may be cALL+[16]. In the context of the non-Hodgkin's lymphomas (NHLs), this reactivity may be useful for the differential diagnosis between follicular lymphoma (FL) and other B-cell disorders (see Table 1.8).

The monoclonal antibody B2 (CD21) recognizes a 140-kdal protein which has two closely related, if not identical, binding sites, one for the C3d receptor CR2 and another for Epstein–Barr virus (EBV). Fingeroth et al.[26] have shown that CR2 is in fact the EBV receptor of human B-lymphocytes. The expression of B2 is restricted to resting B-cells at an intermediate stage of maturation. It is of interest that many B-CLL cases and two-thirds of B-NHLs are B2+[4] whilst hairy cells and plasma cells are B2−[5]. The absence of B2 and the expression of the plasma cell associated antigen PCA-1 on hairy cell leukaemia (HCL) cells suggests that hairy cells are late B-cells[5], a conclusion further supported by the reactivity with FMC7[22, 114] and HC2[76].

Of the monoclonal antibodies that react differentially with certain B-cells, FMC7 has been extensively studied in the authors' laboratory[22]. Table 1.3 summarizes their experience in chronic B-cell disorders. FMC7 is negative in the immature B-cells of non-T-ALL[18]. The most interesting feature of this monoclonal antibody is that it reacts only with a minority of B-CLLs, often in cases with strong SmIg and/or an increased proportion of prolymphocytes, and is consistently

Table 1.3 FMC7 in 250 cases of B-cell leukaemia

Disease	Number	Positive (%)[a]
B-CLL	157	22 (14)
B-PLL	32	28 (88)
HCL	30	30 (100)
LPL[b]	9	8 (89)
NHL/FL	22	11 (50)

[a] Percentage of positive cases; considering only those with 40%
or more FMC7+ lymphocytes.
[b] Includes cases of splenic B-cell lymphoma with villous
lymphocytes (SLVL; see Chapter 7).

positive in B-PLL, HCL and lymphoplasmacytic lymphoma (LPL). Although the properties of the antigen detected by FMC7 are not fully known, it has been suggested that its expression appears to be linked with B-cell maturation[114]. Findings with CD22 parallel, in general, those with FMC7 (e.g. membrane expression in B-PLL, HCL, LPL and B-NHLs) but these reagents do not detect the same antigenic determinants (Table 1.2).

Anti-hairy cell monoclonal antibodies
Several monoclonal antibodies with specificity for hairy cells have now been described[74–76, 94]. Posnett et al. reported two reagents, HC1 and HC2[74] that have recently been characterized further. HC1 reacts only with hairy cells and with no other normal or leukaemic B-cells and, in addition, with endothelial and epidermal basal cells[75]. HC2 is also specific for HCL[74, 76] as also shown by our experience in B-cell malignancies (Table 1.4 and Figure 1.4). In contrast to typical

Table 1.4 HC2 in chronic B-cell leukaemias

Disease	Number	Positive
HCL	30	29
HCL-variant	14	–
B-PLL/B-CLL	35	–
LPL/SLVL[a]	12	–

[a] Splenic lymphoma with villous lymphocytes (see Chapter 7).

HCL, the HCL-variant, a disease with intermediate features between HCL and B-PLL (see Chapter 6) is HC2−. In a few cases of acute myeloid leukaemia (AML) the blasts have also been found to express HC2[74]. HC2 reacts with some B-lymphoblastoid cell lines and with 2% of normal blood lymphocytes[76]. Normal HC2+ cells are more common in T-depleted fractions and bear SmIg of IgG class[76]. B-cell differentiation studies in vitro by means of pokeweed mitogen (PWM) and T-helper factors result in an increase in the number of HC2+ cells after 4–5 days of culture. The HC2+ cells are no longer present after 7 days' culture at the time of maximal plasma cell differentiation[76]. This supports the view that hairy cells are activated B-cells with features of pre-plasma cells as also demonstrated in studies with other monoclonal antibodies[5]. Our observations at the ultrastructural level with the immunogold method have shown that a minority of peripheral blood B-lymphocytes characterized by cytoplasmic villi react with HC1, HC2 and FMC7, therefore suggesting that these cells may be the normal counterparts of hairy cells[85].

Schwarting et al.[94] described a monoclonal antibody, anti-S-HCL-3 (Leu M5, CD11c) which recognizes a complex of 95 and 150 kdal which was present in the majority of cells of 40 cases of hairy cell leukaemia studied and was absent in cells from other B disorders. This monoclonal antibody, however, reacts also with monocytes, macrophages, follicular dendritic cells and 2% of normal lymphocytes. Although this reagent is not strictly specific for hairy cell leukaemia, the authors suggested that if used in combination with a second B-specific monoclonal antibody, which also reacts with hairy cells, it could possibly help to diagnose all cases of this disease[94]. This reagent (CD11c) is also positive in all cases of HCL-variant, although with weaker reactivity than in typical HCL cases. It may also react with circulating cells in some cases of splenic NHL. Very recently a new monoclonal antibody B-ly7[110a] has been shown to be specific for HCL – this has been confirmed in the authors' laboratory and was shown also to react with some of the HCL-variant cases.

Anti-plasma cell monoclonal antibodies
Three reagents which recognize antigens present in secretory B-cells or plasma cells have been described (see Table 1.2). Of these, PC-1 and PCA-1 have been extensively studied in B-cell malignancies and their reactivity has been found to be limited to plasma cell tumours, including myelomatosis, plasma cell leukaemia and Waldenström's macroglobulinaemia[4]. In addition, and as mentioned above, PCA-1 but not PC-1, is positive in hairy cell leukaemia[5]. R1-3 is another monoclonal antibody that reacts with plasma cells as well as with circulating B-lymphocytes in myeloma patients[87]. In the authors' experience R1-3 is positive in plasma cell leukaemia, including some cases in which the cells were morphologically poorly differentiated and difficult to identify as plasmablasts. Thus, it may now be possible to characterize normal and neoplastic plasma cells, not only by the absence of B-cell antigens, e.g. Ia, B4, B1, FMC7, but also by the presence of late antigens demonstrable by PC-1, R1-3 and PCA-1 as well as by the consistent presence of the ubiquitous antigen demonstrated by OKT10 (CD38)[4, 108].

The development of monoclonal antibodies to the late stages of B-cell maturation completes successfully the large battery of reagents now available for the study of B-cell malignancies. It can be predicted confidently that new monoclonal antibodies will continue to be developed, e.g. BL2 which detects a 68-kdal protein[46], and that a more precise characterization of those already available will be forthcoming. At the same time some reagents which created considerable interest in the early stages, e.g. FMC8/BA2 (CD9)[19, 44], may become less useful clinically, despite the fact that there is information about the 24-kdal protein recognized by these monoclonal antibodies, including the localization of its gene in chromosome 12[43].

Monoclonal antibodies to T-cell antigens

The study of T-cell malignancies has benefited greatly from the availability of a wide range of monoclonal antibodies specific for T-cell antigens[14, 31, 40, 83].

Some of these markers are positive with cells throughout most maturation stages (pan-T-markers) or react with cells at particular stages of differentiation, e.g. CD1a on cortical thymocytes. The monoclonal antibodies available for the characterization of normal and neoplastic T-cells are listed in Table 1.5. Some of these reagents are strictly T-cell specific, e.g. CD1a, CD2, CD3, CD4, CD8 etc. whilst others react also with cells of other lineages but are still useful in the context of the T-cell disorders, e.g. CD7, CD11b, CD25 etc.

Table 1.5 Monoclonal antibodies against T-cell antigens

Monoclonal antibody	Specificity	Mol.wt (kdal)	References
CD1a (T6[a]/Leu6[b])	Cortical thymocytes; Langerhans' cells	49	[56, 83]
CD2 (T11/Leu5)	Pan-T; receptor for sheep RBCs	50	[31, 110]
CD3 (T3/Leu4)	Mature T-cells; linked to T-cell receptor; CD3-complex (5 chains)	25, 20, 16	[48, 81]
CD4 (T4/Leu3)	Helper–inducer T-cells	56	[48, 79]
CD5 (T1/Leu1[c])	Pan-T; thymocytes and PB T-cells; B-CLL lymphocytes	67	[48, 57, 60, 78, 86]
CD7 (T16/Leu9[d])	Pan-T; T-cell precursors; thymocytes; PB T-cells	40	[34, 54, 99, 101]
CD8 (T8/Leu2)	Suppressor–cytotoxic T-cells	32	[80]
CD11b (OKM1/Leu15)	Cytotoxic–suppressor cells; NK cells; monocytes; granulocytes	95/165	[17, 49]
CD16 (Leu11)	NK cells; Fc receptor for IgG	50/70	[51]
CD25 (Anti-Tac)	Receptor for IL-2; activated T- and B-cells	55	[53, 105, 106]
CD29 (4B4[e])	Broad; helper CD4+ cells	135	[64a]
CD45R (2H4[e]/GRT2)	T-cell subset (suppressor–inducer)	220/205	[64a]
CD45RO (UCHL1)	T-cell subset (helper)	180	[97a]
CD57 (Leu7)	Cytotoxic T-cells; NK cells	110	[1, 2, 51]
Leu8	Subsets within the CD4 and CD8 lymphocytes; B-cells; monocytes	80	[29, 82]
BE1 and BE2	Sézary cells; T-cell subset	50/78	[11]
T17	Pan-T; 95% PB and thymic T-cells	Unknown	[61, 101]

Abbreviations: as in Table 1.2; IL-2: interleukin-2; NK: natural killer; UCH (T, L): University College Hospital Series[13].

[a] T1–T17: OKT series (Orthoclone).
[b] Leu1–Leu15: Leu series (Becton-Dickinson).
[c] UCHT2, T101, A50.
[d] 3A1, WT1.
[e] Coulterclone.

The first antigen which appears in the membrane during T-cell differentiation is a 40-kdal protein (see Figure 1.1) recognized by several monoclonal antibodies, e.g. 3A1, WT1 and Leu9 of the CD7 group. These reagents are extremely valuable for the identification of immature-T (lymphoblastic) proliferations, including pre-T-ALL (E-rosette negative), T-ALL and T-lymphoblastic lymphoma (T-LbLy)[54, 111]. Experience with CD7 confirms that all thymic-derived leukaemias are

Table 1.6 Pan-T markers in T-cell leukaemias[a]

Membrane phenotype	Positive cases (%)[b]			
	cCD3[c]	CD7	OKT17	E-rosettes
Thymic (TdT+)	100	100	70	70
Post-thymic (TdT−)	100	66	97	80
Overall	100	75	88	77

[a] Negative in other types of leukaemia except CD7 (3A1) which reacts with some AMLs.
[b] More than 25% reactive cells.
[c] Cytoplasmic staining by immunoperoxidase. When tested by immunofluorescence on cell suspensions 16% of thymic-derived ALLs and 73% of post-thymic T-cell leukaemias are CD3+ [77a].

positive. However, the expression of the p40 antigen is not constant in more mature T-cell proliferations (Table 1.6). CD7 is not expressed in non-T (B-lineage) ALL but it may be positive in some acute myeloid leukaemias (AMLs). Therefore, and as with many other reagents, its diagnostic value increases when used as part of a battery of cell markers, e.g. in combination with the assay for TdT the following patterns of reactivity can be observed in acute leukaemia: T-ALL, CD7+, TdT+; non-T-ALL, CD7−, TdT+; AML, CD7−/+, TdT−, with the rider that 20% AML cases may also be TdT+ (see below). Of the mature T-cell malignancies (TdT−, CD1a−), T-PLL is the only one in which CD7 is always positive; the reactivity in other cases, e.g. T-CLL, Sézary syndrome and adult T-cell leukaemia/lymphoma (ATLL), is variable, often being negative. Anti-p40 monoclonal antibodies have been thought to be useful reagents, when linked to ricin or other toxins, for 'purging' bone marrows for the purpose of autotransplantation in T-ALL[66].

OKT17 is a monoclonal antibody (non-clustered) that binds strongly an antigen expressed on T-cells throughout all stages of maturation, except in E-rosette negative (pre-T) blasts. Our experience with this monoclonal antibody (Table 1.6) shows that it is a good pan-T-marker, particularly for mature T-cell proliferations. T17 is not expressed in blasts from non-T-ALLs and AMLs[61]. The combination of CD7, T17 and TdT allows a good discrimination between pre-thymic (TdT+, CD7+, T17−), thymic (TdT+, CD7+, T17+) and post-thymic (TdT−, CD7−/+, T17+) proliferations[61]. Findings with other monoclonal antibodies are more well known. CD4 and CD8 antigens appear during thymic maturation where they are co-expressed with CD1a on cortical thymocytes. Upon further maturation they segregate into the two major T-lymphocyte subsets present in normal peripheral blood: CD3+, CD4+ or 'helper/inducer', and CD3+, CD8+, or 'suppressor/cytotoxic' (Figure 1.5). Mature T-lymphocyte malignancies are often CD4+, or CD8+, with variable expression of the CD3 antigen (see below).

The diagnostic importance of the CD3 complex antigen, which is part of the T-cell receptor (see Chapter 8), has been recognized recently. As for CD22 on B-cells, CD3 is synthesized and expressed first in the cytoplasm of very early T-cells (T-lymphoblasts) and can be demonstrated on fixed cells by immunocytochemical methods (e.g. immunoperoxidase, immunoalkaline phosphatase and also by immunofluorescence). Its demonstration is highly specific for T-cells and probably of greater diagnostic value in acute leukaemia than CD7, as the latter may also react in 20% of AML cases. Nevertheless, the combined finding of cytoplasmic CD3 (cCD3), CD7 and TdT is unique to T-lymphoblastic malignancies.

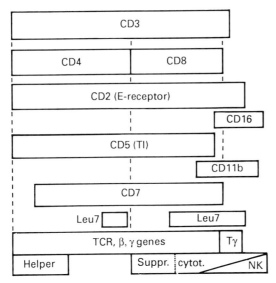

Figure 1.5 Diagram illustrating the major T-cell subsets in the peripheral blood and the overlapping reactivity with several of the monoclonal antibodies described in the text. The figure shows that the two major T-cell subsets CD4 (T4) and CD8 (T8) can be dissected further by some monoclonal antibodies, e.g. CD11b, and that sometimes this helped define T-cell subpopulations with a specific function. It also shows that T-lymphocytes rearrange the genes for the T-cell receptor (TCR) (see also Chapter 8). The figure does not include the further dissection of the CD4+ cells possible with the monoclonal antibodies CD29 (4B4), CD45R (2H4) and CD45RO (UCHL1) (see text)

Immunocompetent (mature or post-thymic) T-lymphocytes are the key components of both humoral and cellular immune response. It is apparent now that the division into two major cell subsets CD4 and CD8 within lymphocytes with phenotype CD3+ only corresponds broadly to the function of these cells (see below). The development of monoclonal antibodies that subdivide further the major subsets permits better definition of discrete functional subsets according to their phenotype (Figure 1.5). These reagents, Leu7 (CD57), Leu11 (CD16) and Leu15/OKM1 (CD11b), have increased the possibility of recognizing distinct T-cell populations. Because the post-thymic T-cell leukaemias are monoclonal expansions of some of these subsets, the unusual phenotypes observed in some cases facilitate the recognition of rare T-cell types which are otherwise difficult to identify in normal blood. Examples of this are the CD4+ cells of ATLL which display suppressor function in vitro. These cells may correspond to a minor subset of radiosensitive CD4+ cells which exert potent feedback suppression upon activation by pokeweed mitogen[100].

The monoclonal antibodies CD57, CD16 and CD11b have been generally regarded as defining cytotoxic cells, in particular natural killer (NK) cells, and have been used to define a third population of human lymphocytes with large granular morphology and Fc receptors for IgG (Tγ cells)[1, 10, 36]. As shown in Figure 1.5 the correspondence with NK function is good with CD16, especially in lymphocytes which are CD16+, CD57−[51]. On the other hand, CD57+, CD3+ cells have a low cytotoxic capacity compared with CD57+, CD3− (CD11b+) cells[2] (Figure 1.5). CD11b may identify the suppressor cells within the CD8 subset; CD8+, CD11b− cells may correspond to cytotoxic T-cells[49].

It has been suggested that the monoclonal antibody Leu8, which recognizes an 80-kdal protein, dissects both the CD4+ and CD8+ cells into functional subsets[28, 32]. Recent studies have disclosed another group of monoclonal antibodies which identify molecules of the common leucocyte antigen (CD45) and which may define functional CD4+ subsets. Two antibodies, 2H4 and GRT22, of the CD45R (restricted) group recognize the high-molecular-weight forms (220/205 kdal) of the common leucocyte antigen (see Table 1.5) and identify the 'naive/virgin' T-cell populations that function as 'suppressor–inducer' cells in vitro. Two other reagents, 4B4 (CD29) and UCHL1 (CD45RO) (see Table 1.5) characterize non-identical 'memory' cells that proliferate to soluble recall antigens and provide help in antigen-specific IgG synthesis. Two mutually exclusive CD4+ subsets have been described in normal peripheral blood: CD45R+, CD29−, UCHL1− (suppressor–inducer) and CD45R−, CD29+, UCHL1+ (helper). It is not clear whether these subsets are separate and derive from a common precursor[64a] or whether they represent different maturational stages within a single lineage but with different functions[13a, 22a]. Despite these findings, in normal CD4+ subsets we have documented a high incidence (47%) of co-expression of CD45R and CD29 in leukaemias of immunologically mature CD4+ lymphocytes[112a].

On a separate issue, UCHL1 is an excellent reagent for use as a T-cell marker in sections of paraffin-embedded tissues (e.g. bone marrow, lymph node etc.), although a negative result does not exclude T-cell lineage.

The importance of the CD3 antigen has been highlighted by evidence that it is part of the T3–T1 complex that constitutes the antigen receptor of human T-lymphocytes[81] (see also Chapter 8). This structure is present in all mature T-cells and will recognize foreign antigens in the presence of major histocompatibility complex gene products – class I in the case of CD3+, CD8+ cells, and class II in the case of CD3+, CD4+ lymphocytes. The monoclonal antibody to the CD3 complex or to a 90-kdal heterodimer constituted by two polypeptide chains linked by a disulphide bond, will block antigen-specific T-cell function and will activate resting T-lymphocytes in the presence of antigen-presenting cells[81].

Monoclonal antibodies against neoplastic T-cells
By analogy to the anti-B-cell monoclonal antibody raised against hairy cells, a few reagents react specifically with some leukaemic T-cell types. These are the monoclonal antibodies BE1 and BE2[11] raised against Sézary cells and SN1[95] and SN2[96] that appear to react exclusively with T-ALL cells. Our experience with BE2, described in Chapter 9 (see Table 9.2), confirms that this is a useful reagent for the characterization of Sézary cells. The monoclonal antibody SN2 is different from other anti-T-cell reagents in that it does not react with normal T-cells or thymocytes. Studies with these 'leukaemia'-specific monoclonal antibodies have been limited and we have to await further work confirming their apparently unique specificity to malignant T-cells.

Monoclonal antibodies against the receptor for interleukin-2 (IL-2)
The monoclonal antibody anti-Tac (CD25)[105, 106] that reacts specifically with the receptor of IL-2[53] has been shown to be of importance, not only for the study of normal T-cells but also as a useful marker for the differential diagnosis of T- and B-cell malignancies. Activated T-cells express, upon stimulation, receptors for IL-2 and are anti-Tac+; normal resting T-lymphocytes are anti-Tac−. The reactivity

with anti-Tac was initially regarded as unique to ATLL, a disease in which the cells are infected with the human T-cell leukaemia virus HTLV-I. Recently it was found that, although with lower density of IL-2 receptors than in ATLL, other neoplastic cells are also positive, notably hairy cells, which, as discussed above, correspond to activated B-lymphocytes. The authors' experience with this monoclonal antibody is summarized in Table 1.7. It is clear from Table 1.7 that CD25 is a useful reagent for cell characterization studies. The observations described in ATLL cells correspond

Table 1.7 CD25 (anti-Tac) in lymphoproliferative disorders

Disease	No. tested	Positive
ATLL	15	14
T-PLL	12	4
CTCL	8	2
T-ALL, T-CLL	26	1
HCL	30	29
HCL-variant	14	0
Other B-cell leukaemias[a]	27	9[b]

[a] B-CLL, B-PLL, non-Hodgkin's lymphoma, plasma cell leukaemia.
[b] Weakly positive in > 30% of cells, mostly B-CLL.

mainly to blood samples. All but one of the typical hairy cell leukaemia cases studied were positive; most cases of HCL-variant are CD25−. Rarely, other T- or B-cell leukaemias show a proportion of positive cells. These may in fact reflect the state of activation of the respective B- and T-lymphocytes. This should not be surprising if it is considered that the stimulation in vitro with specific mitogens results in the development of Tac+ cells in T-PLL (using phytohaemagglutinin) and B-cell CLL and PLL (using Epstein–Barr virus or mitogens).

Monoclonal antibodies reactive with B- and T-cell antigens
There are three monoclonal antibodies: T1/Leu1 (CD5), RFB1 and OKT10 (CD38) which react with antigens normally expressed on early thymocytes and on T-lymphocytes at different stages of maturation, and which are also positive on neoplastic B-cells. This, in turn, has provided useful information for the purposes of diagnosis and classification.

CD5 reacts with a p67 antigen present with increasing density from immature to mature T-lymphocytes[40, 60, 78]. The p67 antigen is consistently demonstrated on B-CLL cells[60] whilst it is frequently absent or inconsistently expressed in cells from other B-cell disorders. CD5 is always negative in hairy cell leukaemia and plasma cell tumours. The cluster CD5 monoclonal antibodies are extremely useful for the phenotypic characterization of the B-CLL lymphocyte: M-rosettes+, SmIg±, CD5+, and for the identification of its cell of origin in normal lymphoid tissues (see Chapter 3). Paradoxically CD5 is often negative in T-CLL cells, particularly in cases with the common phenotype CD3+, CD4−, CD8+. One of the CD5 antibodies, T101, has been used successfully for imaging procedures in

T-cell lymphomas after labelling with indium-111 (^{111}In)[21]. The cells of a non-Hodgkin's lymphoma with intermediate features (mantle-zone or diffuse centrocytic) are also CD5+ (see also Chapter 7).

RFB1 reacts with early haemopoietic precursors of various lineages and persists through the T-lineage up to mature T-cells[14, 40] but it is negative in pre-B-cells and mature B-lymphocytes. This reagent was found by us to be positive in the cells of all cases of B-CLL and HCL[62]. Because RFB1 is strongly expressed on hairy cells, which are CD5−, it is likely that these monoclonal antibodies react with different antigens. This is further supported by the presence of the RFB1 antigen in early myeloid and erythroid cells[14] which are CD5−.

OKT10 (CD38), like RFB1, reacts with immature T-cells and bone marrow precursors[40, 83], and with cells at late stages of B-cell differentiation[108]. Although the CD38 antigen is absent from mature B- and T-cells, it becomes positive upon mitogenic stimulation. The gene for this antigen has recently been assigned to chromosome 4. OKT10 is a useful monoclonal antibody for the characterization of plasma cell dyscrasias, such as lymphoplasmacytic lymphoma (LPL) and myelomatosis (MM). In 10 cases of plasma cell leukaemia studied by the authors, some of them presenting difficulties for the diagnosis by light microscopy morphology, it has been shown that the demonstration of the phenotype SmIg−, Ia−, CD20−, CD19−, CD38+, CyIg+ helped to classify the neoplastic cells as plasma cells.

The monoclonal antibody Ki-1 (CD30)[92], which reacts with Reed–Sternberg cells, has recently been found to react with activated B- and T-cells suggesting that in some types of Hodgkin's disease the typical cells may be of B- or T-cell derivation.

Immunological classification of lymphoid leukaemias

Markers of B-cell malignancies

The most immature cells of the B-lineage are represented by the lymphoblasts of non-T-ALL, disease which includes null, common and pre-B-ALL. The earliest feature of B-cell differentiation in these cells is the rearrangement of the Ig genes[47], and the appearance on the cell membrane of early antigens such as CD19, CD24, CD10 and cytoplasmic CD22[4]. These aspects will be described in more detail in Chapter 2 along with the immunological classification of ALL.

The chronic B-lymphoproliferative disorders are monoclonal proliferations of mature B-lymphocytes. As a rule these diseases affect mainly adults and, in a wide sense, they can include the non-Hodgkin's lymphomas of B-cell type. Here the discussion will be restricted to cases with frequent blood and bone marrow involvement. The contribution of marker studies, chiefly monoclonal antibodies, to the diagnosis of these disorders is summarized in Table 1.8. More information on the membrane phenotype of the various diseases is given in Chapters 3, 5, 6, 7 and 10.

Table 1.8 shows that with a battery of reagents it is possible to characterize precisely the immunological profile of each disease which in turn represents the clonal expansion of B-cells at different stages of maturation. This information adds significant diagnostic power to the morphological and histological analysis which is the basis for the classification of these disorders. The phenotype of B-CLL, which corresponds to a relatively immature B-cell, is quite distinct from the phenotype of

Table 1.8 Membrane markers in chronic B-cell malignancies

Marker(s)	B-CLL	B-PLL	NHL[a]	HCL	MM/WM[b]
M-rosettes	+ +	−	−/+	−/+	−
SmIg[c]	±	+ +	+ +	+ +	−
B1/B4/Ia	+	+	+	+	−
T1(CD5)	+	−/+	−	−	−
B2(CD21)	−/+	+	+	−	−
J5(CD10)	−	−/+	+	−	−
FMC7	−/+	+	+	+	−
Tac/HC2	−[d]	−	−	+[e]	−
PCA-1	−	−	−	+	+
OKT10	−	−	−	−	+

[a] Findings correspond mainly to follicular non-Hodgkin's lymphoma (NHL) with blood and bone marrow involvement.
[b] Myelomatosis (MM), Waldenström's macroglobulinaemia (WM) and plasma cell leukaemia.
[c] Fluorescence intensity.
[d] Anti-Tac weakly positive in some B-CLL (see Table 1.7).
[e] HCL-variant cases are CD25− and HC2− (see Tables 1.4 and 1.7).

late stage B-cells or plasma cells. Some combinations of markers are unique to some diseases, e.g. M-rosettes, CD5, CD23 and weak SmIg in B-CLL; CD21, CD10 and FMC7 in non-Hodgkin's lymphomas; FMC7, CD25, CD11c and PCA-1 in hairy cell leukaemias; and PCA-1, PC-1 and CD38 in plasma cell dyscrasias.

Markers of T-cell malignancies

There are two main groups of T-cell leukaemia/lymphoma according to the stage of maturation of the neoplastic T-cells:

1. Those in which the cells are blasts and have an immature (thymic and pre-thymic) phenotype. These include pre-T-ALL, T-ALL and T-lymphoblastic lymphoma (T-LbLy)[12, 31] and affect mainly children and young adults.
2. Those in which the T-cells are mature (post-thymic) and morphologically well differentiated. These include T-CLL, T-PLL, ATLL and the cutaneous T-cell lymphomas (CTCLs), Sézary syndrome and mycosis fungoides, and affect mainly adults.

A common feature of the immature T-cell malignancies is the presence of TdT in the cell nucleus[15, 31], CD3 in the cytoplasm and the p40 antigen, detected by CD7, on the cell membrane (Table 1.9). The division between pre-T- and T-ALL may be semantic but it defines pre-T-cells as being E-rosette negative; these also express in some cases the cALL antigen. T-ALL cells are slightly more immature than those of T-LbLy[12, 31]; this difference may be useful for the differential diagnosis of cases presenting with an anterior mediastinal mass. T-LbLy cells often have the phenotype of cortical thymocytes (CD1a+, CD4+, CD8+); in a minority of cases they also express membrane CD3[12].

Mature T-cell proliferations are always TdT− and CD1a− (Table 1.10) and have a rather heterogeneous expression of the late T-cell antigens. T-PLL, ATLL and CTCL are nearly always disorders of the CD4+, CD8− subset; T-CLL frequently, but not always, is a disorder of CD8+, CD4−, CD57+ lymphocytes. T-PLL is the only one of these conditions that expresses strongly the p40 antigen (CD7) in

Table 1.9 Membrane phenotype of immature (TdT+) T-cell malignancies

Marker[a]	Pre-T-ALL	T-ALL	T-LbLy
cCD3	+	+	+
CD7	+	+	+
CD5	+/−	+	+
CD2	−	+	+
CD1a	−	−/+	+
mCD3	−	−	−/+

[a] Ordered according to their expression during T-cell maturation.

c = cytoplasmic; m = membrane.

Table 1.10 Membrane phenotype of mature (TdT−, CD1a−) T-cell leukaemias

Monoclonal antibody	T-CLL	T-PLL	ATLL	CTCL
CD2	+	+[a]	+[a]	+[a]
CD3	+	+[a]	+[a]	+
CD4	−[b]	+[c]	+	+
CD5	−[b]	+	+	+
CD7	−	+	−	−
CD8	+[b]	−[c]	−	−
CD25	−	−[d]	+[e]	−[d]
OKT17	+	+	+	+
BE2	−	−	−/+	+

[a] Negative in 20% of cases (low % of E-rosettes; weak membrane staining with CD3).
[b] 15% of T-CLL cases CD5+, CD4+, CD8−.
[c] Some cases CD4−, CD8+ and some CD4+, CD8+.
[d] Positive in some cases (see Table 1.7).
[e] Details in Table 8.3 (see Chapter 8).

almost all cases studied; these, as well as other features, suggest that T-prolymphocytes may be slightly more immature T-cells.

Markers of acute leukaemia

The distinction between ALL (T- and B-lineages) and acute myeloid leukaemia (AML) is now greatly facilitated by the routine use of the TdT assay[15, 39] and some monoclonal antibodies, e.g. My7/MC52 (CD13), My9 (CD33)[32] and 3C5 (CD34)[103], for the diagnosis of AML subtypes, and the reagents discussed earlier for characterizing the various ALL subtypes, chiefly CD19, CD3 and CD7 (Table 1.11). The use of an immunological approach does not preclude, for AML, the use of good morphological preparations and some standard cytochemical methods, e.g. Sudan black B and myeloperoxidase for M1, M2 and M4, and α-naphthyl acetate esterase for the diagnosis of M4 and M5. Further improvements in the classification of AML derive from the recognition of megakaryoblastic leukaemia or M7 by means of monoclonal antibodies specific to platelet glycoproteins[91, 107].

Table 1.11 Distinction between ALL and AML subtypes

Marker[a]	ALL		AML		
	T-ALL	Non-T[b]	M1	M2	M3/4/5
My9 (CD33)[c]	−	−	±/+	+	+
3C5 (CD34)	−	+	+	+/−	−
B4 (CD19)	−	+	−	−	−
TdT	+	+	−/+	−	−
3A1 (CD7)	+	−	±	−	±
CD3	+	−	−	−	−

[a] Only reagents which are of value for the differential diagnosis are included.
[b] Null, common and pre-B-ALL.
[c] Other useful reagents for the diagnosis are monoclonal antibodies of the CD13 group (My7, MCS2). Cases of early AML with negative cytochemistry (hence designated M0) are often shown to be myeloid by monoclonal antibodies of the CD13 or CD33 groups[73a].

Pitfalls in the use of monoclonal antibodies on AML cells
When detecting membrane antigens in AML cells, particularly the monocytic subtypes M4 and M5, there should be an awareness of a number of pitfalls which could render the use of monoclonal antibodies inaccurate. False positive results are common in these cases unless special precautions are taken to avoid the non-specific binding of IgG molecules to the high affinity Fc receptor of monocytic cells. Both the first layer, mouse IgG (McAb), and the second layer, goat or rabbit IgG (fluorescein isothiocyanate – FITC), can stick non-specifically to the Fc receptor. When the problem is the second layer, this is easy to detect because the omission of the monoclonal antibody, which is one of the usual controls, will still render the test positive. The solution to this problem is the use of F(ab)$_2$ fragments of IgG as second layer reagents; this control should always be negative.

The false positivity due to the non-specific binding of the first layer, more common when the monoclonal antibody is of the IgG2 class, is not easy to detect unless many monoclonal antibodies are used and some are unexpectedly positive. The routine use of one or more irrelevant first layers as controls, preferably of the same IgG class as the monoclonal antibody, should suffice to detect the problem. To avoid this non-specific binding of the monoclonal antibody (first layer) it is necessary to block the Fc receptors with human or rabbit sera. A 2% dilution of human AB serum is used routinely; it is possible that the use of aggregated IgG, as applied originally to demonstrate Fc receptors on B-cells, may be even better. In this case one should also be aware that the attachment of AB serum or aggregated IgG will give positive reactions if anti-Ig reagents are used; with monoclonal antibodies the results should usually be negative.

Lymphocyte functional assays

Functional analyses have become increasingly important in view of the well recognized heterogeneity of lymphoid cells (see Figure 1.5). The availability of tests capable of exploring the properties of given lymphocyte subsets has allowed correlations to be made between the phenotypic expression and the function of normal and leukaemic cells.

Table 1.12 T-cell related functions

1. Proliferative response to mitogens (PHA, ConA), antigens or alloantigens (mixed lymphocyte reaction)
2. Helper function
3. Suppressor function
4. Natural killer (NK) capacity
5. Antibody-dependent cell-mediated cytotoxicity (ADCC) or killer (K) function
6. T-cell growth in vitro: colonies, cell lines, clones
7. Release of soluble factors
8. Interaction with other haemopoietic lineages

The most frequently employed in vitro T-cell functional assays are listed in Table 1.12. The development of B-cell functional tests has lagged behind those for T-lymphocytes but new information has become available about culture systems which permit the growth of B-cell colonies and the immortalization of normal and neoplastic B-lymphocytes by means of the Epstein–Barr virus (EBV). We will also refer to methods that examine the interaction between lymphoid cells and myeloid and erythroid precursors, in view of the implication of T-cell proliferations in the pathogenesis of cytopenias and immunoparesis in B- and T-lymphoid leukaemias.

Lymphocyte transformation

Normal circulating T-lymphocytes can be induced to proliferate following various stimuli (Table 1.12). The test most frequently employed is based on their response to plant mitogens, usually phytohaemagglutinin (PHA). This technique is relatively simple and measures the transformation of small lymphocytes to blast cells by morphological means and/or by the uptake of tritiated thymidine during the last few hours of a 3-day culture as an index of DNA synthesis. An optimal T-lymphocyte response to PHA requires the presence of accessory cells, namely monocytes/macrophages, which act via the production of interleukin-1 (IL-1).

Cell proliferation represents the final event of a complex multistep process which activates the responding cells from a resting state or G_0 through G_1, S and G_2 phases leading to mitosis or M phase. Numerous factors are known to contribute to this process. The mitogen or antigen stimulates the lymphocyte to enter G_1; the trigger for DNA synthesis (S phase) is provided by a different signal which is probably a soluble factor. Following activation lymphocytes express on their membrane receptors for T-cell growth factor or interleukin-2 (IL-2) which can be demonstrated by the monoclonal antibody CD25[53, 105]. The release of IL-1 by accessory cells is important in this first stage; some activated lymphocytes then produce IL-2 which triggers the progress through the cell cycle. The T-lymphocyte population responsive to PHA is included within the helper/inducer (CD4+) subset; the suppressor/cytotoxic (CD8+) T-cells respond poorly to PHA.

T-colony growth

Several methods have been used in the last 10 years to obtain the formation in vitro of T-lymphocyte colonies from normal peripheral blood and bone marrow. These include one or two step procedures, pre-incubation with the appropriate mitogen (usually PHA), addition of stimulating factors etc.[24, 27, 55]. The presence of accessory cells or of leucocyte-conditioned media or of a leucocyte-rich underlayer is essential, and this suggests that optimal growth is not obtained in the presence only of the mitogen[27, 55]. Both IL-1 and IL-2, released in culture or added exogenously, play a key role in the formation of T-colonies.

T-colony growth seems to be a property of CD4+, Tμ lymphocytes. This assay has now been applied to the study of lymphoproliferative disorders[27]. A reduced or absent colony forming capacity is a feature of the majority of mature T-cell leukaemias despite the presence of the CD4 antigen on their cells, e.g. in T-PLL and CTCL (see Table 1.10). It is likely that in these disorders the abnormal proliferation involves a subset of CD4+ cells with low colony forming capacity or, alternatively, that an intrinsic functional defect exists in the neoplastic population. T-colony assays have also been employed to investigate the functional behaviour of the residual T-cell population in chronic B-cell leukaemias (see Chapter 3). T-colony growth is usually depressed in both B-CLL and B-PLL whilst it is preserved in most patients with hairy cell leukaemia.

Helper and suppressor function

The ability of T-cells to promote or inhibit the maturation of B-lymphocytes into antibody-producing plasma cells can be assessed in vitro by a number of techniques[88]. The helper assay is based on the co-culture of isolated normal peripheral blood B-cells with the allogeneic T-cell population to be tested in the presence of pokeweed mitogen (PWM) as polyclonal B-cell activator. After 7 days' culture the proportion of viable cells expressing CyIg is scored by immunofluorescence and compared with the control culture which includes only B-cells. The suppressor function is evaluated by adding T-cells, which contain the suppressor cells, to the previous culture and assessing the reduction in the proportion of CyIg-positive cells. There are technical limitations to such a technique which can now be overcome by using methods which measure the release of Ig in the supernatant of cultures by radioimmunoassay or enzyme-linked immunosorbent assay (ELISA) systems[88]. The capacity of T-cells to suppress the proliferative response to PHA or concanavalin A (ConA) has also been used as a measure of T-cell function but it is not clear how this effect correlates with the suppression assessed in a PWM-driven system.

Results with isolated T-cell subsets indicate that the helper function resides mainly within the CD4+ subset whilst the CD8+ fraction contains most suppressor cells[82]. This phenotypic and functional subdivision is in fact an oversimplification. New monoclonal antibodies directed against minority T-cell subsets, e.g. CD45RA or 2H4, CD45RO or UCHL1 and improved separation techniques have permitted a clearer definition of functional behaviour of lymphocyte subpopulations. For this purpose the advent of cell sorting techniques has been of great value. It has now been established that the helper function resides in 20% of CD4+ lymphocytes (see Figure 1.5)[82] and that a small subset of CD4+ cells is also capable of exerting suppressor activity[101]. It has also been shown that the suppressor function exerted by radiosensitive CD8+ cells requires the collaboration of radiosensitive CD4+ cells to induce maximum suppression[100].

This well-documented phenotypic and functional T-cell heterogeneity gained further confirmation from studies on the various forms of T-cell leukaemia (Table 1.13) which are characterized by the clonal expansion of different T-cell subsets. Table 1.13 also illustrates that functional assays are important to characterize more

Table 1.13 Functional heterogeneity in T-cell leukaemias[a]

Phenotype	Function	Leukaemia
CD4	Helper	CTCL, T-PLL
	Suppressor	ATLL (CTCL)
	Pro-suppressor	ALL[b]
	None recognized	T-PLL
CD8	Suppressor	
	K (NK)	T-CLL
CD4−, CD8−, CD11b+	NK (K)	T-CLL

[a] More details are given in the chapters describing the various T-cell disorders.
[b] From Broder et al. [17a].

precisely leukaemic T-cell populations which have, otherwise, a similar membrane phenotype when tested by monoclonal antibodies.

Cytotoxic assays

Natural killer (NK) cells and antibody-dependent killer (K) cells are thought to represent an important defence mechanism against tumours and virus infections. NK cells have the ability to lyse spontaneously different targets including fresh cells and several tumour cell lines, whilst K cells lyse only antibody-coated target cells (ADCCs). Lysis is measured as the percentage of ^{51}Cr released by labelled target cells compared with the spontaneous release in the presence of medium alone (Figure 1.6)[71, 109].

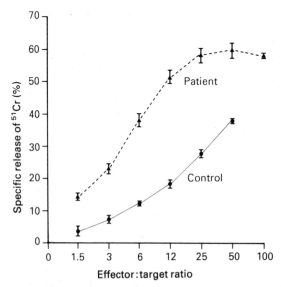

Figure 1.6 Example of the assessment of antibody-dependent cell-mediated cytotoxicity (ADCC) activity with a sample of normal lymphocytes. Killer activity is measured by the release of ^{51}Cr from labelled target cells (p815 mastocytoma cells) sensitized with IgG in an exponential fashion upon the increase of the number of effector (cytotoxic) cells

Although some degree of cytotoxic function is found within the T-cell population (mostly in the CD8 subset), it is generally agreed that this activity resides principally within a non-T-, non-B-cell population of cells named large granular lymphocytes (LGLs) characterized by the presence of azurophilic granules in the cytoplasm[102]. These cells are non-adherent, express receptors for the Fc portion of IgG and are capable of forming E-rosettes (50% of them)[10, 36]. Several monoclonal antibodies (i.e. CD11b, CD57, CD16) react with the majority of human NK and K lymphocytes (see above). The cells in most cases of T-CLL have, in our experience, the morphology and phenotype of LGLs and function in vitro as K and/or NK cells (Table 1.13; see also Chapter 4).

T-cell growth factor and T-cell lines

It has become possible, in the last few years, to promote the long-term proliferation of T-cells. A key event for this development was the discovery of interleukin-2 (IL-2)[65] which is a small molecule of 15 kilodaltons which promotes T-cell growth. The gene of IL-2 has been mapped onto the long arm of chromosome 4[97].

IL-2 can be detected in the supernatant of mitogen-stimulated peripheral blood mononuclear cells. Several methodological modifications have been attempted in order to improve the release of IL-2 and to standardize its production. This has been necessary as the titres of IL-2 may vary greatly from culture to culture. Some of the modifications employed include the use of pooled donors, pooled tonsils, addition of the phorbol diester 12-O-tetradecanoylphorbol-13-acetate (TPA), depletion of adherent cells and culture times between 36 and 48 hours. Considerable amounts of mitogen-free IL-2 can be obtained from some leukaemic T-cell lines. IL-2 can now be produced by molecular DNA recombinant technology and this will facilitate its availability in large amounts and in well-defined titres.

The modalities of long-term culture of normal and leukaemic T-cells may represent a discriminating feature. T-lymphocytes from normal blood can grow in the presence of IL-2 after prior antigen or lectin stimulation[65] and this in turn activates the IL-2 receptor which allows the T-cell to respond to the proliferative stimuli. Some leukaemic T-cells of mature, post-thymic origin, i.e. from ATLL, may grow in the presence of purified (lectin-free) IL-2 alone without the need of mitogenic stimulation[89]. The stimulus in these ATLL cells is probably provided by the presence of HTLV-I in its genome. Certain leukaemic T-cell lines originated from immature T-lymphoblasts have, on the other hand, been grown spontaneously without the addition of exogenous growth factor(s).

T-cell clones

It is now possible to clone T-lymphocytes in vitro following appropriate stimuli and the use of IL-2. This technique has opened new prospects for the study of T-cell subsets because it allows the proliferation, from single cells, of pure T-lymphocyte populations which thus retain specific phenotypes and functions.

Several methods have been used to clone human T-cells. These include the culture of cells obtained from T-cell colonies based on the assumption that they may be clonal or by limiting dilution in the presence of feeder cells, an antigen or a mitogen and IL-2[42, 64, 112]. Almost all circulating T-lymphocytes from normals have clonogenic potential[64]. According to the system and the stimuli used, clones of CD4+ (more frequently) and of CD8+ cells have been described. Functional studies have shown that the majority of such T-cell clones express cytolytic activities, although clones with suppressor or helper functions have also been reported. These clones have also been shown to produce different lymphokines.

The clinical application of these techniques has been so far limited. It has been shown, however, that clones of human killer T-cells can be grown, following sensitization in a mixed lymphocyte culture, against autologous lymphoma B-cells. The cytotoxic activity of these clones seems specific against the autologous lymphoma but not against allogeneic lymphoma B-cells. These findings may lead to a more rational approach of specific immunotherapy in clinical practice via the generation of cytotoxic T-cell clones with specific anti-leukaemia activity.

Release of soluble factors and interactions with other haemopoietic lineages

There is evidence of close interactions between T-lymphocytes and other haemopoietic cells which are mediated by soluble factors released by T-cells. It is now well established that T-lymphocytes produce factors responsible for colony stimulating activity, which promote the growth of granulocyte/macrophage and eosinophilic colonies, as well as burst promoting activity, which induces the growth of erythroid progenitor cells. In addition to IL-2 and γ-interferon, which are secreted by activated T-cells, it has become apparent too that these cells release factors which induce the proliferation or the differentiation of normal B-cells[37].

The characterization of the cells responsible for the release of these cytokines has been possible by the long-term growth in culture of T-cells and T-cell clones. For example CD4+ and CD8+ cell lines derived from normal peripheral blood release soluble factors which promote the growth of myeloid, erythroid and mixed colonies[50]. The production of these lymphokines, which is independent of accessory cells, PHA or serum, demonstrates a close interaction between T-cells and other haemopoietic lineages and suggests a regulatory role by these lymphocytes in the growth of human progenitor cells.

These interactions support the hypothesis of an involvement of T-cells in the pathogenesis of several haematological disorders and/or of some of their complications. For example, there is evidence that T-cells which inhibit haemopoiesis may be present in aplastic anaemia[9, 104]. This has been documented by showing that the in vitro growth of bone marrow myeloid precursors in this disease improves following removal of T-cells[7]. This inhibitory effect can be reproduced by adding T-cells in autologous co-culture experiments or by mixing the patients' lymphocytes with normal allogeneic marrow cells[7, 9, 41]. This effect in aplastic anaemia apears to be due to inhibitory Tγ cells which are CD8+[9]. The existence of inhibitory T-cells in the bone marrow has been documented in 39 of 234 patients (16.6%) with neutropenia and granulocytic hypoplasia[8]. The pathogenic relevance of this finding was confirmed by evidence showing that the sensitivity in vitro of these inhibitory T-cells to corticosteroids correlated with a clinical response to therapy with prednisone.

The possibility that abnormal T-cells could affect the myeloid or erythroid compartments has been investigated in a T-CLL disorder in which the patients are often neutropenic and/or anaemic (see Chapter 4). Whilst information about the effect on the granulocytic precursors is still controversial, there is growing evidence for a pathogenic role of T-cells in the T-CLL cases associated with red cell aplasia. An effect by the 'normal' T-cells has also been implicated in the pathogenesis of the red cell aplasia which occasionally complicates B-CLL[58].

B-colonies

In recent years it has been possible to grow human B-lymphocyte colonies as an extension of work on murine systems[77]. The use of these techniques has, however, been limited and they have not been widely applied to the study of B-cell lymphoproliferative disorders[72]. This assay system is not very reproducible and this results partly from technical problems in isolating pure B-cell populations as well as from difficulties in the characterization of the colony cells grown in agar or methylcellulose. The proliferation of the few residual T-cells in the presence of mitogenic stimuli also creates problems.

Lymphoblastoid B-cell lines

Normal B-cells bearing Epstein–Barr virus (EBV) receptors can be immortalized into lymphoblastoid cell lines following infection in vitro by the virus. Numerous cell lines have been established from Burkitt's lymphoma cells bearing the typical translocation t(8;14) or one of the variants [t(2;8) or t(8;22)]. In a proportion of cases it has been also possible to establish lymphoblastoid cell lines from chronic B-cell leukaemias. These lines, obtained from cases of B-CLL, B-PLL and hairy cell leukaemia, have been shown to retain the same immunological and cytochemical characteristics of the primary cells[25, 38, 90]. The authors have recently succeeded in growing EBV transformed lines from B-PLL cases; all of them appear to stem from the original leukaemic clone, because they maintain the same marker chromosome abnormality, namely t(11;14), 14q+, +12 and/or the identical Ig gene rearrangement configuration[62a]. These B-cell lines represent presently the only assays available for studies on B-cell proliferation and differentiation.

References

1. Abo, T. and Balch, C. M. (1981) A differentiation antigen of human NK and K cells identified by a monoclonal antibody (HNK-1). *Journal of Immunology,* **129**, 1024–1029
2. Abo, T., Cooper, M. C. and Balch, Ch. M. (1982) Characterisation of HNK-1+ (Leu7) human lymphocytes. I. Two distinct phenotypes of human NK cells with different cytotoxic capability. *Journal of Immunology,* **129**, 1752–1757
3. Abramson, C. S., Kersey, J. H. and LeBien, T. W. (1981) A monoclonal antibody (BA-1) reactive with cells of human B-lymphocyte lineage. *Journal of Immunology,* **126**, 83–88
4. Anderson, K. C., Bates, M. P., Slaughenhoupt, B. L., Pinkus, G. S., Schlossman, S. F. and Nadler, L. M. (1984) Expression of human B cell-associated antigens on leukemias and lymphomas: a model of human B cell differentiation. *Blood,* **63**, 1424–1433
5. Anderson, K. C., Boyd, A. W., Fisher, D. C., Leslie, D., Schlossman, S. F. and Nadler, L. M. (1985) Hairy cell leukemia: a tumor of pre-plasma cells. *Blood* **65**, 620–629
6. Anderson, K. C., Park, E. K., Bates, M. P. et al. (1983) Antigens on human plasma cells identified by monoclonal antibodies. *Journal of Immunology,* **130**, 1132–1138
7. Ascensao, J. L., Kay, N. E., Banisadre, M. and Zanjani, E. D. (1981) Cell-cell interaction in human granulopoiesis: role of T lymphocytes. *Experimental Hematology,* **9**, 473–478
8. Bagby, G. C. Jr, Lawrence, H. J. and Neerhout, R. C. (1983) T-lymphocyte-mediated granulopoietic failure: in vitro identification of prednisone-responsive patients. *New England Journal of Medicine,* **309**, 1073–1078
9. Bacigalupo, A., Podesta, M., Mingari, M. C., Moretta, L., Van Lint, M. T. and Marmont, A. (1980) Immune suppression of hematopoiesis in aplastic anemia: activity of Tγ lymphocytes. *Journal of Immunology,* **125**, 1449–1453

10. Ballieux, R. E. and Heijnen, C. J. (1983) Immunoregulatory T cell subpopulations in man: dissection by monoclonal antibodies and Fc receptors. *Immunological Reviews*, **74**, 5–28
11. Berger, C. L., Morrison, S., Chu, A. et al. (1982) Diagnosis of cutaneous T cell lymphoma by use of monoclonal antibodies reactive with tumor-associated antigens. *Journal of Clinical Investigation*, **70**, 1205–1215
12. Bernard, A., Boumsell, L., Reinherz, E. L. et al. (1981) Cell surface characterization of malignant T cells from lymphoblastic lymphoma using monoclonal antibodies: Evidence for phenotypic differences between malignant T cells from patients with acute lymphoblastic leukemia and lymphoblastic lymphoma. *Blood*, **57**, 1105–1110
13. Beverley, P. C. L. (1982) The use of the fluorescence activated cell sorter for the identification and analysis of function of cell subpopulations. In: *Monoclonal Antibodies in Clinical Medicine*, edited by A. J. McMichael and J. W. Fabre, pp. 557–584. London: Academic Press
13a. Beverley, P. C. L., Merkenschlager, M. and Terry, L. (1988) Phenotypic diversity of the CD45 antigen and its relationship to function. *Immunology*, Suppl. 1, 3–5
14. Bodger, M. P., Francis, G. E., Delia, D., Granger, S. M. and Janossy, G. (1981) A monoclonal antibody specific for immature human hemopoietic cells and T lineage cells. *Journal of Immunology*, **127**, 2269–2274
15. Bollum, F. J. (1979) Terminal deoxynucleotidyl transferase as a hematopoietic cell marker. *Blood*, **54**, 1203–1215
16. Braun, M. P., Martin, P. J., Ledbetter, J. A. and Hansen, J. A. (1983) Granulocytes and cultured human fibroblasts express common acute lymphoblastic leukemia-associated antigens. *Blood*, **61**, 718–725
17. Breard, J., Reinherz, E. L., Kung, P. C., Goldstein, G. and Schlossman, S. F. (1980) A monoclonal antibody reactive with human peripheral blood monocytes. *Journal of Immunology*, **124**, 1943–1948
17a. Broder, S., Poplack, D., Whang-Peng, J. et al. (1978) Characterization of a suppressor-cell leukemia. Evidence for the requirement of an interaction of two T cells in the development of human suppressor effector cells. *New England Journal of Medicine*, **298**, 66–72
18. Brooks, D. A., Beckman, I. G. R., Bradley, J., McNamara, P. J., Thomas, M. E. and Zola, H. (1981) Human lymphocyte markers defined by antibodies derived from somatic cell hybrids. IV. A monoclonal antibody reacting specifically with a subpopulation of human B lymphocytes. *Journal of Immunology*, **126**, 1373–1377
19. Brooks, D. A., Bradley, J. and Zola, H. (1982) A differentiation antigen expressed selectively by a proportion of human blood cells: detection with a monoclonal antibody. *Pathology*, **14**, 5–11
20. Brouet, J-C. and Seligmann, M. (1977) Chronic lymphocytic leukaemia as an immunoproliferative disorder. *Clinics in Haematology*, **6**, 169–184
21. Bunn, P. A., Carrasquillo, J. A., Keenan, A. M. et al. (1984) Imaging of T-cell lymphoma by radiolabelled monoclonal antibody. *Lancet*, ii, 1219–1221
21a. Campana, D., Janossy, G., Bofill, M. et al. (1985) Human B-cell development. I. Phenotypic differences of B lymphocytes in the bone marrow and peripheral lymphoid tissue. *Journal of Immunology*, **134**, 1524–1529
22. Catovsky, D., Cherchi, M., Brooks, D., Bradley, J. and Zola, H. (1981) Heterogeneity of B-cell leukemias demonstrated by the monoclonal antibody FMC7. *Blood*, **58**, 406–408
22a. Clement, L. T., Yamashita, N. and Martin, A. M. (1988) The functionally distinct subpopulations of human CD4+ helper inducer T lymphocytes defined by anti-CD45R antibodies derive sequentially from a differentiation pathway that is regulated by activation-dependent post-thymic differentiation. *Journal of Immunology*, **141**, 1464–1470
23. De Mey, J. (1983) Colloidal gold probes in immunocytochemistry. In: *Immunocytochemistry: Practical Applications in Pathology and Biology*, edited by J. M. Polak and S. Van Noorden, pp. 82–112. Bristol: Wright PSG
23a. Defrance, T., Aubry, J. P., Rousset, F. et al. (1987) Human recombinant interleukin 4 induces Fc receptors (CD23) on normal human B lymphocytes. *Journal of Experimental Medicine*, **165**, 1459–1467
24. Fibach, E., Gerassi, E. and Sachs, L. (1976) Induction of colony formation in vitro by human lymphocytes. *Nature*, **259**, 127–128

25. Finerty, S., Rickinson, A. B., Epstein, M. A. and Platts-Mills, T. A. E. (1982) Interaction of Epstein–Barr virus with leukaemic B cells in vitro. II. Cell line establishment from prolymphocytic leukaemia and from Waldenström's macroglobulinaemia. *International Journal of Cancer*, **30**, 1–7

26. Fingeroth, J. D., Weis, J. J., Tedder, T. F., Strominger, J. L., Biro, P. A. and Fearon, D. T. (1984) Epstein–Barr virus receptor of human B lymphocytes is the C3d receptor CR2. *Proceedings of the National Academy of Sciences of the USA*, **81**, 4510–4514

27. Foa, R. and Catovsky, D. (1979) T-lymphocyte colonies in normal blood, bone marrow and lymphoproliferative disorders. *Clinical and Experimental Immunology*, **36**, 488–495

28. Forster, H. K., Gudat, F. G., Girard, M-F. et al. (1982) Monoclonal antibody against a membrane antigen characterizing leukemic human B-lymphocytes. *Cancer Research*, **42**, 1927–1934

29. Gatenby, P. A., Kansas, G. S., Xian, C. Y., Evans, R. L. and Engleman, E. G. (1982) Dissection of immunoregulatory subpopulations of T lymphocytes within the helper and suppressor sublineages in man. *Journal of Immunology*, **129**, 1997–2000

29a. Gordon, J., Flores-Romo, L., Cairns, J. A. et al. (1989) CD23: a multi-functional receptor/lymphokine? *Immunology Today*, **10**, 153–157

30. Greaves, M. F., Hariri, G., Newman, R. A., Sutherland, D. R., Ritter, M. A. and Ritz, J. (1983) Selective expression of the common acute lymphoblastic leukemia (gp100) antigen on immature lymphoid cells and their malignant counterparts. *Blood*, **61**, 628–639

31. Greaves, M. F., Rao, J., Hariri, G. et al. (1981) Phenotypic heterogeneity and cellular origins of T cell malignancies. *Leukemia Research*, **5**, 281–299

32. Griffin, J. D., Linch, D., Sabbath, K., Larcom, P. and Schlossman, S. F. (1984) A monoclonal antibody reactive with normal and leukemic human myeloid progenitor cells. *Leukemia Research*, **8**, 521–534

33. Guy, K., Docherty, L. and Dewar, A. E. (1986) Deficient expression of MHC Class II antigens in some cases of human B-cell leukaemia. *Clinical and Experimental Immunology*, **63**, 290–297

34. Guy, K. and van Heyningen, V. (1983) An ordered sequence of expression of human MHC class-II antigens during B-cell maturation? *Immunology Today*, **4**, 186–189

35. Haynes, B. F., Mann, D. L., Hemler, M. E. et al. (1980) Characterization of a monoclonal antibody that defines immunoregulatory T cell subset for immunoglobulin synthesis in humans. *Proceedings of the National Academy of Sciences of the USA*, **77**, 2914–2918

36. Horwitz, D. A. and Bakke, A. C. (1984) An Fc receptor-bearing, third population of human mononuclear cells with cytotoxic and regulatory function. *Immunology Today*, **5**, 148–153

37. Howard, M., Farrar, J., Hilfiker, M. et al. (1982) Identification of a T cell-derived B cell growth factor distinct from interleukin 2. *Journal of Experimental Medicine*, **155**, 914–923

38. Hurley, J. N., Fu, S. M., Kunkel, H. G., McKenna, G. and Scharff, M. D. (1978) Lymphoblastoid cell lines from patients with chronic lymphocytic leukemia: identification of tumor origin by idiotypic analysis. *Proceedings of the National Academy of Sciences of the USA*, **75**, 5706–5710

39. Jani, P., Verbi, W., Greaves, M. F., Bevan, D. and Bollum, F. (1983) Terminal deoxynucleotidyl transferase in acute myeloid leukaemia. *Leukemia Research*, **7**, 17–29

40. Janossy, G. and Prentice, H. G. (1982) T cell subpopulations, monoclonal antibodies and their therapeutic applications. *Clinics in Haematology*, **11**, 631–660

41. Kagan, W. A., Ascensao, J. L., Fialk, M. A., Coleman, M., Valera, E. D. and Good, R. A. (1979) Studies on the pathogenesis of aplastic anemia. *American Journal of Medicine*, **66**, 444–449

42. Kahle, P., Wernet, P., Rehbein, A., Kumbier, I. and Pawelec, G. (1981) Cloning of functional human T lymphocytes by limiting dilution: impact of killer cells and interleukin 2 sources on cloning efficiencies. *Scandinavian Journal of Immunology*, **14**, 493–502

43. Katz, F., Povey, S., Parkar, M., et al. (1983) Chromosome asignment of monoclonal antibody-defined determinants on human leukemic cells. *European Journal of Immunology*, **13**, 1008–1013

44. Kersey, J. A., LeBien, T. W., Abramson, C. S., Newman, R., Sutherland, R. and Greaves, M. (1981) p24: a human leukemia-associated and lymphohemopoietic progenitor cell surface structure identified with monoclonal antibody. *Journal of Experimental Medicine*, **153**, 726–731

45. Knapp, W., Majdic, O., Bettelheim, P. and Liszka, K. (1982) VIL-A1, a monoclonal antibody reactive with common acute lymphatic leukemia cells. *Leukemia Research*, **6**, 137–147

45a. Knapp, W., Dorken, B., Rieber, P. et al. (1989) Update of CD antigens after the 4th International Workshop. *International Journal of Cancer*, **44**, 190–191

46. Knowles, D. M., Tolidjian, B., Marboe, C. C., Halper, J. P., Azzo, W. and Wang, C. Y. (1983) A new human B-lymphocyte surface antigen (BL2) detectable by a hybridoma monoclonal antibody: Distribution on benign and malignant lymphoid cells. *Blood*, **62**, 191–199

47. Korsmeyer, S. J., Hieter, P. A., Ravetch, J. V., Poplack, D. G., Waldmann, T. A. and Leder, P. (1981) Developmental hierarchy of immunoglobulin gene rearrangements in human leukemic pre-B cells. *Proceedings of the National Academy of Sciences of the USA*, **78**, 7096–7100

48. Kung, P. C., Goldstein, G., Reinherz, E. L. and Schlossman, S. F. (1979) Monoclonal antibodies defining distinctive human T-cell surface antigens. *Science*, **206**, 347–349

49. Landay, A., Gartland, G. L. and Clement, L. T. (1983) Characterization of a phenotypically distinct subpopulation of Leu2+ cells that suppresses T cell proliferative responses. *Journal of Immunology*, **131**, 2757–2761

50. Lanfrancone, L., Ferrero, D., Gallo, E., Foa, R. and Tarella, C. (1985) Release of hemopoietic factors by normal human T cell lines with either suppressor or helper activity. *Journal of Cellular Physiology*, **122**, 7–13

51. Lanier, L. L., Le, A. M., Phillips, J. H., Warner, N. L. and Babcock, G. F. (1983) Subpopulations of human natural killer cells defined by expression of the Leu-7 (HNK-1) and Leu-11 (NK-15) antigens. *Journal of Immunology*, **131**, 1789–1796

52. Lebacq-Verheyden, A. M., Ravoet, A. M., Bazin, H., Sutherland, D. R., Tidman, N. and Greaves, M. F. (1983) Rat AL2, AL3, AL4 and AL5 monoclonal antibodies bind to the common acute lymphoblastic leukaemia antigen (CALLA gp 100). *International Journal of Cancer*, **32**, 273–279

53. Leonard, W. J., Depper, J. M., Uchiyama, T., Smith, K. A., Waldmann, T. A. and Greene, W. C. (1982) A monoclonal antibody that appears to recognise the receptor for human T cell growth factor; partial characterisation of the receptor. *Nature*, **300**, 267–269

54. Link, M., Warnke, R., Finlay, J. et al. (1983) A single monoclonal antibody identified T-cell lineage of childhood lymphoid malignancies. *Blood*, **62**, 722–728

55. Lowenberg, B. and De Zeeuw, H. M. C. (1979) A method for cloning T-lymphocytic precursors in agar. *American Journal of Hematology*, **6**, 35–43

56. McKenzie, I. F. C. and Zola, H. (1983) Monoclonal antibodies to B cells. *Immunology Today*, **4**, 10–15

57. McMichael, A. J., Pilch, J. R., Galfre, G., Mason, D. Y., Fabre, J. W. and Milstein, C. (1979) A human thymocyte antigen defined by a hybrid myeloma monoclonal antibody. *European Journal of Immunology*, **9**, 205–210

58. Mangan, K. F., Chikkappa, G. and Farley, P. C. (1982) T gamma (Tγ) cells suppress growth of erythroid colony-forming units in vitro in the pure red cell aplasia of B-cell chronic lymphocytic leukemia. *Journal of Clinical Investigation*, **70**, 1148–1156

59. Markey, G. M., McConnell, R. E., Alexander, H. D., Morris, T. C. M. and Robertson, J. H. (1983) Identification of cellular immunoglobulins in chronic lymphocytic leukaemia by immunoperoxidase staining. *Journal of Clinical Pathology*, **36**, 1391–1396

60. Martin, P. J., Hansen, J. A., Siadak, A. W. and Nowinski, R. C. (1981) Monoclonal antibodies recognizing normal human T-lymphocytes and malignant human B-lymphocytes: a comparative study. *Journal of Immunology*, **127**, 1920–1923

60a. Mason, D. Y., Stein, H., Gerdes, J. et al. (1987) Value of Monoclonal anti-CD22 (p135) antibodies for the detection of normal and neoplastic B lymphoid cells. *Blood*, **69**, 836–840

61. Matutes, E., Parreira, A., Foa, R. and Catovsky, D. (1985) Monoclonal antibody OKT17 recognises most cases of T-cell malignancy. *British Journal of Haematology*, **61**, 649–656

62. Melo, J. V., Catovsky, D. and Bodger, M. (1984) Reactivity of the monoclonal antibody RFB-1. *Scandinavian Journal of Haematology*, **32**, 417–422

62a. Melo, J. V. et al. (1988) *Clinical and Experimental Immunology*, **73**, 23–28

63. Melvin, S. L. (1979) Comparison of techniques for detecting T-cell acute lymphocytic leukemia. *Blood*, **54**, 210–215

64. Moretta, A., Pantaleo, G., Moretta, L., Cerottini, J-C. and Mingari, M. C. (1983) Direct demonstration of the clonogenic potential of every human peripheral blood T cell. Clonal analysis of HLA-DR expression and cytolytic activity. *Journal of Experimental Medicine*, **157**, 743–754

64a. Morimoto, C., Letvin, N. L., Boyd, A. W. et al. (1985) The isolation and characterisation of the human helper inducer T cell subset. *Journal of Immunology*, **134**, 3762–3769

64b. Morimoto, C., Letvin, N. L., Distaso, J. A., Aldrich, W. R. and Schlossman, S. F. (1985) The isolation and characterisation of the human suppressor inducer subset. *Journal of Immunology*, **134**, 1508–1515

65. Morgan, D. A., Ruscetti, F. W. and Gallo, R. (1976) Selective in vitro growth of T lymphocytes from normal human bone marrows. *Science*, **193**, 1007–1008

65a. Mulligan, S. (1990) Human B cells: differentiation and neoplasia. In *Leukemia and Lymphoma*, in press

66. Myers, C. D., Thorpe, P. E., Ross, W. C. J. et al. (1984) An immunotoxin with therapeutic potential in T cell leukemia: WT1-ricin A. *Blood*, **63**, 1178–1185

67. Nadler, L. M., Anderson, K. C., Marti, G. et al. (1983) B4, a human B lymphocyte-associated antigen expressed on normal, mitogen-activated and malignant B lymphocytes. *Journal of Immunology*, **131**, 244–250

68. Nadler, L. M., Ritz, J., Hardy, R., Pesando, J. M., Schlossman, S. F. and Stashenko, P. (1981) A unique cell surface antigen identifying lymphoid malignancies of B cell origin. *Journal of Clinical Investigation*, **67**, 134–140

69. Nadler, L. M., Stashenko, P., Hardy, R., van Agthoven, A., Terhost, C. and Schlossman, S. F. (1981) Characterization of a human B cell-specific antigen (B2) distinct from B1. *Journal of Immunology*, **126**, 1941–1947

70. Nadler, L. M., Takvorian, T., Botnick, L. et al. (1984) Anti-B1 monoclonal antibody and complement treatment in autologous bone marrow transplantation for relapsed B-cell non-Hodgkin's lymphoma. *Lancet*, **ii**, 427–431

71. Ortaldo, J. R., Oldham, R. K., Cannon, G. C. and Herberman, R. B. (1977) Specificity of natural cytotoxic reactivity of normal human lymphocytes against a myeloid leukemia cell line. *Journal of the National Cancer Institute*, **59**, 77–82

72. Perri, R. T. and Kay, N. E. (1982) Monoclonal CLL B-cells may be induced to grow in an in vitro B-cell assay system. *Blood*, **59**, 247–249

73. Polli, N., O-Brien, M., Tavares de Castro, J., Matutes, E., San Miguel, J. F. and Catovsky, D. (1985) Characterization of blast cells in chronic granulocytic leukaemia in transformation, acute myelofibrosis and undifferentiated leukaemia. I. Ultrastructural morphology and cytochemistry. *British Journal of Haematology*, **59**, 277–296

73a. Pombo de Oliveira, M. S. (1988) Early expression of MCS2 (CD13) in the cytoplasm of blast cells from acute myeloid leukaemia. *Acta Haematologica*, **80**, 61–64

74. Posnett, D. N., Chiorazzi, N. and Kunkel, H. G. (1982) Monoclonal antibodies with specificity for hairy cell leukemia cells. *Journal of Clinical Investigation*, **70**, 254–261

75. Posnett, D. N., Marboe, C. C., Knowles II, D. M., Jaffe, E. A. and Kunkel, H. G. (1984) A membrane antigen (HC1) selectively present on hairy cell leukemia cells, endothelial cells, and epidermal basal cells. *Journal of Immunology*, **132**, 1–3

76. Posnett, D. N., Wang, C-Y., Chiorazzi, N., Crow, M. K. and Kunkel, H. G. (1984) An antigen characteristic of hairy cell leukemia cells is expressed on certain activated B cells. *Journal of Immunology*, **133**, 1635–1640

77. Radnay, J., Goldman, I. and Rozenszajn, L. A. (1979) Growth of human B-lymphocyte colonies in vitro. *Nature*, **278**, 351–353

77a. Rani, S. (1988) Different expression of CD3 and CD22 in leukemic cells according to whether tested in suspension or fixed on slides. *Hematologic Pathology*, **2**, 73–78

78. Reinherz, E. L., Kung, P. C., Goldstein, G. and Schlossman, S. F. (1979) A monoclonal antibody with selective reactivity with functionally mature thymocytes and all peripheral human T-cells. *Journal of Immunology*, **123**, 1312–1317

79. Reinherz, E. L., Kung, P. C., Goldstein, G. and Schlossman, S. F. (1979) Further characterization of the human inducer T cell subset defined by monoclonal antibody. *Journal of Immunology*, **123**, 2894–2896

80. Reinherz, E. L., Kung, P. C., Goldstein, G. and Schlossman, S. F. (1980) A monoclonal antibody reactive with the human cytotoxic/suppressor T cell subset previously defined by a heteroantiserum termed TH2. *Journal of Immunology*, **124**, 1301–1307

81. Reinherz, E. L., Meuer, S. C. and Schlossman, S. F. (1983) The human T cell receptor: analysis with cytotoxic T cell clones. *Immunological Reviews*, **74**, 83–112

82. Reinherz, E. L., Morimoto, C., Fitzgerald, K. A., Huzzey, R. E., Daley, J. F. and Schlossman, S. F. (1982) Heterogeneity of human T4+ inducer T cells defined by a monoclonal antibody that delineates two functional subpopulations. *Journal of Immunology*, **128**, 463–468

83. Reinherz, E. L. and Schlossman, S. F. (1980) The differentiation and function of human T lymphocytes. *Cell*, **19**, 821–827

84. Ritz, J., Pesando, J. M., Notis-McConarty, J., Lazarus, H. and Schlossman, S. F. (1980) A monoclonal antibody to human acute lymphoblastic leukaemia. *Nature*, **283**, 583–585

85. Robinson, D. S. F., Posnett, D. N., Zola, H. and Catovsky, D. (1985) Normal counterparts of hairy cells and B-prolymphocytes in the peripheral blood. An ultrastructural study with monoclonal antibodies and the immunogold method. *Leukemia Research*, **9**, 335–348

86. Royston, I., Majda, J. A., Baird, S. M., Meserve, B. L. and Griffiths, J. C. (1980) Human T-cell antigens defined by monoclonal antibodies: the 65,000 Dalton antigen of T-cells (T65) is also found on chronic lymphocytic leukemia cells bearing surface immunoglobulin. *Journal of Immunology*, **125**, 725–731

87. Ruiz-Arguelles, G. J., Katzmann, J. A., Greipp, P. R., Gonchoroff, N. J., Garton, J. P. and Kyle, R. A. (1984) Multiple myeloma: circulating lymphocytes that express plasma cell antigens. *Blood*, **64**, 352–356

88. Rümke, H. C., Terpstra, F. G., Out, T. A., Vossen, J. M. and Zeijlemaker, W. P. (1981) Immunoglobulin production by human lymphocytes in a microculture system: culture conditions and cellular interactions. *Clinical Immunology and Immunopathology*, **19**, 338–350

89. Ruscetti, F. W. and Gallo, R. C. (1981) Human T-lymphocyte growth factor and function of T lymphocytes. *Blood*, **57**, 379–394

90. Sairenji, T., Spiro, R. C., Reisert, P. S. et al. (1983) Analysis of transformation with Epstein–Barr virus and phenotypic characteristics of lymphoblastoid cell lines established from patients with hairy cell leukemia. *American Journal of Hematology*, **15**, 361–374

91. San Miguel, J. F., Tavares de Castro, J., Matutes, E. et al. (1985) Characterization of blast cells in chronic granulocytic leukaemia in transformation, acute myelofibrosis and undifferentiated leukaemia. II. Studies with monoclonal antibodies and terminal transferase. *British Journal of Haematology*, **59**, 297–309

92. Schwab, U., Stein, H., Gerdes, J. et al. (1982) Production of a monoclonal antibody specific for Hodgkin and Sternberg–Reed cells of Hodgkin's lymphoma and a subset of normal lymphoid cells. *Nature*, **299**, 65–67

93. Schuit, H. R. E., Hijmans, W. and Jansen, J. (1984) Surface bound or cytoplasmic immunoglobulins: interpretation of the immunofluorescence observed in cytocentrifuge slides of human lymphocytes. *Clinical and Experimental Immunology*, **56**, 694–700

94. Schwarting, R., Stein, H. and Wang, C. Y. (1985) The monoclonal antibodies S-HCL 1 (Leu-14) and S-HCL3 (Leu-M5) allow the diagnosis of hairy cell leukaemia. *Blood*, **65**, 974–983

95. Seon, B. K., Negoro, S. and Barcos, M. P. (1983) Monoclonal antibody that defines a unique human T-cell leukemia antigen. *Proceedings of the National Academy of Sciences of the USA*, **80**, 845–849

96. Seon, B. K., Negoro, S., Barcos, M. P., Tebbi, C. K., Chervinsky, D. and Fukukawa, T. (1984) Monoclonal antibody SN2 defining a human T cell leukemia-associated cell surface glycoprotein. *Journal of Immunology*, **132**, 2089–2095

97. Siegal, L. J., Harper, M. E., Wong-Staal, F., Gallo, R. C., Nash, W. G. and O'Brien, S. J. (1984) Gene for T-cell growth factor: location on human chromosome 4q and feline chromosome B1. *Science*, **223**, 175–178

97a. Smith, S. H., Brown, M. H., Rowe, D. et al. (1986) Functional subsets of human helper inducer cells defined by new monoclonal antibody UCHL1. *Immunology*, **58**, 63–70

98. Stashenko, P., Nadler, L. M., Hardy, R. and Schlossman, S. F. (1980) Characterization of a human B lymphocyte-specific antigen. *Journal of Immunology*, **125**, 1678–1685

99. Tax, W. J. M., Willems, H. W., Kibbelaar, M. D. A. et al. (1981) Monoclonal antibodies against human thymocytes and T lymphocytes. *Protides of the Biological Fluids*, **29**, 701–704

100. Thomas, Y., Rogozinski, L., Irigoyen, O. H. et al. (1981) Functional analysis of human T cell subsets defined by monoclonal antibodies. IV. Induction of suppressor cells within the OKT4+ population. *Journal of Experimental Medicine*, **154**, 459–467

101. Thomas, Y., Rogozinski, L., Irigoyen, O. H. et al. (1982) Functional analysis of human T cell subsets defined by monoclonal antibodies. V. Suppressor cells within the activated OKT4+ population belong to a distinct subset. *Journal of Immunology,* **128**, 1386–1390

102. Timonen, T., Ortaldo, J. R. and Herberman, R. G. (1981) Characteristics of human large granular lymphocytes and relationship to natural killer and K cells. *Journal of Experimental Medicine,* **153**, 564–582

103. Tindle, R. W., Nichols, R. A. B., Chan, L. C., Campana, D., Catovsky, D. and Birnie, G. D. (1985) A novel monoclonal antibody BI-3C5 recognises myeloblasts and non-B non-T lymphoblasts in acute leukemias and CGL blast crises, and reacts with immature cells in normal bone marrow. *Leukemia Research,* **9**, 1–9

104. Torok-Storb, B. J., Sieff, C., Storb, R., Adamson, J. and Thomas, E. D. (1980) In vitro tests for distinguishing possible immune-mediated aplastic anemia from transfusion-induced sensitization. *Blood,* **55**, 211–215

105. Uchiyama, T., Broder, S. and Waldmann, T. A. (1981) A monoclonal antibody (anti-Tac) reactive with activated and functionally mature human T cells. I. Production of anti-Tac monoclonal antibody and distribution of Tac (+) cells. *Journal of Immunology,* **126**, 1393–1397

106. Uchiyama, T., Nelson, D. L., Fleisher, T. A. and Waldmann, T. A. (1981) A monoclonal antibody (anti-Tac) reactive with activated and functionally mature human T cells. II. Expression of Tac antigen on activated cytotoxic killer T cells, suppressor cells, and on one of two types of helper T cells. *Journal of Immunology,* **126**, 1398–1403

107. Vainchenker, W., Deschamps, J., Vastin, J. et al. (1982) Two monoclonal antibodies as markers of human megakaryocyte maturation. Immunofluorescent staining and platelet peroxidase detection in megakaryocyte colonies and in vivo cells from normal and leukemic patients. *Blood,* **59**, 514–521

108. Van Camp, B., Thielemans, C., Dehou, M. F., de Mey, J. and de Waele, M. (1982) Two monoclonal antibodies (OKIa1 and OKT10) for the study of the final B cell maturation. *Journal of Clinical Immunology,* **2**(suppl), 67S–74S

109. Van Oers, M. H. J., Zeijlemaker, W. P. and Schellekens, P. Th. A. (1977) Separation and properties of EA-rosette-forming lymphocytes in humans. *European Journal of Immunology,* **7**, 143–150

110. Van Wauwe, J., Goossens, J., Decock, W., Kung, P. and Goldstein, G. (1981) Suppression of human T cell mitogenesis and E rosette formation by the monoclonal antibody OKT11A. *Immunology,* **44**, 865–871

110a. Vissar, L., Shaw, A., Slupsky, J., Vos, H. and Poppema, S. (1989) Monoclonal antibodies reactive with hairy cell leukemia. *Blood,* **74**, 320–325

111. Vodinelich, L., Tax, W., Bai, Y., Pegram, S., Capel, P. and Greaves, M. F. (1983) A monoclonal antibody (WT1) for detecting leukemias of T-cell precursors (T-ALL). *Blood,* **62**, 1108–1113

112. Woods, G. M. and Lowenthal, R. M. (1984) Cellular interactions and IL2 requirements of PHA-induced human T-lymphocyte colonies. *Experimental Hematology,* **12**, 301–308

112a. Warner, I., Matutes, E. and Catovsky, D. (1990) *British Journal of Haematology* (in press)

112b. Yukawa, K., Kikutani, H., Owaki, H. et al. (1987) A B-cell specific differentiation antigen CD23 is a receptor for IgE (FCR) on lymphocytes. *Journal of Immunology,* **138**, 2576–2580

113. Zola, H., McNamara, P. J., Moore, H. A. et al. (1983) Maturation of human B lymphocytes – studies with a panel of monoclonal antibodies against membrane antigens. *Clinical And Experimental Immunology,* **52**, 655–664

114. Zola, H., Moore, H. A., Hohmann, A., Hunter, I. K., Nikoloutsopoulos, A. and Bradley, J. (1984) The antigen of mature human B cells detected by the monoclonal antibody FMC7; studies on the nature of the antigen and modulation of its expression. *Journal of Immunology,* **133**, 321–326

Chapter 2

Acute lymphoblastic leukaemia

Introduction

Acute lymphoblastic leukaemia (ALL) results from the neoplastic proliferation of immature lymphoid cells, or lymphoblasts, which characterize the early stages of differentiation of the B- and T-cell lineages. ALL is the most common malignancy in children and constitutes 80% of the leukaemias up to the age of 15 years. In adults (over 15 years of age), ALL is relatively less common and constitutes 15–20% of all cases of acute leukaemia.

There has been a significant progress in the treatment of this disease, particularly in children, and a greater understanding of the nature of its proliferating cells. This in turn has contributed to a better diagnosis and has facilitated the design of treatment protocols with due consideration of the prognostic features.

Whilst the outlook for childhood ALL has improved dramatically in the last 15 years, since the pioneering work of Pinkel and the concepts of 'total therapy' and central nervous system (CNS) prophylaxis[95], the results of treatment in adult ALL have lagged behind[40, 51, 105]. Although the reasons for this difference are not completely clear, some features of adult ALL, e.g. the higher incidence of Philadelphia chromosome positive (Ph+) cases[118, 119] and of the L2 morphological type[5, 6], may have a contributory role. This chapter will review the advances in diagnosis, classification and treatment and will discuss the new information derived from the use of monoclonal antibodies and molecular genetics concerning the biology of lymphoblasts.

Clinical features

Presenting symptoms in childhood ALL are often more dramatic than those of adults. The more frequent ones are fever and pallor in 60% of cases, purpura or other bleeding manifestations in 50% of cases and bone pain and/or arthralgia in 30% of cases. Bone pain is caused by subperiosteal bone infiltration. A correct diagnosis could sometimes be delayed while unnecessary investigations for rheumatic fever are being pursued. Less commonly dry cough, dyspnoea, facial oedema and other symptoms associated with superior vena cava obstruction resulting from an anterior mediastinal (thymic) mass (AMM), a feature of T-ALL, may be first manifestations of the disease.

The most common physical signs of ALL are hepatosplenomegaly, in two-thirds of cases, and lymphadenopathy in half of them. Enlarged mediastinal lymph nodes, particularly the presence of an AMM can be demonstrated on a chest X-ray as a widening of the mediastinum with anterior localization, best seen in lateral views, in 5–7% of cases[23].

The presence of isolated splenomegaly in patients in remission does not necessarily indicate a leukaemic relapse and may reflect an immunological reaction to the leukaemia[75] or be related to viral illnesses, such as cytomegalovirus infections or, rarely, could be the conseqeunce of hepatic fibrosis caused by cytotoxic drugs, e.g. methotrexate.

Haematological findings

The blood count shows anaemia, Hb < 10 g/dl and/or thrombocytopenia, platelets $< 100 \times 10^9$/l, in over 80% of cases. The white blood cell (WBC) count is variable; in half of the cases it is $> 10 \times 10^9$/l with a predominance of blasts showing lymphoid morphology in the peripheral blood (PB) films. The height of the presenting WBC count is the most important prognostic factor of the disease, both in children and adults (see below).

Anaemia and thrombocytopenia are a direct result of the diffuse and heavy bone marrow infiltration by lymphoblasts. Occasionally a very low platelet count may be a feature of disseminated intravascular coagulation (DIC), which has been described in cases of ALL presenting with a high WBC count, particularly T-ALL. Other manifestations of DIC, such as low fibrinogen and fibrin degradation products, may be observed in such cases.

The morphological appearance of the bone marrow lymphoblasts constitutes the basis for the FAB (French–American–British) classification of ALL[5, 6] (see below). The bone marrow is obtained by aspirate in all cases. A trephine bone marrow biopsy specimen may be necessary in cases presenting with associated myelofibrosis or whenever an adequate sample cannot be obtained by aspiration. Bone marrow samples are also used to monitor disease activity and to document complete remission (CR) or relapse status. Most protocols recommend, for this purpose, bone marrow aspirations at regular intervals, e.g. every 2 or 3 months. The need of this routine bone marrow aspirate in childhood ALL has been examined by the Children's Cancer Study Group[103]. The yield of an unpredicted bone marrow relapse that was not suspected by clinical findings, e.g. CNS involvement or other extramedullary disease, or PB counts, circulating blasts, Hb < 10 g/l, platelets $< 100 \times 10^9$/l, WBC $< 2.5 \times 10^9$/l, was less than 1% of all the bone marrow aspirates in that study.

Morphological classification

The FAB group defined morphological criteria for the classification of ALL in three types: L1, L2 and L3, according to the appearances of the lymphoblasts in films from bone marrow aspirates. The initial description[5], which was thought to be slightly imprecise for purposes of reproducibility, was later revised and semiquantitative criteria, compounded in a scoring system, were proposed[6].

L1 cells have high nucleo-/cytoplasmic (N/C) ratio, inconspicuous nucleoli, regular nuclear membrane outline and are, overall, small – less than twice the size of a small lymphocyte (Figure 2.1a). L2 cells, in contrast, have a low N/C ratio,

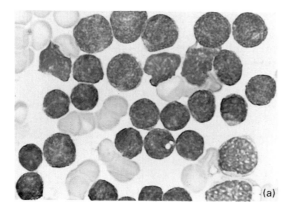

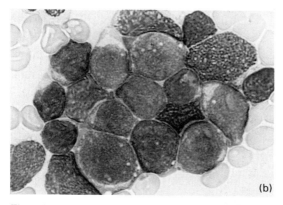

Figure 2.1 Bone marrow appearances in ALL. (a) L1 type (score +2); (b) L2 type (score −3). × 1200, reduced to 62% on reproduction

often have a prominent nucleolus, regular or irregular nuclear outline and tend to be larger than L1 blasts (Figure 2.1b). The difference between a typical L1 blast and a typical L2 cell is illustrated in Figure 2.2, which accentuates the main morphological features described above.

In order to improve the distinction between L1 and L2 cells the FAB group proposed a simple scoring system[6] which is positive, i.e. 0, 1 or 2, in L1 and negative, i.e. −1 to −4 in L2. *Two features score as positive*: a high N/C ratio (cytoplasm occupies less than 20% of the surface area of the cell) and a small or ill-defined nucleolus, both in ≥75% of cells. *Four features score as negative*: low N/C ratio (cytoplasm occupies more than 20% of the surface area of the cells), one or more prominent nucleoli and irregular nuclear membrane outline, in ≥25% of blasts, and the presence of ≥50% large cells.

L3 cells resemble closely those seen in aspirates or lymph node imprints from Burkitt's lymphoma, the main features being a deep basophilic cytoplasm often asociated with marked vacuolation (Figure 2.3); numerous mitotic figures are found as a rule in the bone marrow of L3 cases. L3 morphology is seen mainly in B-ALL which is characterized by the presence of immunoglobulins on the cell membrane and the characteristic chromosome abnormality t(8;14) (see below).

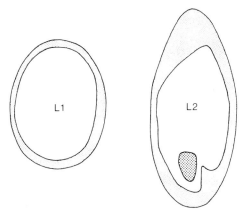

Figure 2.2 Diagrammatic representation of L1 and L2 cells. The main differences are: the larger size, the presence of a prominent nucleolus and the lower N/C ratio in L2 cells

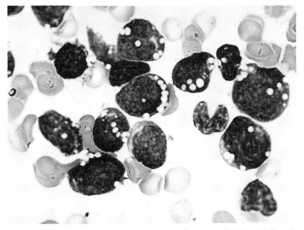

Figure 2.3 Bone marrow appearances of a case of ALL-L3 (Burkitt type). × 1200, reduced to 69% on reproduction

With the exception of L3, the FAB type does not correlate with the immunological classification of ALL. Blasts of T-ALL often have a markedly irregular or convoluted nucleus and tend to be of variable size. A proportion of them is small with a hyperchromatic nucleus[73]. As the only criterion for L2 is the irregular nuclear membrane, T-ALL cases score more often as L1 than as L2.

Cell morphology seems to correlate well with age and prognosis. The incidence of L2 increases with age and almost all cases over 50 years of age are of L2 morphology. Overall, 50–60% of adult cases have L2 blasts whilst in children only 15–25% of cases are of the L2 type. Conversely, the proportion of L1 is significantly higher in children (75–85% of cases) than in adults (30–40% of cases). L3 is rare, with an incidence of 1–3% in children and 2–5% in adults.

Several studies have shown that L2 morphology is associated with a worse prognosis than L1. In adults, L2 cases have a lower complete remission rate, although it is difficult to show that this finding is independent of the patient's age. A large study by the Children's Cancer Study Group[79], using a modification of the original FAB criteria close to the revised proposals [6], showed that blast morphology was a good predictor of survival and remission duration. The best prognosis was seen in L1 cases and the worst in L3.

Cell kinetic and cytofluorometric studies have shown that L2 is associated with a higher incidence of aneuploidy (70.6%) than L1 (34%) and a higher proportion of cells in S phase (12.4% in L2 and 5.8% in L1)[116]. Thus the morphological types L1, L2 and L3 correlate with important clinical and biological parameters. The reproducibility of the classification also depends to a large extent on the utilization of optimal peripheral blood and bone marrow preparations which are essential prerequisites for any morphological evaluation.

Granular ALL

Lymphoblasts with azurophilic granules have been described in a minority of cases. These blasts are PAS+ (periodic acid–Schiff) and myeloperoxidase negative and have a lymphoid phenotype. Five cases of children with common-ALL (cALL) were described by Stein et al.[115]: four cases were L1 and one L2. Ultrastructural examination disclosed membrane-bound radiolucent inclusions. Cytochemistry and membrane phenotype may be necessary in these cases to exclude acute myeloid leukaemia.

Hand-mirror variant

A minority of blasts may show the so called hand-mirror configuration in 15% of ALLs[68, 107]. This is the morphological expression of cell motility with the handle or uropod representing the posterior portion of the moving cell. The significance of this phenomenon is not clear. Hand-mirror blasts are seen only in the bone marrow and not in the peripheral blood. The presence of these cells, even in high proportions, does not correlate with bad prognosis in childhood ALL[107].

A study by Liso et al.[68] in nine adult ALLs with 12–57% hand-mirror cells noted, as other reports, that such patients may have a relatively long survival despite not achieving complete remission. Although no correlation with cell markers was observed in this study, four of the nine cases had a strong acid phosphatase reaction localized to the uropod area; three of these cases had cALL.

From the published data and the authors' own observations it seems that hand-mirror cells are more common in adult cases[68], are probably seen more frequently in relapsed bone marrow and are not necessarily associated with T-ALL, bur further studies with the newer monoclonal antibodies are necessary. Hand-mirror cells are not artefacts of the bone marrow preparations because they can be demonstrated by electron microscopy and by phase contrast and time lapse microcinematography[68].

Cytochemistry

Lymphoblasts are negative with the cytochemical reactions for myeloid cells, myeloperoxidase and Sudan black B, typical of myeloblasts, and lack the characteristic NaF-sensitive α-naphthyl acetate esterase (ANAE) of monoblasts[5]. Only in rare cases of biphenotypic acute leukaemia (see below) is it possible to demonstrate the coexistence of lymphoblasts with granulocyte or monocyte precursors which may be myeloperoxidase or ANAE positive. Stass et al. [113] have recently reported that Sudan black B positivity in 5% or more blasts, but with negative myeloperoxidase, may be seen in 1.6% of cases with genuine ALL. Stass et al. concluded that the Sudan black reaction may not be as specific as the myeloperoxidase reaction for the diagnosis of acute myeloid leukaemia (AML). A single case has still not been observed by the present authors that by all criteria was ALL with a positive sudanophilia.

The two cytochemical methods which have been more widely used in ALL are PAS and acid phosphatase.

PAS

A granular reaction of magenta colour has for a long time been associated by haematologists with lymphoid cells. The PAS reaction can be seen as fine or coarse granules or single positive blocks. The PAS in lymphoblasts represents intracellular glycogen as can be shown by the digestion of this substance with diastase. Although characteristic of ALL, some other types of acute leukaemia, chiefly the monocytic type of AML (M5), may in fact show a strong PAS reaction. The glycogen content of lymphoblasts is known to change with the phases of the cell cycle, increasing in G_0-G_1 and decreasing markedly in the S phase. Presumably for that reason, cases of ALL with a low proliferative rate such as common-ALL (cALL) often have L1 morphology and PAS+ blasts, usually with single blocks of reaction product; 70–80% of cALL cases are PAS+ [44]. ALL cases with a greater proliferative rate (see below), e.g. T-ALL and B-ALL (L3), are as a rule weakly PAS+ or PAS−. A block positivity is less frequent in adult ALL and this may relate to the higher frequency of L2 morphology and null-cell phenotype (B-lineage, but not cALL).

Several studies have shown a correlation between the PAS reaction and prognosis. When this is analysed in greater detail it can be seen that PAS negativity is associated with features of bad prognosis, e.g. T-ALL and B-ALL and/or high WBC count. Although the relationship between the PAS reaction and the immunological subtypes of ALL is by no means clear, its diagnostic value in the context of ALL, having excluded the possibility of acute myeloid leukaemia by other methods, still deserves some attention.

Acid phosphatase

A strong localized paranuclear acid phosphatase reaction in 70% or more blasts (Figure 2.4) has been described as characteristic of T-ALL and many studies have confirmed the authors' original observations [18,19]. Acid phosphatase activity is also a feature of fetal thymocytes and most mature T-cell leukaemias (see Chapter 5). The acid phosphatase in T-lymphoblasts is predominantly localized in the membranes of the Golgi zone and in a few lysosomal granules in its vicinity. The correlation between acid phosphatase and T-cell markers in ALL is close to 100% when cases of pre-T-ALL (negative E-rosettes) are included. A few early reports, including the authors', described the typical acid phosphatase reaction in a minority of 'non-T'-ALL cases with anterior mediastinal masses [4, 19]. Clearly, the definition of T-ALL in such studies did not include the T-specific monoclonal antibodies CD7 and cCD3 (see Chapter 1) which detect the very early cases of

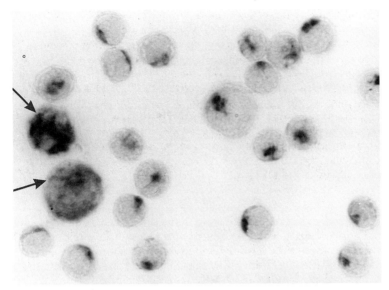

Figure 2.4 Localized cytochemical reaction for acid phosphatase in lymphoblasts from a case of T-ALL. Note also the diffuse reaction pattern in two monocytes (arrows). × 1200, reduced to 86% on reproduction

T-ALL, including pre-T-ALL. Many of those acid phosphatase positive cases would have now been considered of T-lineage. Because of the above association it is not surprising that acid phosphatase positivity has been found to correlate with bad prognosis because this reaction tends to be seen more often in cases with high WBC and T-cell markers. T-lymphoblastic lymphoma (T-LbLy), a disorder closely related to T-ALL, is also characterized by a positive acid phosphatase reaction demonstrable on histological sections or tumour imprints.

Other acid hydrolases

In addition to acid phosphatase other hydrolytic enzymes have been investigated in ALL, namely ANAE, β-glucuronidase and N-acetyl-β-glucosaminidase[4]. ANAE tends to follow the pattern of acid phosphatase but it reacts with a lower proportion of T-ALL cases. The ANAE reaction product is localized or takes the form of several cytoplasmic 'dots'. The activity of the four acid hydrolases becomes more abundant during T-cell maturation and they can be used as 'pan-T' cytochemical markers in the T-lymphoproliferative disorders (see Chapter 5). In ALL, 20–30% of non-T cases may show β-glucuronidase and N-acetyl-β-glucosaminidase activity. Furthermore, all these enzymes are also positive in some acute myeloid leukaemias, so they are not strictly specific for lymphoblasts. Basso et al.[4] examined a series of 120 children with non-B-, non-T-ALL (the only markers used were E-rosette and SmIg) with four acid hydrolases and found that the duration of the first remission was always longer when the blasts were negative for all the enzyme reactions, particularly β-glucuronidase. The prognosis in that series was inversely correlated with the number of positive reactions; the worst prognosis was observed in cases which were simultaneously positive for acid phosphatase and

ANAE (5 of 10 had an anterior mediastinal mass and 4 of 10 had WBC $> 100 \times 10^9/l$) or for β-glucuronidase and N-acetyl-β-glucosaminidase.

The isoenzymes of acid phosphatase, ANAE and N-acetyl-β-glucosaminidase (hexosaminidase) have been studied by biochemical methods in order to examine the possibility of specific disease patterns[37]. The isoenzymes demonstrated in leukaemic lymphoblasts are, in general, no different from those found in normal blood cells. Nevertheless, a finding previously reported by Ellis et al.[30], the presence of a hexosaminidase with intermediate mobility (between A and B) in cALL (23 of 27 cases) and absent in T-ALL was confirmed in the study of Gaedicke and Drexler[37]. The intermediate isoenzyme was demonstrated in the latter study in 8 of 11 cALLs and was not seen in 12 T-ALL samples; 3 of 6 acute myeloid leukaemias, however, also showed that pattern although as a very faint band[37].

Adenosine deaminase

The levels of adenosine deaminase (ADA), the enzyme responsible for the conversion of adenosine to inosine during purine degradation, are increased in many lymphoid cells, chiefly thymocytes and T-lymphocytes. ADA activity is high in ALL and also in AML cells. In contrast to the DNA polymerase terminal transferase (TdT), ADA levels are higher in T-ALL than in cALL blasts[25]. The availability of a potent ADA inhibitor, 2'-deoxycoformycin, has prompted clinical studies on the effect of this agent in the treatment of refractory and relapsed T-ALL[96].

Immunological classification

Studies with conventional B- and T-markers

The knowledge that lymphoid cells can be classified on the basis of membrane antigens which characterize lymphocyte subsets with defined functional properties has opened a new era in the classification of ALL. Three groups of ALL were identified initially[15]: T-ALL in which the lymphoblasts are capable of forming E-rosettes[58, 110], the rare B-ALL in which the cells express SmIg and a larger group on non-T-, non-B-ALL.

A further advance was contributed by the discovery that the majority of non-T-, non-B-ALL blast cells displayed the common-ALL (cALL) antigen. This antigenic determinant, with a molecular weight of 100 kilodaltons, was recognized by a polyclonal antiserum prepared by immunizing rabbits with ALL blast cells coated with anti-lymphocyte antibodies[41]. At the same time the diagnostic role of the nuclear enzyme TdT became apparent. The demonstration of TdT represents an important tool in the distinction between ALL and AML (see Chapter 1). All forms of ALL, with the exception of B-ALL, show TdT activity, the highest levels, when measured biochemically, being found in cALL[12, 24, 25, 52, 54, 72].

A subsequent development in the classification of ALL was the discovery that cells from 20% of cALL have μ chains in the cytoplasm (Cyμ), a feature of pre-B-lymphocytes[14, 121]. This was the first indication that a proportion of cALL, classified since as pre-B, was already committed to the B-cell lineage.

The early recognition of the T-cell origin of some ALLs by the formation of E-rosettes was later confirmed by the reactivity with polyclonal antisera directed against human T-lymphocyte antigens (HUTLAs) obtained by immunizing rabbits with human or monkey thymocytes or human T-cell lines[9, 117]. At the same time it was shown that preincubation of ALL cells with a thymic factor may enhance the proportion of E+ blasts[2].

Studies with monoclonal antibodies

The possibility of a more precise characterization of ALL blasts has improved further with the advent of monoclonal antibodies that have largely confirmed the classification based on conventional techniques[32, 38, 44]. Several of the monoclonal antibodies directed against T-cell antigens present in cells at different stages of intrathymic maturation were found to be useful in the analysis of ALL (see Chapter 1). More recently the production of monoclonal antibodies which are specific for B-cell antigens has enabled a better analysis of B-lineage ALL.

Immunological subtypes of ALL

T-ALL
Monoclonal antibodies have confirmed the immature nature of T-lymphoblasts, also suggested by the high levels of TdT, and have revealed a previously unrecognized heterogeneity in this disease. These studies have demonstrated that in T-ALL, unlike the chronic T-cell leukaemias, the neoplastic cells express a thymic phenotype (Figure 2.5). Monoclonal antibodies have been useful in the

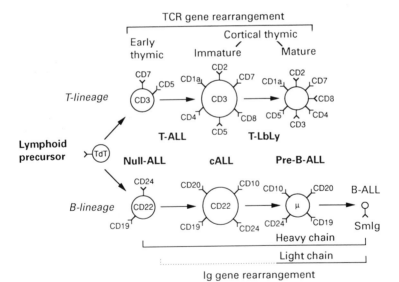

Figure 2.5 Classification of ALL bases on immunological and molecular studies showing that lymphoblasts belong to either the T- or B-cell compartment. T-lineage includes cases with early and late thymic phenotypes. T-ALL has often an immature membrane phenotype whilst T-lymphoblastic lymphoma (T-LbLy) represents a malignancy of cortical thymocytes. Non-T-ALL cells, including null-ALL, are committed to the B-cell differentiation pathway. Molecular studies at the Ig gene level, show that B-ALL, pre-B-ALL, cALL and null-ALL have evidence of heavy chain rearrangement; 20–40% of cases may also have light chain gene rearrangement. The size of the circles represents the approximate incidence of the ALL subtypes within the T- and B-cell lineages. Rearrangement of the T-cell receptor (TCR) β-chain gene is an early event on the T-cell lineage (discussed in Chapter 8)

Table 2.1 Immunological classification of ALL

Disease	TdT	CD3 (cyt)	CD7[a] (p40)	CD2 (E-ros)	HLA-DR	CD19 (B4)	CD24 (BA1)	CD10[b] (gp100)	Cytμ	SmIg
Pre-T-ALL	+	+	+	−	−	−	−	−	−	−
T-ALL	+	+	+	+	−	−	−	−	−	−
Null-ALL[c]	+	−	−	−	+	+	+/−	−	−	−
cALL	+	−	−	−	+	+	+	+	−	−
Pre-B-ALL	+	−	−	−	+	+	+	+	+	−
B-ALL	−	−	−	−	+	+	+	−[d]	−	+

[a] Monoclonal antibodies 3A1, WT1, Leu9 etc. (see Chapter 1).
[b] Monoclonal antibodies J5, AL2, VIL-1, BA3 etc.
[c] Early B-lineage ALL or 'pre' pre-B-ALL.
[d] Occasionally positive.

identification of pre-T-ALL which constitutes 20–25% of T-lineage ALL, and which otherwise would have been classified as null-ALL (Table 2.1). These cases could be assigned to the T-cell lineage on the basis of the positivity with monoclonal antibodies of the CD3 (cCD3), CD7 and CD5 groups[32, 33, 48, 54a, 99a] and, in some cases, also against the CD1a thymic antigen (see Chapter 1). Monoclonal antibodies against the p40 antigen (CD7) and the CD3 complex (cCD3) recognize T-ALL at all levels of maturation (Table 2.1) thus allowing the diagnosis of most cases.

The use of several monoclonal antibodies has permitted a better definition of the early and late stages of T-cell differentiation[101]. Early or pre-T-ALL cases are E−, TdT+, cCD3+, CD7+ and weakly express the p67 (CD5) antigen. Other markers such as CD1a, CD4 and CD8 appear at a slightly later stage in variable combinations. A scheme based on the available information of the membrane expression in T-ALL and T-LbLy is illustrated in Figure 2.5.

The clinical relevance of using numerous anti-T monoclonal antibodies to analyse the precise level of cell differentiation in T-ALL still needs to be established because it is not certain whether there are differences in prognosis between cases with an early or a late phenotype. The incidence of T-ALL according to the different reports ranges between 15% and 30%, both in adults and in children[15, 44, 117, 120] (Table 2.2). An Italian multicentre study on 190 cases of ALL reported a lower incidence of T-ALL in children than in adults, 11% and 26% respectively[32]. The highest incidence of T-ALL is found in adolescents[110] and young adults; the disease is rare over the age of 35 years.

Table 2.2 Incidence of ALL subtypes according to age

Age group[a]	T-ALL	Null-ALL	cALL (pre-B-ALL)	B-ALL
Adults	20%	20%	60% (20%)[b]	1%
Children	15%	10%	75% (20%)[b]	1%

[a] Usual age for separating children from adults is 15 years.
[b] Percentage of cALL positive cases.

Common-ALL

Several monoclonal antibodies which react with the cALL antigen (gp100, CD10) have now been produced (see Chapter 1). The reactivity of these reagents is comparable with that of the polyclonal antiserum. About 75% of childhood ALLs are cALL+[32, 44] whilst the proportion of cALL+ cases is lower in adults[32, 44] (Table 2.2).

The availability of several monoclonal antibodies which react with early B-cells has shown that almost all cases of cALL are recognized by one or more of these reagents such as B4 (CD19), BA1 (CD24) and cCD22[32, 34, 54a, 57, 66, 85] (see also Chapter 1). These findings confirm that blast cells in cALL are committed along the B-differentiation pathway. This has been further demonstrated by the induction of some B-cell antigens, i.e. CD20 and CD24 in cALL+ cells following incubation with the phorbol diester 12-*O*-tetradecanoylphorbol-13-acetate (TPA)[27, 34, 86]. The combination of extensive phenotypic analysis with more precise DNA studies seems to provide good evidence for the B-cell origin of most non-T cases. The monoclonal antibody B4 (CD19), which has been reported to recognize 95% of non-T-ALL whilst being negative on T-lymphocytes, myeloid cells, erythrocytes and platelets, reacts with an early B-cell antigen and is of value in the characterization of cALL[85] (see also Chapter 1). Based on the reactivity of various B-cell-related monoclonal antibodies, the order in which these are expressed on B-lineage ALL cells is proposed in Figure 2.5. Whilst CD19 and cCD22 appear to react with all cALL cases, CD24 recognizes 90% of these cases (both in adults and in children)[32, 57], and CD20 only 30–50% of cases[85]. The last marker to appear is Cyμ and it is often associated with the expression of the cALL antigen[32, 85]. Although cALL can be found throughout all ages, a characteristic peak incidence is seen in small children.

A major advance in our understanding of the nature of the cALL antigen (CD10) has been reported lately (reviewed by LeBien and McCormack[66a]). The gene coding for CD10 has been cloned and the amino acid sequence was found to be identical to that of the membrane-associated enzyme neutral endopeptidase (NEP) found in humans and other species. NEP is also known as a metalloendopeptidase (since it uses zinc as a cofactor) or as enkephalinase (enkephalin is one of the many substrates) and may be important in neutrophil function and chemotaxis (neutrophils are CD10+). The function of CD10/NEP on lymphoid cells still needs clarification and its natural substrate has not yet been identified[66a]. Further advances in this area are likely to be forthcoming and they may possibly have a bearing on elucidating the pathogenesis of the most common form of leukaemia in childhood.

Null-ALL

This corresponds most often to B-lineage cells which do not express the cALL (CD10) antigen but which are HLA-DR, CD19, cCD22, and TdT+. The number of cases diagnosed as null-ALL has decreased over the years as a result of improved methods for cell characterization. Null-ALL can also be designated as 'early' B-ALL and includes B-lineage cases (cCD22+, CD19+, CD24+, but CD10−) and very rare acute leukaemias of uncertain lineage. The proportion of null-ALL cases which cannot be further classified is of the order of 5% in children and slightly higher in adults. Attempts to induce the expression of more mature B-markers, i.e. CD10, CD20 and CyIg, using differentiation agents, have been difficult in these cells, although the authors have recently succeeded in inducing CD10, CD19 and

CD24 in the blasts of a 6-month-old child classified as null-ALL. Some cases may correspond to stem-cell leukaemias and a few others may show early features of myeloid differentiation which can be demonstrated by myeloid-specific monoclonal antibodies, e.g. CD13 and CD33.

Null-ALL appears to have a characteristic age distribution; it is relatively frequent within childhood ALL cases under the age of 1, and tends to increase in older adults.

Gene rearrangement analysis and correlation with membrane phenotype

It is now well established that the pathway of B-cell differentiation into mature Ig-producing lymphocytes is a multistep process, the first known event of which seems to be a gene rearrangement at the DNA level[11, 100]. The pattern of gene rearrangement first involves the heavy chain gene and thereafter proceeds to the light chains, κ prior to λ. This discovery has been of value in the identification of the B-cell origin of some human leukaemias and is also a reliable marker to establish the clonal nature of a given lymphoid population[1]. A gene reorganization can be detected only if the population examined is monoclonal and thus the DNA rearrangement pattern is unique for that particular neoplasm. Each B-lymphocyte has, in fact, an individual pattern of rearrangement and a polyclonal B-cell expansion would give rise to multiple different rearrangements which would not be visible on a Southern blot. Molecular studies at the DNA level have therefore contributed to the characterization of human lymphoid leukaemias, particularly ALL[34, 62, 63]. Analyses carried out on relatively large series of patients have demonstrated that practically all cases of cALL show evidence of heavy chain gene rearrangement[34, 62] (Table 2.3). A rare case of cALL with a germ-line DNA configuration has been reported[34]. Light chain gene rearrangement occurs in 30–40% of cALL cases, with κ more frequently rearranged than λ. A germ-line Ig configuration has been observed in most cases of T-ALL, but some have shown rearrangement of the heavy chain genes[35, 59]. In some cases of pre-T-ALL the cALL antigen may be found on the leukaemic cells. DNA studies on fresh and leukaemic T-cell lines suggest that the occasional expression of the cALL antigen is not associated with evidence of Ig gene rearrangement[62], thus excluding B-lineage commitment. It is worth noting that the cALL antigen may be found on a proportion of human thymic cells[92].

An attempt has been made to correlate the pattern of Ig gene rearrangement with the expression of B-cell markers in non-T-ALL[34]. Our analysis showed that at least one additional B-cell marker (CD24, CD20 or CyIg) can be found in addition to CD10 (gp100) in all cALL cases in which there is evidence of Ig gene rearrangement. Studies at the DNA level are of particular relevance to null-ALL cells which often express few B-cell antigens (except CD10). The reports confirm that most of these cases show evidence of Ig heavy chain gene rearrangement[29, 34, 62, 85]. The authors have demonstrated Ig heavy chain rearrangement in 13 cases of null-ALL (with expression of CD19, CD24 or other B-cell antigens); in 5 of them the κ or light chain gene was also rearranged or deleted[34a].

It is likely that the combined use of DNA and membrane marker studies will define the cell origin of all cases of ALL. The importance of combining immunological analyses to molecular studies is stressed by the finding of an Ig heavy chain gene rearrangement in occasional cases of acute myeloid leukaemia[47], in T-cell lines and some cases of T-ALL[35, 46, 59, 62, 104]. In

Table 2.3 Heavy and light chain Ig gene organization in lymphoid leukaemias

	T-ALL		Null-ALL		cALL		B-CLL		B-PLL		HCL		T-CLL/ T-PLL	
	H	L	H	L	H	L	H	L	H	L	H	L	H	L
DNA analysis Incidence (%)	G 100[b]	G 100	R 100	R[a] 25	R 100[c]	R 30–40	R 100	R 100	R 100	R 100	R 100	R 100	G 100[d]	G 100

Abbreviations: H: heavy chain; L: light chain; R: rearranged; G: germ-line.

[a] In the majority of cases κ light chain rearrangements.
[b] Cases with heavy chain gene rearrangement reported [35, 46, 59, 62].
[c] One germ-line case reported [34].
[d] Exceptional cases of chronic T-cell leukaemias and a proportion of TdT+ AML with rearrangement of the heavy chain gene have been observed by the authors.

chronic lymphoid leukaemias of indisputed B-cell origin, i.e. B-CLL, B-PLL and hairy cell leukaemia, the lymphocytes always have a rearranged Ig heavy chain pattern[36, 50, 63], including a rare case of B-PLL with negative SmIg and CyIg but positive with other B-cell markers[77] and cases of B-CLL with an unexpected co-expression of T-cell markers[82a]. The rearrangement of the Ig light chain genes occurs in all these cases, reflecting the more mature nature of the neoplastic cells. The demonstration of Ig gene rearrangement has also been of great value in establishing the presence of clonal B-cell populations in lymphomatous tissues of otherwise uncertain nature[1]. Furthermore, Ig gene rearrangements have been described in the lymphoid blast crises of chronic myeloid leukaemia[3, 35]. The available information on the Ig gene configuration in acute and chronic lymphoid leukaemias is summarized in Table 2.3. Recent studies demonstrating the rearrangement of the genes (β, γ, δ) of the T-cell receptor in T-ALL and other T-cell malignancies are discussed fully in Chapter 8.

Cell kinetics

Early studies using tritiated thymidine in vitro to assess the percentage of S phase cells, or labelling index (LI), have shown that in ALL there is no difference between the LI of peripheral blood and bone marrow cells – mean 5.6% and 6.8%, respectively[39]. This contrasts with findings in acute myeloid leukaemia where the LI of bone marrow cells is always higher than of blood blasts – mean 10.7% and 4.4%, respectively[39].

Recent studies have used flow cytometry with fluorescent dyes (acridine orange or propidium iodide) for the analysis of DNA stem-line ploidy and cell cycle distribution. The frequency of aneuploidy (DNA content different from normal) and the percentage of S phase cells varies according to the immunological subtype of ALL. The proliferative rate (S phase cells) is low in cALL, high in T-ALL and very high in B-ALL[69]. The incidence of DNA aneuploidy is significantly higher in L2 than in L1 cases – 71% and 34%, respectively[116]. L2 ALL was also shown to have a higher proliferation rate than L1 – 12.4% and 5.8% S phase cells, respectively[116].

Hyperdiploidy is a common finding in standard risk childhood ALL. Although this can be demonstrated accurately by the more laborious chromosome techniques[122], flow cytometry can demonstrate hyperdiploidy (corresponding to $\geqslant 53$ chromosomes) with relative ease. Children with hyperdiploid lymphoblasts responded better to treatment than those with diploid or slightly increased DNA content[70]. Similar findings shown by chromosome studies[107a, 109, 111, 118] have helped to identify a group of children with a low probability of relapse[70]. Flow cytometry is an important complement of chromosome studies and has the advantage that results can be obtained in all cases. However, this technique is unable to detect balanced chromosome translocations or to identify cases with minimal changes in chromosome numbers (e.g. from 44 to 48).

Prognostic factors

It is now recognized that patterns of relapse and survival in ALL are greatly influenced by a number of prognostic features which are listed in Table 2.4. These

Table 2.4 Prognostic factors in ALL at presentation[a]

Feature	Good	Bad
WBC ($\times 10^9$/l) [44]	<10	>50
Age (years)	2–10	<2, >14 (>50 in adults)
Sex	Female	Male
Karyotype [119]	>50 chromosomes [70, 107a, 109, 111]	Translocations[b]
Morphology [79]	L1	L2, L3
Immunophenotype [44]	cALL [21] (excluding pre-B)	B-ALL, pre-B [28] and T-ALL [117]
Organomegaly	None	AMM [23], lymphadenopathy, hepatomegaly
CNS leukaemia	Absent	Present
Cytochemistry [4]	PAS+	AP+, PAS−
Labelling index	Low	High [69]

[a] Listed in order of importance and relate to the effect on remission induction, remission duration and probability of relapse (bone marrow, CNS and testicular). *Key references in brackets.*
[b] t(4;11); t(9;22); t(8;14) [7a, 119].

Abbreviations: AMM: anterior mediastinal mass; AP: acid phosphatase; CNS: central nervous system.

factors have been better defined in childhood ALL but some, like WBCs, are significant in all age groups. The importance of a given prognostic factor depends on whether it is shown to be statistically significant in many studies and whether it has independent value by multivariate analysis. Some, like T-ALL, are strongly associated with poor prognosis because of their relationship with several unfavourable features such as high WBC count (often $> 100 \times 10^9$/l), male sex (M:F ratio 4:1) and an anterior mediastinal mass (AMM; 50% of cases). The independent effect of an AMM has been disputed. Some studies[23] concluded that in itself it does not carry a bad prognosis, but for its relationship to high WBC count, male sex, age over 10 years and frequent association with lymphadenopathy.

The importance of prognostic factors also relates to the type of treatment given as has been well illustrated in West German studies[65]. For example, the significance of thymic involvement was very strong in an early study using a non-intensive regimen. In later studies, the BFM protocol (1970–76)[102], the effect of an AMM almost disappeared as a result of more intensive and better therapy. A worse prognosis of boys with ALL has been documented in many trials which showed higher rates of bone marrow relapse as well as the characteristic complication of this group – testicular relapse (see below).

The effect of race on the survival of childhood ALL has been shown by several studies. Black children in the USA[28] and Asian children in the UK seem to fare worse than White children treated by similar protocols. The reason for these differences has been a matter of debate. Some have argued that socioeconomic factors, including poor nutrition and/or difficulties in communication, were responsible. Against this is the observation that the incidence of particular types of ALL is often different in these groups, e.g. Black children have a lower incidence of cALL and a relatively higher frequency of T-ALL. On the other hand, changes in phenotype from B-ALL to cALL attributable to socioeconomic changes were reported from Israel[99].

The importance of karyotype as an independent risk factor was demonstrated by the Third International Workshop[119]. The very good prognosis of children with a modal chromosome number greater than 50 has been confirmed by other studies[70, 107a, 109, 111].

In addition to T-ALL, another group defined by marker studies and associated with worse prognosis is pre-B-ALL. The Pediatric Oncology Group observed that children with pre-B disease (cALL with Cyμ) have a shorter remission duration than others with non-T-ALL who were similarly treated[28]. Although WBC count was the most important prognostic variable in that study, the pre-B phenotype was still important when it was corrected for WBC counts.

Nowadays the design of treatment protocols takes into account the prognostic features listed in Table 2.4. Usually they are compounded in groups defining low or standard risk, intermediate or medium, and high-risk cases. Others have defined 'scores' to allocate patients in each treatment arm; the BFM group uses a diagram which defines the risk according to the peripheral blood blast cell count and the liver and spleen sizes[65]. It is clear that with improvements in treatment some of the features listed in Table 2.4 may cease to have clinical significance and it is possible that some others will become important in the future.

Special features of some ALL subtypes

In addition to the groups defined by morphology, markers, prognostic factors and cytogenetics (see below), some ALL subtypes merit special comment because of their close relation with childhood non-Hodgkin's lymphomas (NHLs), their distinct clinical behaviour and/or their biological implications.

The relationship of ALL to childhood non-Hodgkin's lymphomas

One important area in need of clarification is the relationship of T-ALL and B-ALL to the corresponding NHL. Childhood NHLs are diffuse high grade malignancies which, with few exceptions, fall in three histological types:

1. Lymphoblastic (LbLy), the majority corresponding to T-LbLy.
2. Undifferentiated or non-lymphoblastic (Burkitt's and non-Burkitt's), the majority of which are of B-cell type.
3. Large cell or immunoblastic, which is less common and could be of B-, T- or undefined cell type and is often Ki-1+ (CD30+).

NHL cases with an early B-cell phenotype (null or cALL) are very rare. At least half of the cases are of T-cell type (T-LbLy) and the rest have a mature B-phenotype (SmIg+), with few of macrophage or undetermined lineage. There is a great overlap betweeen the concepts of leukaemia and lymphoma, especially in paediatric practice. Leukaemia refers to a disorder that starts and affects chiefly the bone marrow and almost always involves the blood. Lymphoma refers to a malignancy arising from extramedullary sites (usually lymph nodes) although the neoplastic infiltration may rapidly spread to the blood and bone marrow.

T-ALL and T-LbLy

A significant overlap exists between these two closely related disorders. T-ALL has an anterior mediastinal mass (AMM) or thymic tumour in 50% of cases[23, 44, 110, 117], whilst this is a feature of 95% of cases of T-LbLy. In clinical studies the separation is based on the degree of bone marrow involvement, 5% or 25% of blasts being the upper limits usually considered for a diagnosis of LbLy. Above those values or when blasts are found in the circulation the diagnosis is always ALL.

Analysis of the presenting features of T-ALL has suggested that this disease may, in fact, start outside the bone marrow, in particular because the initial haemoglobin and platelet counts are higher than in B-lineage (non-T)-ALL[44, 110]. Lymphadenopathy and hepatosplenomegaly, reflecting widespread tumour progression, are more common in T-ALL than in T-LbLy, whilst pleural effusions reflecting perhaps local spread and/or disruption of lymphatic channels are more frequent in the latter condition. Both tumours have similar age incidence (10–30 years) and predominate in males. Morphology, convoluted or non-convoluted blasts, and cytochemistry, strong paranuclear acid phosphatase reaction[18, 19, 114], are also features in common. On the other hand, an important difference which may, in turn, be responsible for the different clinical behaviour of these T-cell tumours has been observed in the membrane phenotype of the lymphoblasts (see also Chapter 1). Cells in T-ALL have immature features and include the pre-T-ALL group in which an AMM is not common; cells in T-LbLy often correspond to cortical thymocytes, express T6 (CD1a) and co-express T4 (CD4) and T8 (CD8) which is an infrequent finding in T-ALL; both tumours are E+(CD2+) TdT+, cCD3+, CD7+ and share other T-antigens[58, 110, 117]. It is possible that, although in both diseases the cells are of thymic origin, the membrane characteristics may influence the leukaemic evolution. It is well known that in cases presenting with an AMM the tumour may evolve into a florid T-ALL within days or weeks[26]. In fact the rate of leukaemic progression in T-LbLy may be as high as 70%. The prognosis of T-ALL is probably worse than that of T-LbLy but this may largely depend on its greater tumour burden. Staging systems used for NHL and analysis of prognostic factors in T-ALL may help to apply the best possible treatment strategies for these aggressive T-cell tumours.

B-ALL (L3) and Burkitt's lymphoma
The relationship of B-ALL and Burkitt's NHL is closer than that between T-ALL and T-LbLy. The similarities include morphology (L3 or Burkitt cell type), B-cell markers (SmIg etc.) and chromosome translocations, chiefly t(8;14) in 80% of cases[31, 81]. The different clinical presentations may relate to environmental factors. Burkitt's lymphoma is a well-recognized entity of equatorial Africa, an area of holoendemic malaria[74] (see also Chapter 7). The incidence of diffuse bone marrow involvement in this tumour is low and its presentation as ALL is rare; late marrow involvement can be seen in 16% of cases. Non-endemic Burkitt's lymphoma has a higher incidence of bone marrow involvement (see Table 7.7, Chapter 7) and it is in non-African countries where a presentation as acute leukaemia is often seen.

B-ALL rarely presents as widespread disease with abdominal masses; more frequently it has mainly blood and bone marrow involvement. Flandrin et al.[31] described six European patients with B-ALL who presented with a WBC count of 6.9–29 × 10^9/l, with 1–50% blasts in the peripheral film, and 90–100% L3 blasts in the bone marrow. The main clinical features were hepatosplenomegaly and bone lesions; only one patient later developed a jaw tumour. B-ALL has an extremely bad prognosis and the treatment may be complicated by a 'tumour lysis' syndrome with a number of metabolic abnormalities, principally hyperkalaemia. The authors have treated three patients with B-ALL with t(8;14), two of whom presented without any organ enlargement. Despite an intense chemotherapy protocol two of them developed early CNS disease, a feature of B-ALL, and later bone marrow relapse and died less than 6 months after diagnosis. The third patient received an allogeneic bone marrow transplantation whilst in remission and has remained well 3 years after this procedure.

Adult ALL

One of the striking facts about ALL in adult patients (≥ 15 years of age) is the overall poor prognosis when compared with childhood ALL even when many clinical and laboratory features are not very different between these disorders. Complete remissions in adult ALL series have, until recently, rarely been recorded in over 80% of cases[40, 51, 105], at a time when the complete remission rate is close to 100% in children. There are features found with a higher incidence in adult ALL which may contribute to the poor prognosis of this disease compared with childhood ALL; these are: L2 morphology[6], the Ph chromosome[8, 17, 106, 118], lack of hyperdiploidy (L. Secker-Walker, personal communication) and a null-phenotype. In most recent studies 30–40% of adults with ALL were alive at 3 years; this figure compares unfavourably with the results in children where 70–80% of cases are expected to be alive at 3 years.

The authors have reviewed a series of 69 adult patients treated at Hammersmith Hospital over a 10-year period (1974–84)[75a]. The overall 5-year survival in this series was 21% and the remission rate 78%. When examining prognostic variables it was observed that age and WBC count had the greatest influence in prognosis. Morphology was important but it was related to age, the incidence of L2 being 77% in patients over 35 years whilst in those aged less than 35 years it was 58%. The best prognosis, 42% actuarial survival at 5 years, was seen in young patients, less than 35 years, who presented with WBC count less than $10 \times 10^9/l$. This group constituted less than 25% of the cases of that series.

Mixed or biphenotypic leukaemias

The wider use of monoclonal antibodies and a detailed analysis by cytochemical methods have disclosed, in the last few years, the existence of the so-called biphenotypic or mixed acute leukaemias. The coexistence of blasts from different lineages, e.g. lymphoid and myeloid, is generally recognized in Ph+ chronic granulocytic leukaemia (CGL), a disorder affecting the pluripotential stem cell. Awareness of a similar situation in ALL with t(4;11) is also becoming apparent (see below). In addition to these conditions, a number of well-documented cases presenting as ALL or acute myeloid leukaemia (AML) with double markers or involving more than one lineage are increasingly being reported[68a, 83, 88, 112].

Three types of situation have been documented. First, there are cases in which two or more distinct populations of blasts can be recognized constituting real 'mixtures'[93a]. In these cases, as in CGL blast crises, some blasts are lymphoid (e.g. TdT+, MPO−, My9−) and others myeloid (myeloblasts or monoblasts). Depending on the treatment given one or other blast cell type may predominate later in the evolution of the disease. Secondly, there is a similar double population but with only one of them apparent at diagnosis and being responsible for the diagnosis of ALL or AML. Following treatment and complete remission a phenotypic shift is then demonstrated[76, 92a]. Stass et al.[112] reported such a shift in 6 out of 89 children (6.7%) with relapsed acute leukaemia: 4 ALLs relapsed as AML and 2 AMLs relapsed as ALL. The authors have observed a patient diagnosed as AML on the basis of cytochemistry (Sudan black +, myeloperoxidase +) but with TdT+, cALL− blasts, who achieved remission with anti-AML therapy and one year after presentation relapsed with a cALL phenotype (TdT+, cALL+, MPO−, Sudan black−). A second complete remission was obtained, now with anti-ALL therapy, and has continued for over 9 months [76]; the patient eventually relapsed with ALL cells in the ovaries and died of widespread disease. Interestingly four of the patients of Stass et al. [112] achieved a second remission by switching to the therapy appropriate to the predominant blast cell type. Thirdly, there are cases in which the cells co-express myeloid or lymphoid markers, more commonly TdT, CD19 and CD10 in 'AML' and CD33 and CD13 in 'ALL' [12a, 71a]. This situation may reflect the infidelity of the markers rather than a truly dual population. Because of this the evidence for overlapping features should only be acceptable when more than one specific reagent is present in the 'wrong' cell lineage. Studies at the DNA level may be relevant to define the real nature of the blasts, particularly in this latter group of patients [68a]. In the authors' experience no true genomically biclonal acute leukaemia (i.e. one blastic population rearranged and one blastic population germ line) has so far been documented. The authors have observed a child who at presentation was diagnosed as TdT+ AML and who relapsed as cALL and in whom the blasts showed on the two occasions an identical rearrangement of the Ig and TCR γ-genes on the entire population. In addition to the non-specificity of certain monoclonal antibodies [42a] it is important to consider here the problem of non-specific binding to Fcγ receptors in monoblasts referred to in Chapter 1.

The significance of the biphenotypic phenomenon, also illustrated by cases with t(9;22) and t(4;11), is that the leukaemic process involves early stem cells with potential for differentiation into myeloid and lymphoid lineages [42a]. The clinical relevance of these findings and the implications for treatment, as illustrated above, makes it necessary to study and document carefully such cases so that their true nature could be further elucidated. The clinical importance of the expression of 'myeloid' antigens in ALL has been stressed in adult patients in an American study [111a] which described the highest incidence (33%) of this phenomenon. Although this report by Sobol et al. [111a] included as ALLs some cases with negative B- and T-markers, which should have been considered as AML-MO [93a, 95a], in the group of B-lineage ALL with positive myeloid antigens, the complete remission rate was significantly lower (29% vs 71%) and the survival shorter (median 8.1 months vs >26 months) compared with the group of B-lineage ALL without myeloid markers. The incidence of myeloid markers in ALL has been lower in other studies, about 10–20% [12a, 54a, 95a]. The large Australian study of Bradstock et al. [12a] could not confirm the worse prognosis for childhood and adult ALL cases with biphenotypic features.

Treatment

There has been significant progress in the outlook of children with ALL in the last 25 years; the progress has been less dramatic in adult ALL. The advances in therapy have been manifold but a few important landmarks can be singled out: the concept of 'total therapy' and CNS prophylaxis [95], the cytoreductive role of

L-asparaginase during induction therapy, the use of methotrexate at intermediate or high dosages to overcome drug resistance and cross the blood–CNS barrier[82], the periodic reinductions with vincristine and prednisolone, the intensive consolidation protocols of the West German BFM group[65, 102], and the advent of new agents and combinations, such as teniposide (VM-26) and cytosine arabinoside (Ara-C), and mitozantrone. Evidence of this progress is reflected in the figures of 50–70% 5-year disease-free survival which are currently obtained in children with ALL[65, 89].

The recognition of prognostic features (see Table 2.4) has helped to tailor protocols according to risk categories. It is known that more intensive regimens have carried with them a greater risk of morbidity and even mortality for patients in complete remission. The major progress has come from pilot studies which were subsequently tested in large multicentre trials. Childhood ALL clearly shows the benefits of treating patients as part of study protocols that ask critical questions. Experience in the UK has shown that the quality of care and the overall results are better for patients treated in specialized centres according to well-defined guidelines. Despite the progress a number of unresolved questions remain, namely: the optimal regimen for CNS prophylaxis, whether testicular relapse can be prevented by local measures or with intensified systemic therapy, the optimal duration of maintenance therapy, the ways to improve the treatment of adult ALL and the role of bone marrow transplantation for poor prognosis groups. The strategy for the treatment of ALL is based on five phases: remission induction, early intensification or consolidation, CNS prophylaxis, cytoreduction or reinduction, and maintenance therapy.

Remission induction

Vincristine and prednisone or prednisolone have become the established first line of therapy for ALL. These two agents alone can induce complete remission in 90% of children with ALL rapidly and without toxicity. A higher complete remission rate (95–98%) and a greater cell kill is achieved when one or two other drugs are added in the first few weeks of therapy – commonly l-asparaginase and/or an anthracycline, daunorubicin or doxorubicin. Whilst the addition of the enzyme l-asparaginase has been shown to improve the long-term outcome, the value of adding an anthracycline in this early phase is still being investigated. The important long-term advantages of intensifying the induction therapy should be weighed against the higher incidence of serious complications which sometimes could be fatal. The addition of daunorubicin will prolong the period of neutropenia and may cause infections more easily. The addition of doxorubicin will cause more mucositis and overall worse complications than daunorubicin. L-Asparaginase delays the haemopoietic recovery and has its own side effects such as anaphylaxis, hyperglycaemia, hypofibrinogenaemia and other metabolic abnormalities, which can be seen in 10–20% of patients, depending on the source of the enzyme. For example in the UKALL trials fewer complications were documented with asparaginase from *Erwinia* sp. than when the enzyme from *Escherichia coli* was used.

The use of daunorubicin during the induction phase in adult-ALL has been shown to be associated with a higher complete remission rate in many studies. One study by the Cancer and Leukemia Group B showed an 84% complete remission rate in patients given daunorubicin and 47% when daunorubicin was not used[40].

When daunorubicin was added to the latter group the complete remission rate improved to 76%. Disappointingly, the long-term outcome of both groups of adult patients, 25% disease free at 3 years, was no different[40].

Consolidation

The first 4 weeks of remission induction treatment are followed by an intensification phase that includes alternative agents to those used during induction. This programme starts usually when complete remission has been obtained and/or at least when the recovery of the blood counts has taken place. The BFM studies have used an intensive 4-week protocol which included cyclophosphamide, 6-mercaptopurine, Ara-C, methotrexate given intrathecally and cranial irradiation[65, 112]. In the BFM study (1976–79), high-risk patients received, in addition, a reinduction (reinforcement) course with dexamethasone, vincristine, doxorubicin, Ara-C, 6-thioguanine and intrathecal methotrexate. This further intensification resulted in a significant improvement in the proportion of high-risk cases, from 46% to 65%, with prolonged continuous complete remission and a decrease in the importance of the bad prognosis associated with T-ALL. These more intensive programmes were associated initially with a 6.7–7.5% mortality in complete remission, but lately this incidence decreased to 3.8–4.9% as a result of greater supportive care measures, which are essential for the undertaking of this type of treatment[65].

The UKALL X trial is testing, in children and adults, the value of one or two identical intensification courses with seven drugs: vincristine, prednisolone, daunorubicin, 6-thioguanine, etoposide, Ara-C and intrathecal methotrexate.

Methotrexate, given as an intravenous infusion at intermediate doses $(500\,mg/m^2)$ followed by Leucovorin (folinic acid) rescue is also used as consolidation therapy[82]. In some studies, this regimen together with intrathecal methotrexate was used as CNS prophylaxis to replace cranial irradiation. The incidence of bone marrow and testicular relapse seems to decrease significantly with methotrexate infusions but not the incidence of meningeal leukaemia. It is possible that this modality, which has little toxicity, could be used as consolidation preceding cranial irradiation which so far has been shown to be the most effective way of preventing CNS disease. Current trials are testing the value of high doses $(2\,g/m^2$ or higher) as consolidation therapy and for CNS prophylaxis.

CNS prophylaxis

The concept of the CNS as a sanctuary site, which is prevented by the blood–CSF barrier from receiving effective concentrations of the drugs used in the treatment of ALL, was the key for one of the major advances in the therapy of this disease. The studies of Pinkel at St Jude Hospital[95] led the way by demonstrating the benefits of using craniospinal irradiation once bone marrow remission was achieved. Not only did the incidence of meningeal leukaemia decrease 10 times, from 50% to 5%, but the benefits in survival were also significant.

Several methods have been used to prevent meningeal complications: periodic intrathecal methotrexate, craniospinal irradiation/cranial irradiation at 2400 or 1800 cGy combined with four to six intrathecal injections of methotrexate, infusions of methotrexate at intermediate dosages combined with intrathecal methotrexate, and combinations of methotrexate, Ara-C and hydrocortisone given intrathecally. Most protocols also incorporate early intrathecal injections of methotrexate during remission induction. Each procedure has advantages and disadvantages. The trend towards reducing the doses of cranial irradiation to 1800 cGy followed the reports of long-term neuropsychological sequelae, CT scan changes (dilatation of ventricles, intracerebral calcification etc.) and growth retardation, in children cured of their leukaemia. Methotrexate alone given intrathecally can cause acute reactions such as mild nausea, fever, headaches and vomiting, and cause a somnolence syndrome seen 5–7 weeks post-cranial irradiation[7]. Major complications, including subacute necrotizing leucoencephalopathy, are seen after treatment of meningeal leukaemia[56] or when systemic methotrexate is given at doses higher than 40 mg/m^2 intravenously. Methotrexate intrathecally or by infusion should not be given, for that reason, after the completion of cranial irradiation.

The Children's Cancer Study Group showed that 1800 cGy is as effective as 2400 cGy in preventing CNS disease[91], although the higher dose may be more effective for children with a high WBC count[102]. It is of course not proven that the lower dose is not associated with long-term toxicity or that slightly lower doses may not be equally effective. There is good evidence that it is the combination of cranial irradiation and intrathecal methotrexate that is associated with neurological problems, particularly when used for established CNS disease[7]. Methotrexate alone given for a short period, e.g. six doses, is not effective in preventing CNS leukaemia[89].

Adequate concentrations of methotrexate in the CSF when given by 24-hour intravenous infusions followed by folinic acid (Leucovorin) rescue can be obtained with doses of 1000 mg/m^2[7]. Using intermediate doses, e.g. 500 mg/m^2, the CNS prophylaxis is not so effective unless accompanied by intrathecal injections. Even so this method alone is less effective for CNS prophylaxis. The best regimen of administrating intrathecal methotrexate is by calculating the dose according to age and CNS volume and not by body size: dosages currently used are 5 mg for less than 1 year of age, 7.5 mg for 1–2 years, 10 mg for 2–3 years and 12.5 mg over 3 years. Despite prophylactic measures, CNS leukaemia may occur in 3–5% of cases, increasing to 10% in high-risk cases in parallel with the WBC.

The incidence of meningeal leukaemias in adult ALL is the same as in children. Therefore prophylactic measures are an essential part of the management of adults where problems of long-term sequelae have not been so well documented.

Maintenance therapy

Long-term maintenance has been established as an essential part in the management of ALL. Early studies showed that methotrexate was an important component of this treatment, and later that 6-mercaptopurine was incorporated in such programmes. Whilst there is the need for a relatively prolonged period of maintenance, the precise effect of this continuous therapy and, in particular, the optimal duration are not clear. Presumably this type of regimen is useful for slowly proliferating ALL with a proportion of blasts coming out of the G$_0$ phase at regular intervals.

One of the UKALL trials in the 1970s showed that 19 months' maintenance was not adequate and that maintenance for 36 months was better. Since then most studies have used between 2 and 3 years of maintenance. Analysis of the St Jude Hospital results in the late 1970s showed that 2.5 years were probably adequate for female patients. A comparison between 3 and 5 years' maintenance[90] showed no major differences in survival, although again boys had twice as many relapses as girls. A slightly higher incidence of bone marrow relapse rate was observed in those treated for 3 years but this was not reflected in a worse survival. Encouragingly, in this study, after randomization at 3 years, the proportion of children who remained disease free was greater than 80% in both groups.

Conventional maintenance programmes include methotrexate which is best given once a week orally or preferably, because of irregular absorption by mouth, by intramuscular injections. 6-Mercaptopurine is given continuously on a daily schedule. The value of reinduction courses with vincristine and prednisone are not proven[65] but these are included in most protocols. Some studies in adults incorporate daunorubicin during reinductions[105].

It is possible that in the next few years the concept of maintenance therapy may change as a result of the more intensive regimens used for consolidation. However, it is likely that the traditional maintenance approach for 2–2.5 years will continue until such time as randomized trials show that such prolonged therapy may not be necessary. The authors are not aware that this question is being considered at present by the leading groups, although BFM studies comparing 1.5 and 2 years of overall duration, which include the 7 months of intensive induction/consolidation therapy, are in progress at present[65].

Pattern of relapse

The aim of treatment in ALL is to obtain long periods of disease-free survival which can be considered equivalent to clinical cures. In fact, although late relapses do occur, they are extremely rare after the initial treatment has stopped for 4–5 years. There are important differences in outcome regarding the timing of a relapse. When this occurs in the first 2–3 years, while the patient is still on treatment, the prognosis is poor because it is the manifestation of resistant disease. Relatively late relapses, particularly if they do not involve the bone marrow, have the possibility of a second prolonged remission. Nevertheless, if the primary treatment has been adequate and intensive enough, a relapse always indicates a degree of resistance by cells that have survived the initial treatment. Besides the bone marrow, the primary sites of relapse are the CNS, or meningeal leukaemia, and the testis, or testicular relapse. Less frequent sites for extramedullary relapse are the ovaries and the eye (iris and anterior ocular chamber or the optic nerve)[84].

Bone marrow relapse

A report by Chessells et al.[22] summarizes the fate of children experiencing a bone marrow relapse after treatment has been stopped. When relapse occurs within the first 6 months of stopping therapy, 80% will achieve a second complete remission but of short duration (median 6 months). In those who relapse after 6 months, the complete remission rate is 100% and the remission duration longer (median 2 years). However, it has become apparent that 88% will relapse again, which in one-third occurs in the CNS. Thus the long-term outcome for bone marrow relapse is extremely poor. Only two children out of the 34 reported (6%) were alive without relapse 5 years from the first episode of bone marrow relapse and one of them was suffering from leucoencephalopathy[22].

Although there is consensus about using first-line drugs during the primary treatment and making all the curative efforts the first time round, the need still exists to consider treatment for a patient in bone marrow relapse. Careful analysis of the drugs employed initially should reveal whether any one can still be used without toxicity, this being particularly relevant in the case of the anthracyclines. Clearly the treatment programme should be substantially more intensive than the initial one; the only remote possibility of success relies on the use of new agents and/or new combinations not previously used. It is not clear yet whether bone marrow transplantation can claim a high salvage rate in this type of patient.

Meningeal leukaemia

As CNS prophylaxis is now an integral part of the curative efforts in ALL, the high incidence of this complication (50–60% of cases) is a feature of the past. Nevertheless, between 3% and 7% of cases may experience a CNS relapse after adequate prophylactic measures.

The manifestations of meningeal leukaemia are often florid: severe headaches, easy vomiting and other clinical features of raised intracranial pressure. Unilateral facial nerve palsy is frequent in T-ALL and may not always relate to meningeal involvement. In some cases the neurological examination suggests lower motor neurone paralysis probably due to leukaemic infiltration of the seventh nerve. The diagnosis of CNS involvement requires a lumbar puncture, measurement of the CSF pressure and examination of the CSF, including a WBC count and careful morphological analysis of cytospin slides stained with Romanovsky dyes. A diagnosis is usually made with a cell count greater than 50 per μl but a count of 5 cells per μl may suffice provided leukaemic cells are unequivocally recognized on the slides. In doubtful cases the use of anti-TdT or monoclonal antibodies may help to distinguish a reactive pleocytosis, which will show monocytes and T-lymphocytes (always TdT−), from a lymphoblastic infiltrate. Knowledge of the phenotype of the original leukaemic cells may help use of the most relevant reagents in the small specimens often obtained. Immunocytochemical methods, e.g. immunoperoxidase, are superior to analysis of cell suspensions for this purpose.

There is no satisfactory treatment for meningeal leukaemia, but long-term remissions and sometimes clinical cures can be achieved with craniospinal irradiation or long-term programmes of intrathecal injections using methotrexate alone or in rotation with Ara-C. To facilitate the intrathecal administration of these drugs, Ommaya subcutaneous reservoirs connected to the lateral ventricle have been used. Prolonged administration of methotrexate into the CSF after cranial irradiation for established leukaemic meningitis carries a high risk of leucoencephalopathy which is, as a rule, fatal[56]. This devastating complication characterized by dementia, tremor, ataxia, convulsions and coma is the result of a demyelinating process associated with areas of necrosis in the temporal and parietal lobes. Although the major cause of this complication has been suggested as methotrexate, the predisposing effect of cranial irradiation and the underlying meningeal leukaemia are equally important.

Testicular relapse

After the breakthrough of CNS prophylaxis and the longer survivals observed in childhood ALL, it became apparent that boys were faring worse than girls and that a proportion of them, 8–30%, were relapsing first in the testis. With the use of more intensive protocols, in particular the use of intermediate doses of methotrexate[82], the incidence of this complication seems to be falling recently to less than 5%[65].

If testicular leukaemia is only treated locally it is often followed by a systemic relapse. Thus the view has grown that this complication is not an isolated event, but probably represents the 'tip of the iceberg' and that the testes are not a true sanctuary site as the CNS. Evidence for a blood–testicular barrier is not good and histology of the testis suggests that the drugs administered systemically probably reach that organ in adequate concentrations.

There are two types of testicular relapse: early and late[10]. Early relapse is seen during maintenance therapy in 1–2% of boys with high-risk factors, is as a rule bilateral and reflects inadequate overall control of the leukaemia. As a result it is always associated with bad prognosis. Late relapse occurs when off therapy, it is often unilateral and, in contrast to early relapse, may not carry a poor prognosis. Following local irradiation (2400 cGy), systemic reinduction therapy and maintenance for 2 years, the majority of patients may experience prolonged remissions. In a series from St Jude Hospital[98] 10 of 12 children were in bone marrow remission with a median of 4 years, 9 of them remaining off therapy for 13–18 months. Similar results were obtained in a study from the Hopsital for Sick Children in London.

Until recently most trials recommended carrying out a bilateral testicular biopsy at the time of completing maintenance therapy. If a positive biopsy was obtained, treatment proceeded as described above. The value of this early detection of testicular leukaemia was investigated in a trial of 238 boys with biopsies carried out, in half of them, at the end of the first 1 or 1.5 years of treatment[98]. No significant differences in outcome in both groups of children were observed in this study. Thus, the authors concluded that the routine testicular biopsy at the end of maintenance therapy needs to be re-evaluated. Only one positive biopsy with occult disease was found out of 106 boys tested; on the other hand 6 children with a negative biopsy subsequently developed overt testicular relapse.

The need to prevent testicular involvement by prophylactic irradiation has few advocates. Although the incidence of isolated testicular relapse may decrease in this way, the overall prognosis does not improve. Furthermore, a significant decrease in the incidence of this complication is seen now with more effective chemotherapy regimens, which confirms the view that testicular disease is rarely an isolated event.

Infectious complications

A number of infectious problems can occur during the management of ALL patients. Bacterial infections associated with neutropenia are less common than in acute myeloid leukaemia because bone marrow hypoplasia is not a prerequisite for complete remission in ALL. However, the newer more intensive consolidation protocols could induce short periods of severe neutropenia ($< 0.5 \times 10^9$/l) which may lead to Gram-negative sepsis as often seen in acute myeloid leukaemia.

The most severe infections in children are caused by viruses and are a consequence of immunosuppression. These viral illnesses are responsible for a significant morbidity and a 3–5% mortality in patients in complete remission. The most common fatal infections are interstitial pneumonitis; in one of the MRC UKALL trials 40% of them were caused by measles. These lung infections develop suddenly with fever, tachypnoea, hypoxaemia and bilateral infiltrates in the chest X-ray. In the past such episodes were caused by *Pneumocystis carinii* but this is now prevented by the prophylactic use of co-trimoxazole (Septrin) which is given in a three times a week schedule during the whole period of treatment. The management and prevention of viral complications in children with ALL involves a great deal of alertness by paediatricians regarding contacts at home and at school, information on current epidemics and the possibility of using passive prophylaxis with γ-globulin preparations, preferably if available with a high titre of antibodies, against measles or varicella-zoster.

A severe and often fatal illness seen in children with ALL, described as 'haemophagocytic syndrome', often results from abnormal or defective responses to infections caused by some DNA viruses, e.g. Epstein–Barr virus or the herpes virus. This syndrome has been wrongly reported in the literature as a 'malignant' transformation or evolution of the primary ALL. The correct interpretation is critical in such cases because adequate supportive measures and anti-viral therapy may reverse an almost fatal condition. The authors have witnessed the full recovery of a 6-year-old child with ALL in complete remission from a haemophagocytic syndrome associated with a parainfluenzal infection who presented with pancytopenia, fever and active erythrophagocytosis in the bone marrow.

Bone marrow transplantation

The improved prognosis of low risk ALL has made it necessary that the early experience with bone marrow transplantation (BMT) in this disease has been limited to patients in second or subsequent remissions. For this reason, in addition to the problems common to this procedure which are the cause of morbidity and mortality close to 30%, the experience of bone marrow transplantation in ALL has been less encouraging than in other diseases, namely acute myeloid leukaemia (AML) and chronic granulocytic leukaemia (CGL) in chronic phase. The major problem in ALL has been a high relapse rate, close to 50%, which suggests that refractory disease may be difficult to eliminate following high dose cyclophosphamide and total body irradiation.

The results of a survey carried out by the European Group for BMT described the results in 192 ALL patients who were recipients of bone marrow from HLA-identical siblings (allogeneic BMT). Patients with non-T-ALL (B-lineage) did better than those with T-ALL, and those transplanted in first complete remission did significantly better than those transplanted in second or third complete remission[124]. Relapses at 2 years were low in first complete remission ALL (both types) and were high, 32% and 48% for transplants in second complete remission in non-T- and T-ALL respectively. It is clear from the good results obtained in first complete remission that careful patient selection will be a critical step for further advances. The definition of high risk based on prognostic features, although in need of constant review, still suggests that patients with B-ALL, T-ALL presenting with high WBC count, adults with high WBC count, L2 morphology and/or null-ALL, as well as cases of any age with chromosome translocations, are candidates for BMT if a suitable donor is available. The fact that in the comparisons made with salvage chemotherapy, BMT always came out better and the fact that a minority (about 20%) of long-term survivors in those transplanted after a second relapse do exist, suggest that this procedure can still be used as a last resort in this disease. A recent update from the International BMT Registry[3a] reported data on 690 patients. The actuarial 5-year leukaemia-free survival for allogeneic BMT performed in first complete remission was 42% and 26% when carried out in second remission. Results were better in children than in adults. A number of disease- and transplant-related variables were analysed and these may be useful for assessing the best indications for BMT in ALL.

A further development in the treatment of ALL and other acute leukaemias is the use of autologous bone marrow transplantation, when HLA-matched donors are not available (this being the case in over two-thirds of cases). This procedure can be part of the initial therapeutic strategy, e.g. in bad prognosis cases such as those with t(9;22) or t(4;11), or can be used later to treat patients during second or subsequent remissions. Advantages of autologous bone marrow transplantation are the lack of graft-vs-host disease, wider availability of this procedure (compared with allogeneic BMT) and overall fewer complications. Disadvantages are the lack of a 'graft-vs-leukaemia' effect, which is associated with allogeneic BMT and graft-vs-host reaction, and the possibility of reinfusing bone marrow which still contains viable leukaemia cells. To avoid the latter, a number of methods (drugs, monoclonal antibodies) for 'purging' the bone marrow before reinfusion are being explored at the present time.

Chromosome abnormalities

Significant progress has taken place in the study of chromosome abnormalities in human leukaemia. Information derived from the new findings is relevant to the diagnosis, prognosis and pathogenesis of the malignant process. Specific karyotypic abnormalities are now demonstrated in all types of human leukaemia: AML, ALL, B-cell and T-cell leukaemias. In the chronic lymphoid leukaemias the use of specific B- or T-cell mitogens is essential to obtain metaphases of the neoplastic cells. In ALL metaphases are obtained directly or, preferably, after short-term culture without mitogens. Traditionally ALL chromosomes are known to be fuzzy and sometimes difficult to identify with banding techniques. Recently, improved methods have facilitated the study of karyotypic abnormalities in bone marrow cells from ALL[122, 123]. As a result of the improved methodology three major sets of findings have emerged:

1. The strong prognostic value of qualitative and quantitative chromosome abnormalities[107a, 109, 119].

Table 2.5 Chromosome translocations in specific types of ALL

t(9;22) (q34;q11)	Ph+ ALL[a]
t(4;11) (q21;q14–23)	Null-ALL
t(1;19) (q23;p13)	Pre-B-ALL
t(11;14) (p13;q11)	T-ALL(E+)
t(8;14) (q24;q32)	B-ALL
t or del(12p)	Common-ALL

[a] Null, common, pre-B- and, rarely, T-ALL.

2. The correlation of some abnormalities with the membrane phenotype of the blast cells[118, 123] (Table 2.5).
3. The existence of distinct forms of ALL, associated with bad prognosis, which are defined by specific abnormalities, namely, t(9;22) or Ph+ ALL[8, 17, 97, 106], t(4;11)[30, 61, 67, 87, 93, 108] and t(8;14) or Burkitt-type (L3) B-ALL[31, 64, 81].

These important clinical correlations are further strengthened by evidence that chromosome aberrations, particularly specific breakpoints, may relate directly or indirectly to the pathogenesis of the malignant process via the activation or translocation of oncogenes[60, 80].

Incidence and relation to prognosis

Cytogenetic abnormalities can be demonstrated in 70% of ALL cases and may be structural or numerical in nature[118].

The most common structural abnormalities are: t(9;22)(q34;q11) or Ph chromosome, found in 12% of cases (5% of childhood ALL and 18% of adult ALL); t(4;11)(q21;q14–23), observed in 5% of cases, with equal frequency in children and adults, including cases of 'congenital' ALL (aged less than 6 months), where three-quarters of cases with abnormal karyotypes have this abnormality; t(8;14)(q24;q32), including 8q−(q24), seen in 5%; 14q+ usually with the breakpoints at q32; 6q−, with variable breakpoints commonly at bands q15 and/or q21, resulting in terminal or interstitial deletions. The incidence of 6q− is 4.6% of all cases and 10% of those with chromosome abnormalities, with equal frequency in children and adults but with more males than females affected.

The most common numerical abnormalities are: hyperdiploidy, which includes two groups, with 47–50 chromosomes (8% of cases) and with more than 50 chromosomes (9% of cases); pseudodiploidy, a heterogeneous group of cases with a modal number of 46 chromosomes but with numerical (gain and loss) or structural abnormalities (different from those described above) (12% of cases); and hypodiploidy, less than 46 chromosomes with the more common modal number being 45 or 44 (6% of cases). Within the latter group, a distinct, but rare type of abnormality, near-haploid with 26–28 chromosomes, has been recognized, frequently affecting adolescent girls with very bad prognosis (median survival 10 months)[13, 55, 118].

The importance of banded chromosome analysis in predicting survival in ALL was clearly established in the Third International Workshop[119]. A more recent analysis of the data on 329 cases[7a] showed that achievement and duration of complete remission and overall survival is different in the various chromosome groups. Karyotype was shown to be an independent prognostic factor, even when other important factors, like WBC count and FAB type, were considered. The differences were marked in childhood ALLs, where the group with more than 50 chromosomes was shown to have the best prognosis, with 70% remaining in first complete remission for over 5 years. These findings were shown independently in other studies[70, 107a, 109] and, as discussed above, the presence of hyperdiploidy can also be demonstrated by flow cytometry in a high proportion of cases[70]. Children with a normal karyotype, those with modal numbers of 47–50 and with 6q− were also in the good prognostic category. In contrast, the translocations t(9;22), t(4;11) and t(8;14) were strongly associated with short survival, both in children and adults[7a,119].

Correlation with immunophenotype (Table 2.5)

It has now become apparent, in the last few years, that some chromosome abnormalities are found in specific groups of cases defined by the membrane phenotype. The first one recognized was the Burkitt translocation t(8;14)(q24;q32) or its variants t(2;8)(p12 or 13;q24) and t(8;22)(q24;q11), found in B-ALL, characterized by SmIg with the monoclonal expression of light chains (κ or λ). Other associations shown later are: t(1;19)(q23;p13) seen in 23–30% of pre-B-ALL cases[16, 123]; t(11;14)(p13;q11) found in 25% of E-rosette positive T-ALL[123] (this abnormality is distinct from t(11;14)(q13;q32) found in B-PLL and other mature B-cell malignancies); and translocations or deletions of chromosome 12 (p12) seen in cALL[123].

Clearly, further sophistication, both of chromosome analysis and immunophenotyping, may result in new associations which, together with known findings in acute myeloid leukaemias, suggest a possible casual relationship betwen specific breakpoints with the development of particular types of acute leukaemia.

A classification based precisely on the correlations between morphology, immunology and cytogenetics (MIC) has in fact been proposed with the aim of defining more objectively discrete disease entities within the spectrum of ALL[30a] and acute myeloid leukaemia[109a].

Philadelphia-positive ALL

It is now well recognized that Philadelphia-positive (Ph+) CGL (chronic granulocytic leukaemia) represents the neoplastic transformation of a pluripotent stem cell which differentiates preferentially to the myeloid lineage during the chronic phase of the disease. Acute blast transformation is a regular event and it is well known that all haemopoietic lineages may be involved. The blast crisis in 20% of cases has all the morphological, phenotypic[43] and molecular features of B-lineage ALL, usually cALL[3, 35]. A number of cases in which the blast cells have characteristics of T-lymphoblasts have also been documented[45, 49, 53]. Whilst the occurrence of a 'lymphoid blast-crisis' during the chronic phase of CGL was a readily accepted concept, the significance of a similar chromosome abnormality t(9;22)(q34;q11), in patients presenting with acute leukaemia, most commonly ALL[8], has been a matter of great interest mainly with respect to the relationship of Ph+ ALL and Ph+ CGL[17].

The presence of a Ph chromosome in de novo ALL is now well documented[118]. This disease could occur in children[97] or adults[8], but it is four times more frequent in the latter. Patients tend to present with splenomegaly (90%), lymphadenopathy (40%) and WBC count over 50 × 10^9/l (40%)[119]. Complete remission rates are lower than in ALL of similar age, and median survivals are short (median 14 months) in children and adults[8, 97, 119]. As in the lymphoid blast-crisis of CGL, the blasts of Ph+ ALL are as a rule of B-lineage, more commonly cALL and, rarely, may show T-cell features[53, 71, 78]. There are several lines of evidence to suggest Ph+ ALL probably represents the early development of a lymphoid blast-crisis on an underlying CGL. This phenomenon is already recognized as such when it develops with other types of blast cells, e.g. myeloblasts or megakaryoblasts. The relationship of the two disorders is supported by the well-documented cases[17] which after complete remission 'revert' to a chronic phase of CGL. The time to develop this chronic phase has varied from 1.5 to 36 months (median 6 months) and it is well recognized that this phase may not be easily detected during maintenance therapy for ALL. Three such cases have been studied at the Hammersmith Hospital; one died in myeloid blast crisis[17]: two others received a bone marrow transplantation, during the chronic phase, of whom one relapsed as ALL and subsequently died and the other is alive in complete remission (Ph−) more than 3 years later. A further argument is the existence of patients in whom a 'silent' chronic phase is documented, before the development of ALL, by haematological data when blood counts are carried out for intercurrent conditions. We have observed two such cases, one in which counts consistent with Ph+ CGL were supported by chromosome analysis one year before Ph+ ALL developed without, at this stage, any morphological evidence of the preceding CGL. Another case developed a lobar pneumonia and his high WBC count was interpreted as a 'leukaemoid reaction'. Two months later Ph+ ALL was diagnosed and chromosome studies in the bone marrow showed cells with: (1) double Ph, corresponding to the lymphoblasts, (2) one Ph chromosome, corresponding to the CGL chronic phase, and (3) Ph−, corresponding to the residual normal cells, still present presumably because the leukaemic process developed too rapidly for them to disappear completely.

One of the arguments used to support the separation of the two disorders is the absence, in Ph+ ALL, of the characteristic additional chromosome abnormalities seen in the blast crises of CGL[118]. Studies in the authors' laboratory[94] have shown that in the lymphoid blast-crisis of CGL there is also a lack of the typical abnormalities seen during the clonal evolution of CGL, namely trisomy 8, trisomy 19 and isochromosome 17q, which are a feature of myeloid transformations. However, the presence of a double Ph chromosome is found in all types of blast crisis. As in other acute leukaemias, the type of chromosome abnormality observed in CGL in addition to t(9;22), correlates with the cell lineage involved in the leukaemic process.

New studies suggest that the molecular basis for the Ph abnormality is not the same in the two types of Ph+ leukaemia. In fact only in a minority of Ph+ ALLs the breakpoint on the long arm of chromosome 22 occurs within the same 5.8-kilobase region, known as breakpoint cluster region (bcr), as in classic CGL, but in most the breakpoint is different. Furthermore, recent evidence shows that a novel protein (p190) is expressed in Ph+ ALL in contrast with the p210 protein product of the bcr-abl fusion gene in Ph+ CGL[20, 64, 68a]. Current studies have shown that most, if not all, children with Ph+ ALL have a breakpoint in chromosome 22 outside the breakpoint cluster region, as defined in CGL, whilst around 50% of Ph+ adult ALLs have this type of DNA rearrangement. In the remaining adults with Ph+ ALL a breakpoint cluster region rearrangement (as in CGL) is demonstrated by Southern blot analysis. It is not clear yet whether the Ph+/bcr− ALL cases with a p190 protein product are clinically different from those which are Ph+/bcr+ and have a p210 protein product, and whether only the latter cases correspond to CGL presenting in lymphoblastic crisis and are the ones which, after complete remission, may revert to a disease indistinguishable from the chronic phase of CGL. Further insights into the molecular mechanisms that are involved in the pathogenesis of both Ph+ and Ph− CGL and Ph+ ALL are rapidly developing. (For recent reviews see Heisterkamp et al.[48a] and Hirsch-Ginsberg et al.[50a].)

ALL with translocation t(4;11)

This abnormality (Figure 2.6) is associated with distinct clinical features: young age, high WBC count, hepatosplenomegaly and lymphadenopathy, poor response

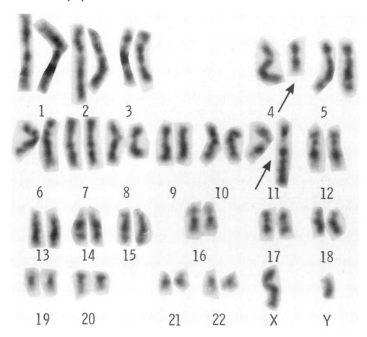

Figure 2.6 Karyotype showing the translocation t(4;11) obtained from the bone marrow of a 16-year-old boy with null-ALL (L1) who presented with a WBC count over $50 \times 10^9/l$. No myeloid features were observed by light microscopy or ultrastructural cytochemistry

to therapy, responses of short duration and, overall, short survival[61, 67, 87, 93, 108]. Although initially classified as L1 or L2 ALL, careful immunological and cytochemical analysis reveals that, in addition to features of early B-cell commitment[29], it is possible to show evidence of myeloid differentiation, often with myelomonocytic characteristics, in a proportion of the blast cells[87, 93]. This bilineage differentiation (lymphoid and myeloid) and the absence of the cALL antigen (null-ALL blasts) suggest the involvement of a pluripotential stem cell in this disorder. This is further confirmed by a case recently described which exhibited early T-cell features[68b]. Thus, t(4;11) is similar in this respect to t(9;22), which results in the Ph chromosome. Clonal evolution is also frequent in cases with t(4;11) and this further underlines the reasons for a worse prognosis.

Burkitt-type ALL

The rare B-ALL with L3 morphology[31] is almost always associated with three reciprocal translocations: t(8;14) (Figure 2.7), in 80% of cases, and the variants t(2;8) and t(8;22) in the remainder. Identical abnormalities are a feature of Burkitt's lymphoma in African children. Additional abnormalities are seen in two-thirds of cases and these often involve chromosome 1, which frequently shows a partial duplication of the long arm. The types of secondary changes are also similar both in L3 ALL and in Burkitt's lymphoma. A feature of clinical interest in these patients is the presentation with bilateral hypoaesthesia of the mandibular region, a symptom that the authors have observed in a young adult with B-ALL (L3) and t(8;14), and suggests the involvement of the sensory root of the trigeminal

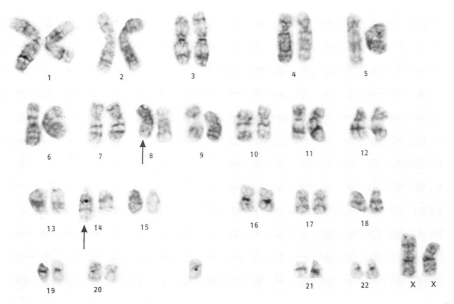

Figuyre 2.7 Karyotype from a case of B-ALL (L3) showing the typical chromosome translocation t(8;14) plus an extra marker chromosome

nerve. Rarely t(8;14) or the variant translocations have been reported in other B-cell malignancies without L3 morphology.

The chromosome breakpoints in the two variant translocations include the regions of the immunoglobulin light chain genes, 2p12 for κ and 22q11 for λ. There is therefore good correspondence between the light chain gene involved in the translocation and the light chain expressed on the cell surface and, with only one exception, the cells of all cases with t(2;8)(p12;q24) expressed κ and those with t(8;22)(q24;q11) expressed λ.

The survival of L3 ALL patients is very short – a median of 4 months was reported in the Third Chromosome Workshop[7a, 119]. If complete remission can be achieved these patients are candidates for bone marrow transplantation if a suitable donor is available.

Chromosome translocations and oncogenes

An important series of discoveries has demonstrated a close relationship between the localization of certain oncogenes (genes that upon activation or amplification can cause cancer) and the breakpoints of chromosomes frequently involved in translocations in leukaemias and lymphomas. These abnormalities affect a limited number of chromosome regions[80] and include inversions, duplications, deletions or reciprocal translocations. The relationship with certain oncogenes, notably c-myc in B-ALL and Burkitt's lymphoma and c-abl in Ph+ CGL and ALL, suggest that these changes are of critical importance in the pathogenesis of human malignancies.

Studies in Burkitt's lymphoma have shown that the juxtaposition of c-myc (localized in 8q24) and one of the three Ig gene loci is a regular event leading to the high expression of *c-myc* (gene activation) from the translocated allele[60]. The use of in situ hybridization techniques has demonstrated that *c-myc* translocates from chromosome 8 to a region of chromosome 14 (q32) adjacent to the genes encoding for the constant region of the Ig heavy chain. This transposition joins these two genes head to head, and is different from that seen in the variant translocations where the break of chromosome 8 takes place below the tail end of the *c-myc* gene, which therefore remains in that chromosome. Here the genes encoding for the constant region of κ (in 2p11) and λ (in 22q11) light chains translocate to chromosome 8 close to the *c-myc* gene with a head-to-tail orientation. Despite this variability, at the molecular level, in the 8q24 breakpoint the two coding exons of *c-myc* are always intact and this may be important for its activation. A similar Ig/*c-myc* juxtaposition also takes place regularly in a murine plasmacytoma with t(12;15), where *c-myc* is located in chromosome 15 and the Ig heavy chain gene in chromosome 12[60]. As in t(8;14) the breakpoint in chromosome 15 is located upstream of the *c-myc* gene.

In Ph+ leukaemia, the t(9;22) results in the translocation of the oncogene *c-abl* from 9q34 to chromosome 22. Whilst in CGL the breakpoints on chromosome 22 cluster over a small 5.8-kilobase region (*bcr*) on band q11, in Ph+ ALL this may not always be the case[20, 50a, 64] (see also above). The *c-sis* oncogene, located in 22q12.3 translocates to chromosome 9 in t(9;22), but there is no evidence that this gene is expressed in CGL.

From the evidence discussed above, it is clear that the study of translocations associated with ALL provides important clues to understanding the mechanisms of neoplastic transformation in leukaemias and lymphomas.

Epidemiology

There has been increasing interest in the study of the epidemiology of ALL, in particular the differences in the incidence of the immunologically defined subtypes in different parts of the world[42, 74, 99]. Several factors, possibly interrelated, may contribute to explain these differences, chiefly geographical, genetic or ethnic and socioeconomic. In Western industrialized countries (Europe and USA) the peak incidence of ALL for the last 30 years has been between the ages of 1 and 5 years. In Africa, India and Japan the peak occurs later, usually after the age of 10 years. This absence of an early peak and the relatively higher incidence of T-ALL in the same countries suggest that cALL may be associated with higher living standards and urban development. An international epidemiological study organized by the Leukaemia Research Fund Centre[42] using standardized reagents for leukaemia cell phenotyping has confirmed that T-ALL has a relatively higher incidence (30–45%) in Africa (Nigeria, Kenya etc.) and India contrasting with the figure of 12.5% consistently observed in the UK for the last 10 years[42].

Differences observed between ethnic groups in some countries point to genetic and/or socioeconomic factors as being important to the exclusion of geographical considerations. For example, studies in the south of the USA (Memphis) and South Africa revealed a lower incidence of cALL in Black children with a corresponding higher incidence of T-ALL. The effect of socioeconomic factors is supported by the experience of the Gaza Strip in Israel, where Burkitt's lymphoma was more prevalent in Arabs and Oriental Jews in the 1960s, but which was superseded, taking into account socioeconomic developments, by more cases of ALL, mainly

T-ALL (30–35%), affecting the same population of children. In contrast, the incidence of T-ALL was lower (10%) in Ashkenazi children[74, 99]. This pattern – high incidence of Burkitt's lymphoma and low frequency of ALL – is characteristic of Equatorial Africa, where it may be predicted that social changes could revert this trend[74]. Further, higher levels of development may be associated with a transition from a relatively high incidence of T-ALL to the present pattern in the West in which cALL predominates. From the various surveys it is apparent too that all types of leukaemia are seen in different parts of the world but with the differences in incidence noted above. Similarly the clinical features of the various forms of the disease are no different in the various countries, e.g. the association of T-ALL with high WBC count, anterior mediastinal masses, male sex and poorer prognosis. Factors such as malnutrition and high infant mortality may contribute to some of the observed differences. The latter of course are not confined only to ALL. For example, the chloromatous presentation of acute myeloid leukaemia in children is more common in Nigeria and Turkey than in other European countries or the USA.

Although many of the above points are still a matter of debate and of different interpretations, it is clear that studies on the epidemiology of acute leukaemia may throw light on a better understanding of the pathogenesis of this malignancy.

References

1. Arnold, A., Cossman, J., Bakshi, A., Jaffe, E. S., Waldmann, T. A. and Korsmeyer, S. J. (1983) Immunoglobulin-gene rearrangements as unique clonal markers in human lymphoid neoplasms. *New England Journal of Medicine,* **309,** 1593–1599

2. Astaldi, G., Cavdar, A. and Topuz, U. (1977) Thymic hormone and T-cell maturation in acute leukaemias. A preliminary study. *Blood Cells,* **3,** 623–635

3. Bakshi, A., Minowada, J., Arnold, A. et al. (1983) Lymphoid blast crises of chronic myelogenous leukemia represent stages in the development of B-cell precursors. *New England Journal of Medicine,* **309,** 826–831

3a. Barrett, A. J., Horowitz, M. M., Gale, R. P. et al. (1989) Marrow transplantation for acute lymphoblastic leukemia: factors affecting relapse and survival. *Blood,* **74,** 862

4. Basso, G., Agostini, C., Cocito, M. G. et al. (1984) Non-T, non-B childhood acute lymphoblastic leukemia. Correlation between cytochemical markers and first complete remission. *Cancer,* **54,** 981–985

5. Bennett, J. M., Catovsky, D., Daniel, M-T. et al. (FAB Co-operative group) (1976) Proposals for the classification of the acute leukaemias. *British Journal of Haematology,* **33,** 451–458

6. Bennett, J. M., Catovsky, D., Daniel, M. T. et al. (FAB Co-operative Group) (1981) The morphological classification of acute lymphoblastic leukaemia: concordance among observers and clinical correlations. *British Journal of Haematology,* **47,** 553–561

7. Bleyer, W. A. (1981) Neurologic sequelae of methotrexate and ionizing radiation: a new classification. *Cancer Treatment Reports,* **65** (suppl. 1), 89–98

7a. Bloomfield, C. D., Goldman, A. I., Alimena, G. et al. (1986) Chromosome abnormalities identify high-risk and low-risk patients with acute lymphoblastic leukemia. *Blood,* **67,** 415–420

8. Bloomfield, C. D., Peterson, L. C., Yunis, J. J. and Brunning, R. D. (1977) The Philadelphia chromosome (Ph^1) in adults presenting with acute leukaemia: a comparison of Ph^1+ and Ph^1− patients. *British Journal of Haematology,* **36,** 347–358

9. Borella, L., Sen, L. and Casper, J. T. (1977) Acute lymphoblastic leukemia (ALL) antigens detected with antisera to E rosette-forming and non-E rosette-forming ALL blasts. *Journal of Immunology,* **118,** 309–315

10. Bowman, W. P., Aur, R. J. A., Hustu, H. O. and Rivera, G. (1984) Isolated testicular relapse in acute lymphocytic leukemia of childhood: categories and influence on survival. *Journal of Clinical Oncology*, **2**, 924–929

11. Brack, C., Hirami, M., Lenhard-Schuller, R. and Tonegawa, S. (1978) A complete immunoglobulin gene is created by somatic recombination. *Cell*, **15**, 1–14

12. Bradstock, K. F., Hoffbrand, A. V., Ganeshaguru, K. et al. (1981) Terminal deoxynucleotidyl transferase expression in acute non-lymphoid leukaemia: an analysis by immunofluorescence. *British Journal of Haematology*, **47**, 133–143

12a. Bradstock, K. F., Kirk, J., Grimsley, P. G., Kabral, A. and Hughes, W. G. (1989) Unusual immunophenotypes in acute leukaemias: incidence and clinical correlations. *British Journal of Haematology*, **72**, 512–518

13. Brodeur, G. M., Williams, D. L., Look, A. T., Bowman, W. P. and Kalwinsky, D. K. (1981) Near-haploid acute lymphoblastic leukemia: a unique subgroup with a poor prognosis? *Blood*, **58**, 14–19

14. Brouet, J. C., Preud'homme, J. L., Penit, C., Valensi, F., Rouget, P. and Seligmann, M. (1979) Acute lymphoblastic leukemia with pre-B-cell characteristics. *Blood*, **54**, 269–273

15. Brouet, J-C., Valensi, F., Daniel, M-T., Flandrin, G., Preud'homme, J-L. and Seligmann, M. (1976) Immunological classification of acute lymphoblastic leukaemias: evaluation of its clinical significance in a hundred patients. *British Journal of Haematology*, **33**, 319–328

16. Carroll, A. J., Crist, W. M., Parmley, R. T., Roper, M., Cooper, M. D. and Finley, W. H. (1984) Pre-B cell leukemia associated with chromosome translocation 1;19. *Blood*, **63**, 721–724

17. Catovsky, D. (1979) Ph[1]-positive acute leukaemia and chronic granulocytic leukaemia: one or two diseases? *British Journal of Haematology*, **42**, 493–498

18. Catovsky, D., Goldman, J. M., Okos, A., Frisch, B. and Galton, D. A. G. (1974) T-lymphoblastic leukaemia: a distinct variant of acute leukaemia. *British Medical Journal*, **2**, 643–646

19. Catovsky, D., Greaves, M. F., Pain, C., Cherchi, M., Janossy, G. and Kay, H. E. M. (1978) Acid phosphatase reaction in acute lymphoblastic leukaemia. *Lancet*, **i**, 749–751

20. Chan, L. C., Karhi, K. K., Rayter, S. I. et al. (1987) A novel abl protein expressed in Philadelphia chromosome positive acute lymphoblastic leukaemia. *Nature*, **325**, 635–637

21. Chessells, J. M., Hardisty, R. M., Rapson, N. T. and Greaves, M. F. (1977) Acute lymphoblastic leukaemia in children: classification and prognosis. *Lancet*, **ii**, 1307–1309

22. Chessells, J., Leiper, A. and Roger, D. (1984) Outcome following late marrow relapse in childhood acute lymphoblastic leukemia. *Journal of Clinical Oncology*, **2**, 1088–1091

23. Chilcote, R. R., Coccia, P., Sather, H. N. et al. (1984) Mediastinal mass in acute lymphoblastic leukemia. *Medical and Pediatric Oncology*, **12**, 9–16

24. Coleman, M. S., Greenwood, M. F., Hutton, J. J. et al. (1978) Adenosine deaminase, terminal deoxynucleotidyl transferase (TdT) and cell surface markers in childhood acute leukemia. *Blood*, **52**, 1125–1131

25. Coleman, M. S., Hutton, J. J., De Simone, P. and Bollum, F. J. (1974) Terminal deoxynucleotidyl transferase in human leukemia. *Proceedings of the National Academy of Sciences of the USA*, **71**, 4404–4408

26. Cooke, J. V. (1932) Mediastinal tumor in acute leukemia. *American Journal of Diseases of Childhood*, **44**, 1153–1177

27. Cossman, J., Neckers, L. M., Arnold, A. and Korsmeyer, S. J. (1982) Induction of differentiation in a case of common acute lymphoblastic leukemia. *New England Journal of Medicine*, **307**, 1251–1254

28. Crist, W., Boyett, J., Roper, M. et al. (1984) Pre-B cell leukemia responds poorly to treatment: a pediatric oncology group study. *Blood*, **63**, 407–414

29. Crist, W. M., Cleary, M. L., Grossi, C. E. et al. (1985) Acute leukemias associated with the 4;11 chromosome translocation have rearranged immunoglobulin heavy chain genes. *Blood*, **66**, 33–38

30. Ellis, R. B., Rapson, N. T., Patrick, A. D. and Greaves, M. F. (1978) Expression of hexosaminidase isoenzymes in childhood leukemia. *New England Journal of Medicine*, **298**, 476–480

30a. First MIC Cooperative Study Group (1986) Morphologic, immunologic and cytogenetic (MIC) working classification of acute lymphoblastic leukemias. *Cancer Genetics and Cytogenetics*, **23**, 189–197

31. Flandrin, G., Brouet, J. C., Daniel, M. T. and Preud'homme, J. L. (1975) Acute leukemia with Burkitt's tumor cells: a study of six cases with special reference to lymphocyte surface markers. *Blood*, **15**, 183–188

32. Foa, R., Baldini, L., Cattoretti, G. et al. (1985) Multimarker phenotypic characterization of adult and childhood acute lymphoblastic leukaemia: an Italian multicentre study. *British Journal of Haematology*, **61**, 251–259

33. Foa, R., Caligaris Cappio, F., Campana, D. et al. (1983) Relevance of monoclonal antibodies in the diagnosis of unusual T-cell acute lymphoblastic leukaemia. *Scandinavian Journal of Haematology*, **30**, 303–307

34. Foa, R., Migone, N., Saitta, M. et al. (1984) Different stages of B-cell differentiation in non-T acute lymphoblastic leukemia. *Journal of Clinical Investigation*, **74**, 1756–1763

34a. Foa, R., Migone, N., Basso, G. et al. (1986) Molecular and immunological evidence of B-cell commitment in 'null' acute lymphoblastic leukaemia. *International Journal of Cancer*, **38**, 317–323

35. Ford, A. M., Molgaard, H. V., Greaves, M. F. and Gould, M. J. (1983) Immunoglobulin gene organisation and expression in haemopoietic stem cell leukaemia. *EMBO Journal*, **2**, 997–1001

36. Foroni, L., Catovsky, D., Rabbitts, T. H. and Luzzatto, L. (1984) DNA rearrangements of immunoglobulin genes correlate with phenotypic markers in B-cell malignancies. *Molecular Biology and Medicine*, **2**, 63–79

37. Gaedicke, G. and Drexler, H. G. (1984) Leukemic cell differentiation in childhood leukemias. Analysis by enzyme markers. *European Journal of Pediatrics*, **142**, 157–164

38. Gavosto, F. (1983) Immunobiological features of acute lymphoblastic leukaemia. *Haematologica*, **68**, 1–19

39. Gavosto, F. and Masera, P. (1975) Different cell proliferation models in myeloblastic and lymphoblastic leukaemia. Contribution of cell kinetics to the classification of acute leukaemias. *Blood Cells*, **1**, 217–222

40. Gottlieb, A. J., Weinberg, V., Ellison, R. R. et al. (1984) Efficacy of daunorubicin in the therapy of adult acute lymphocytic leukemia: A prospective randomized trial by Cancer and Leukemia Group B. *Blood*, **64**, 267–274

41. Greaves, M. F., Brown, G., Rapson, N. T. and Lister, T. A. (1975) Antisera to acute lymphoblastic leukemia cells. *Clinical Immunology and Immunopathology*, **4**, 67–84

42. Greaves, M. F. and Chan, L. C. (Guest editors) (1985) Epidemiology of leukaemia and lymphoma. Report of the Leukaemia Research Fund International Workshop. Oxford, 1984. *Leukemia Research*, **9**, 661–832

42a. Greaves, M. F., Chan, L. C., Furley, A. J. W., Watt, S. M. and Molgaard, H. V. (1986) Lineage promiscuity in hemopoietic differentiation and leukemia. *Blood*, **67**, 1–11

43. Greaves, M. and Janossy, G. (1978) Patterns of gene expression and the cellular origins of human leukaemias. *Biochimica et Biophysica Acta*, **516**, 193–230

44. Greaves, M. F., Janossy, G., Peto, J. and Kay, H. (1981) Immunologically defined subclasses of acute lymphoblastic leukaemia in children: their relationship to presentation features and prognosis. *British Journal of Haematology*, **48**, 179–197

45. Griffin, J. D., Tantravahi, R., Canellos, G. P. et al. (1983) T-cell surface antigens in a patient with blast crisis of chronic myeloid leukemia. *Blood*, **61**, 640–644

46. Ha, K., Minden, M., Hozumi, N. and Gelfand, E. W. (1984) Immunoglobulin μ-chain gene rearrangement in a patient with T cell acute lymphoblastic leukemia. *Journal of Clinical Investigation*, **73**, 1232–1236

47. Ha, K., Minden, M., Hozumi, N. and Gelfand, E. W. (1984) Immunoglobulin gene rearrangement in acute myelogenous leukemia. *Cancer Research*, **44**, 4658–4660

48. Haynes, B. F., Metzgar, R. S., Minna, J. D. and Bunn, P. A. (1981) Phenotypic characterization of cutaneous T cell lymphoma. Use of monoclonal antibodies to compare with other malignant T cells. *New England Journal of Medicine*, **304**, 1319–1323

48a. Heisterkamp, N., Jenkins, R., Thibodeau, S., Testa, J. R., Weinberg, K. and Groffen, J. (1989) The bcr gene in Philadelphia chromosome positive acute lymphoblastic leukemia. *Blood*, **73**, 1307–1311

49. Hermann, F., Ludwig, W-D. and Kolecki, P. (1984) Blast crisis in CML showing early T-lymphoblastic transformation. *British Journal of Haematology*, **56**, 175–176

50. Hieter, P. A., Korsmeyer, S. J., Waldmann, T. A. and Leder, P. (1981) Human immunoglobulin κ light-chain genes are deleted or rearranged in λ-producing B cells. *Nature*, **290**, 368–372

50a. Hirsch-Ginsberg, C., Childs, C., Chang, K.-S. et al. (1988) Phenotypic and molecular heterogeneity in Philadelphia chromosome-positive acute leukemia. *Blood*, **71**, 186–195

51. Hoelzer, D., Thiel, E., Loffler, H. et al. (1984) Intensified therapy in acute lymphoblastic and acute undifferentiated leukemia in adults. *Blood*, **64**, 37–47

52. Hoffbrand, A. V., Ganeshaguru, G., Janossy, G. et al. (1977) Terminal deoxynucleotidyl-transferase levels and membrane phenotypes in diagnosis of acute leukaemia. *Lancet*, **ii**, 520–523

53. Jacobs, P. and Greaves, M. (1984) Ph¹-positive T lymphoblastic transformation. *Leukemia Research*, **8**, 737–739

54. Janossy, G., Hoffbrand, A. V., Greaves, M. F. et al. (1980) Terminal transferase enzyme assay and immunological membrane markers in the diagnosis of leukaemia: a multiparameter analysis of 300 cases. *British Journal of Haematology*, **44**, 221–234

54a. Janossy, G., Coustan-Smith, E. and Campana, D. (1989) The reliability of cytoplasmic CD3 and CD22 antigen expression in the immunodiagnosis of acute leukemia: a study of 500 cases. *Leukemia*, **3**, 170–181

55. Kaneko, Y. and Sakurai, M. (1980) Acute lymphocytic leukemia (ALL) with near-haploidy – a unique subgroup of ALL? *Cancer Genetics and Cytogenetics*, **2**, 13–18

56. Kay, H. E. M., Knapton, P. J., O'Sullivan, J. P. et al. (1972) Encephalopathy in acute leukaemia associated with methotrexate therapy. *Archives of Disease in Childhood*, **47**, 344–354

57. Kersey, J., Goldman, A., Abramson, C. et al. (1982) Clinical usefulness of monoclonal antibody phenotyping in childhood acute lymphoblastic leukaemia. *Lancet*, **ii**, 1419–1423

58. Kersey, J. H., Sabad, A., Gajl-Peczalska, K., Yunis, E. J. and Nesbit, M. E. (1973) Acute lymphoblastic leukemic cells with T (Thymus-derived) lymphocyte markers. *Science*, **182**, 1355–1356

59. Kitchingman, G. R., Rovigatti, U., Mauer, A. M., Melvin, S., Murphy, S. B. and Stass, S. (1985) Rearrangement of immunoglobulin heavy chain genes in T cell acute lymphoblastic leukemia. *Blood*, **65**, 725–729

60. Klein, G. and Klein, E. (1985) Evolution of tumours and the impact of molecular oncology. *Nature*, **315**, 190–195

61. Kocova, M., Kowalczyk, J. R. and Sandberg, A. A. (1985) Translocation 4;11 acute leukemia: three case reports and review of the literature. *Cancer Genetics and Cytogenetics*, **16**, 21–32

62. Korsmeyer, S. J., Arnold, A., Bakhshi, A. et al. (1983) Immunoglobulin gene rearrangement and cell surface antigen expression in acute lymphocytic leukemias of T cell and B cell precursor origins. *Journal of Clinical Investigation*, **71**, 301–313

63. Korsmeyer, S. J., Greene, W. C., Cossman, J. et al. (1983) Rearrangement and expression of immunoglobulin genes and expression of Tac antigen in hairy cell leukemia. *Proceedings of the National Academy of Sciences of the USA*, **80**, 4522–4526

64. Kuzrock, R., Shtalrid, M., Romero, P. et al. (1987) A novel c-abl protein product in Philadelphia-positive acute lymphoblastic leukaemia. *Nature*, **325**, 631–635

65. Lampert, F., Henze, G., Langermann, H-J., Schellong, G., Gadner, H. and Riehm, H-J. (1984) Acute lymphoblastic leukemia: current status of therapy in children. *Recent Results in Cancer Research*, **93**, 159–181

66. LeBien, T., Kersey, J., Nakazawa, S., Minato, K. and Minowada, J. (1982) Analysis of human leukemia/lymphoma cell lines with monoclonal antibodies BA-1, BA-2 and BA-3. *Leukemia Research*, **6**, 299–305

66a. LeBien, T. W. and McCormack, R. T. (1989) The common acute lymphoblastic leukemia antigen (CD10) – Emancipation from a functional enigma. *Blood*, **73**, 625–635

67. Levin, M. D., Michael, P. M., Garson, O. M., Tiedemann, K. and Firkin, F. C. (1984) Clinicopathological characteristics of acute lymphoblastic leukaemia with the 4;11 chromosome translocation. *Pathology*, **16**, 63–66

68. Liso, V., Specchia, G., Pavone, V. et al. (1983) Acute lymphoblastic leukaemia hand-mirror cells. Study of nine cases. *Blut*, **47**, 297–306

68a. Lo Coco, F., Basso, G. and Francia di Celle, P. (1990) Molecular characterization of Ph1+ hybrid acute leukemia. *Leukemia Research*, in press

68b. Lo Coco, F., Francia di Celle, P., Alimena, G. et al. (1989) Acute lymphoblastic leukemia with the 4; 11 translocation exhibiting early T-cell features. *Leukemia, 3,* 79–82

69. Look, A. T., Melvin, S. L., Williams, D. L. et al. (1982) Aneuploidy and percentage of S-phase cells determined by flow cytometry correlate with cell phenotype in childhood acute leukemia. *Blood, 60,* 959–967

70. Look, A. T., Robertson, P. K., Williams, D. L. et al. (1985) Prognostic importance of blast cell DNA content in childhood acute lymphoblastic leukemia. *Blood, 65,* 1079–1086

71. Louwagie, A., Criel, A., Verfaillie, C. M. et al. (1985) Philadelphia-positive T-acute lymphoblastic leukemia. *Cancer Genetics and Cytogenetics, 16,* 297–300

71a. Ludwig, W-D., Bartram, C. R., Harbott, J. et al. (1989) Phenotypic and genotypic heterogeneity in infant acute leukemia. I. Acute lymphoblastic leukemia. *Leukemia, 3,* 431–439

72. McCaffrey, R., Harrison, T. A., Parkman, R. and Baltimore, D. (1975) Terminal deoxynucleotidyl transferase activity in human leukemic cells and in normal thymocytes. *New England Journal of Medicine, 292,* 775–780

73. McKenna, R. W., Parkin, J. and Brunning, R. D. ((1979) Morphological and ultrastructural characteristics of T-cell acute lymphoblastic leukemia. *Cancer, 44,* 1290–1297

74. Magrath, I. T., O'Conor, G. T. and Ramot, B. (1984) Editors. *Pathogenesis of Leukemias and Lymphomas.* New York: Raven Press

75. Manoharan, A., Catovsky, D., Goldman, J. M., Lauria, F., Lampert, I. A. and Galton, D. A. G. (1980) Significance of splenomegaly in childhood acute lymphoblastic leukaemia in remission. *Lancet, i,* 449–452

75a. Marcus, R. E., Catovsky, D., Johnson, S. A. et al. (1986) Adult acute lymphoblastic leukaemia: a study of prognostic features and response to treatment over a ten year period. *British Journal of Cancer, 53,* 175–180

76. Marcus, R., Matutes, E., Drysdale, H. C. and Catovsky, D. (1985) Phenotypic conversion of TdT+ adult AML to CALLA+ ALL. *Scandinavian Journal of Haematology, 35,* 343–347

77. Melo, J. V., Foroni, L., Brito-Babapulle, V. et al. (1985) Prolymphocytic leukemia of B-cell type: rearranged immunoglobulin (Ig) genes with defective Ig production. *Blood, 60,* 391–398

78. Miller, B. A., Reid, M. M., Nell, M. et al. (1984) T-cell acute lymphoblastic leukaemia with late developing Philadelphia chromosome. *British Journal of Haematology, 56,* 139–146

79. Miller, D. R., Leikin, S., Albo, V., Sather, H. and Hammond, D. (1981) Prognostic importance of morphology (FAB classification) in childhood acute lymphoblastic leukaemia (ALL). *British Journal of Haematology, 48,* 199–206

80. Mitelman, F. (1984) Restricted number of chromosomal regions implicated in aetiology of human cancer and leukaemia. *Nature, 310,* 325–327

81. Mitelman, F., Andersson-Anvret, M., Brandt, K. et al. (1979) Reciprocal 8;14 translocation in EBV-negative B-cell acute lymphocytic leukemia with Burkitt-type cells. *International Journal of Cancer, 24,* 27–33

82. Moe, P. J., Seip, M., Finne, P. H. and Kolmannskog, S. (1984) Intermediate dose methotrexate in childhood acute lymphocytic leukemia. *European Paediatric Haematology and Oncology, 1,* 113–118

82a. Morabito, F., Tassinari, A., Callea, V. et al. (1987) Germ-line configuration of the T-cell receptor beta chain gene in B-cell chronic lymphoproliferative disorders which co-express T-cell antigens. *European Journal of Haematology, 39,* 412–417

83. Morgan, M. A. M., Scott, C. S., Tavares de Castro, J. et al. (1985) Biphenotypic leukaemia: a case of mixed T lymphoblastic and myeloblastic leukaemia. *Journal of Clinical Pathology, 38,* 575–581

84. Murray, K. H., Paolino, F., Goldman, J. M., Galton, D. A. G. and Grindle, C. F. J. (1977) Ocular involvement in leukaemia. Report of three cases. *Lancet, i,* 829–831

85. Nadler, L. M., Korsmeyer, S. J., Anderson, K. C. et al. (1984) B cell origin of non-T cell acute lymphoblastic leukemia. A model for discrete stages of neoplastic and normal pre-B cell differentiation. *Journal of Clinical Investigation, 74,* 332–340

86. Nadler, L. M., Ritz, J., Bates, M. P. et al. (1982) Induction of human B cell antigens in non-T cell acute lymphoblastic leukemia. *Journal of Clinical Investigation, 70,* 433–442

87. Nagasaka, M., Maeda, S., Maeda, H. et al. (1983) Four cases of t(4;11) acute leukemia and its myelomonocytic nature in infants. *Blood, 61,* 1174–1181

88. Neame, P. B., Soamboonsrup, P., Browman, G. et al. (1985) Simultaneous or sequential expression of lymphoid and myeloid phenotypes in acute leukemia. *Blood,* **65,** 142–148

89. Nesbit, M. E., Sather, H., Robison, L. L. et al. (1982) Sanctuary therapy: a randomized trial of 724 children with previously untreated acute lymphoblastic leukemia. A report from Children's Cancer Study Group. *Cancer Research,* **42,** 674–680

90. Nesbit, M. E., Sather, H. N., Robison, L. L., Ortega, J. A., Hammond, G. D. and the Children's Cancer Study Group (1983) Randomized study of 3 years versus 5 years of chemotherapy in childhood acute lymphoblastic leukemia. *Journal of Clinical Oncology,* **1,** 308–316

91. Nesbit, M. E., Sather, H. N., Robison, L. L. et al. (1981) Presymptomatic central nervous system therapy in previously untreated childhood acute lymphoblastic leukaemia: comparison of 1800 rad and 2400 rad. A report for Children's Cancer Study Group. *Lancet,* **i,** 461–466

92. Neudorf, S. M. L., LeBien, T. W. and Kersey, J. H. (1984) Characterization of thymocytes expressing the common acute lymphoblastic leukemia antigen. *Leukemia Research,* **8,** 173–179

92a. Nosaka, T., Ohno, H., Doi, S. et al. (1988) Phenotypic conversion of T lymphoblastic lymphoma to acute biphenotypic leukemia composed of lymphoblasts and myeloblasts. *Journal of Clinical Investigation,* **81,** 1824–1828

93. Parkin, J. L., Arthur, D. C., Abramson, C. S. et al. (1982) Acute leukemia associated with the t(4;11) chromosome rearrangement: ultrastructural and immunologic characteristics. *Blood,* **60,** 1321–1331

93a. Parreira, A., Pombo de Oliveira, M. S., Matutes, E., Foroni, L., Morilla, R. and Catovsky, D. (1988) Terminal deoxynucleotidyl transferase positive acute myeloid leukaemia: an association with immature myeloblastic leukaemia. *British Journal of Haematology,* **69,** 219–224

94. Parreira, L., Kearney, L., Rassool, F. et al. (1986) Correlation between chromosomal abnormalities and blast phenotype in the blast crisis of Ph positive CGL. *Cancer Genetics and Cytogenetics,* **22,** 29–34

95. Pinkel, D. (1971) Five-year follow-up of 'total therapy' of childhood lymphocytic leukemia. *Journal of the American Medical Association,* **216,** 648–652

95a. Pombo de Oliveira, M. S., Matutes, E., Rani, S., Morilla, R. and Catovsky, D. (1988) Early expression of MCS2 (CD13) in the cytoplasm of blast cells from acute myeloid leukaemia. *Acta Haematologica,* **80,** 61–64

96. Prentice, H. G., Russel, H. N., Lee, N. et al. (1981) Therapeutic selectivity of and prediction of response to 2'-deoxycyformycin in acute leukaemia. *Lancet,* **ii,** 1250–1254

97. Priest, J. R., Robison, L. L., McKenna, R. W. et al. (1980) Philadelphia chromosome positive childhood acute lymphoblastic leukaemia. *Blood,* **56,** 15–22

98. Pui, C-H., Dahl, G. V., Bowman, W. P. et al. (1985) Elective testicular biopsy during chemotherapy for childhood leukaemia is of no clinical value. *Lancet,* **ii,** 410–412

99. Ramot, B., Ben-Bassat, I., Brecher, A., Zaizov, R. and Modan, M. (1984) The epidemiology of childhood acute lymphoblastic leukaemia and non-Hodgkin's lymphoma in Israel between 1976 and 1981. *Leukemia Research,* **8,** 691–699

99a. Rani, S., De Oliveira, M. S. P. and Catovsky, D. (1988) Different expression of CD3 and CD22 in leukemic cells according to whether tested in suspension or fixed on slides. *Hematologic Pathology,* **2,** 73–78

100. Ravetch, J. V., Siebenlist, U., Korsmeyer, S., Waldmann, T. and Leder, P. (1981) Structure of the human immunoglobulin μ locus: characterization of embryonic and rearranged J and D genes. *Cell,* **27,** 583–591

101. Reinherz, E. L., Kung, P. C., Goldstein, G., Levey, R. H. and Schlossman, S. F. (1980) Discrete stages of human intrathymic differentiation: analysis of normal thymocytes and leukemic lymphoblasts of T-cell lineage. *Proceedings of the National Academy of Sciences of the USA,* **77,** 1588–1592

102. Riehm, H., Langermann, H-J., Gadner, H., Odenwald, E. and Henze, G. (1980) The Berlin childhood acute lymphoblastic leukemia therapy study, 1970–1976. *American Journal of Pediatric Hematology/Oncology,* **2,** 299–306

103. Rogers, P. C., Bleyer, W. A., Coccia, P. et al. (1984) Yield of unpredicted bone-marrow relapse diagnosed by routine marrow aspiration in children with acute lymphoblastic leukaemia. A report from the Children's Cancer Study Group. *Lancet,* **i,** 1320–1322

104. Rovigatti, U., Mirro, J., Kitchingman, G. et al. (1984) Heavy chain immunoglobulin gene rearrangement in acute nonlymphocytic leukemia. *Blood*, **63**, 1023–1027
105. Sanchez-Fayos, J., Outeirino, J., Villalobos, E. et al. (1985) Acute lymphoblastic leukaemia in adults: results of a 'total-therapy' programme in 47 patients over 15 years old. *British Journal of Haematology*, **59**, 689–696
106. Sandberg, A. A., Morgan, R., Kipps, T. J., Hecht, B. K. and Hecht, F. (1985) The Philadelphia (Ph) chromosome in leukemia. II. Variant Ph translocations in acute lymphoblastic leukemia. *Cancer Genetics and Cytogenetics*, **14**, 11–21
107. Schumacher, H. R., Champion, J. E., Thomas, W. J., Pitts, L. L. and Stass, S. A. (1979) Acute lymphoblastic leukemia – hand mirror variant. An analysis of a large group of patients. *American Journal of Hematology*, **7**, 11–17
107a. Secker-Walker, L. M., Chessells, J. M., Stewart, L., Swansbury, G. J., Richards, S. and Lawler, S. D. (1989) Chromosomes and other prognostic factors in acute lymphoblastic leukaemia: a long-term follow-up. *British Journal of Haematology*, **72**, 336–342
108. Secker-Walker, L. M., Stewart, E. L., Chan, L., O'Callaghan, U. and Chessells, J. M. (1985) The (4;11) translocation in acute leukaemia of childhood: the importance of additional chromosomal aberrations. *British Journal of Haematology*, **61**, 101–111
109. Secker-Walker, L. M., Swansbury, G. H., Hardisty, R. M. et al. (1982) Cytogenetics of acute lymphoblastic leukaemia in children as a factor in the prediction of long-term survival. *British Journal of Haematology*, **52**, 389–399
109a. Second MIC Cooperative Study Group (1988) Morphologic, immunologic and cytogenetic (MIC) working classification of acute myeloid leukemias. *Cancer Genetics and Cytogenetics*, **30**, 1–15
110. Sen, L. and Borella, L. (1975) Clinical importance of lymphoblasts with T markers in childhood acute leukemia. *New England Journal of Medicine*, **292**, 828–832
111. Smets, L. A., Slater, R. M., Behrendt, H., Van't Veer, M. B. and Homan-Blok, J. (1985) Phenotypic and karyotypic properties of hyperdiploid acute lymphoblastic leukaemia of childhood. *British Journal of Haematology*, **61**, 113–123
111a. Sobol, R. E., Mick, R., Royston, I. et al. (1987) Clinical importance of myeloid antigen expression in adult acute lymphoblastic leukemia. *New England Journal of Medicine*, **316**, 1111–1117
112. Stass, S., Mirro, J., Melvin, S., Pui, C-H., Murphy, S. B. and Williams, D. (1984) Lineage switch in acute leukemia. *Blood*, **64**, 701–706
113. Stass, S. A., Pui, C-H., Melvin, S. et al. (1984) Sudan black B positive acute lymphoblastic leukaemia. *British Journal of Haematology*, **57**, 413–421
114. Stein, H., Peterson, N., Gaedicke, G., Lennert, K. and Landback, G. (1976) Lymphoblastic lymphoma of convoluted or acid phosphatase type. A tumor of T precursor cells. *International Journal of Cancer*, **17**, 292–295
115. Stein, P., Peiper, S., Butler, D., Melvin, S., William, D. and Stass, S. (1983) Granular acute lymphoblastic leukemia. *American Journal of Clinical Pathology*, **79**, 426–430
116. Suarez, C., Miller, D. R., Steinherz, P. G., Melamed, M. M. and Andreeff, M. (1985) DNA and RNA determination in 111 cases of childhood acute lymphoblastic leukaemia (ALL) by flow cytometry: correlation of FAB classification with DNA stemline and proliferation. *British Journal of Haematology*, **60**, 677–686
117. Thiel, E., Rodt, H., Huhn, D. et al. (1980) Multimarker classification of acute lymphoblastic leukemia: evidence for further T subgroups and evaluation of their clinical significance. *Blood*, **56**, 759–772
118. Third International Workshop on Chromosomes in Leukemia, 1980 (1981) Chromosomal abnormalities in acute lymphoblastic leukemia: structural and numerical changes in 234 cases. *Cancer Genetics and Cytogenetics*, **4**, 101–110
119. Third International Workshop on Chromosomes in Leukemia (1983) Chromosomal abnormalities and their clinical significance in acute lymphoblastic leukemia. *Cancer Research*, **43**, 868–873
120. Van der Reijden, H. J., van Wering, E. R., van de Rijn, J. M. et al. (1983) Immunological typing of acute lymphoblastic leukaemia. *Scandinavian Journal of Haematology*, **30**, 356–366
121. Vogler, L. B., Crist, W. M., Bockman, D. E., Pearl, E. R., Lawton, A. R. and Cooper, M. D. (1978) Pre-B-cell leukemia. A new phenotype of childhood lymphoblastic leukemia. *New England Journal of Medicine*, **298**, 872–878

122. Williams, D. L., Harris, A., Williams, K. J., Brosius, M. J. and Lemonds, W. (1984) A direct bone marrow chromosome technique for acute lymphoblastic leukemia. *Cancer Genetics and Cytogenetics,* **13**, 239–257

123. Williams, D. L., Look, A. T., Melvin, S. L. et al. (1984) New chromosomal translocations correlate with specific immunophenotypes of childhood acute lymphoblastic leukemia. *Cell,* **36**, 101–109

124. Zwaan, F. E., Hermans, J., Barrett, A. J. and Speck, B. (1984) Bone marrow transplantation for acute lymphoblastic leukaemia: a survey of the European Group for bone marrow transplantation. *British Journal of Haematology,* **58**, 33–42

Chapter 3

B-cell chronic lymphocytic leukaemia

Introduction

Chronic lymphocytic leukaemia (CLL) is the most common of the chronic leukaemias with an incidence higher than that of chronic granulocytic leukaemia (CGL) in Western populations, particularly over the age of 50 years[51]. Within the lymphoproliferative disorders the incidence of CLL is 70%, with most cases (98.5%) being of B-cell type or B-CLL[8].

The peak incidence of CLL is between 60 and 80 years (Figure 3.1); cases below the age of 40 are extremely rare. Thus, in Asian and African countries where the life expectancy of the population is lower than in Europe, CLL is relatively uncommon[51]. Racial factors may also be important as judged by the low incidence of B-CLL in Japan where life expectancy is as high as in Western countries. A splenomegalic form of CLL affecting females below the age of 50 has recently been recognized in Nigeria[124].

Compared with other leukaemias CLL shows a consistently higher incidence of males than females. The usual M:F ratio is 2:1[9, 103]; in the MRC CLL 1 trial in

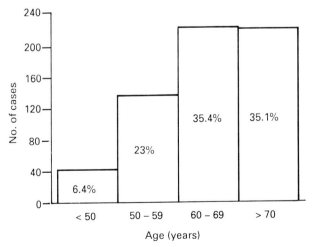

Figure 3.1 Histogram of the relative incidence of B-CLL by age groups based on data from 660 patients entered into the MRC CLL trial 1[18a]

which 645 patients were entered, the ratio was 1.8:1[18a]; in a retrospective large Canadian series it was 1.7:1[115]. The M:F ratio decreases with increasing age[18a].

CLL was described in the 1960s as an accumulative disease of the immunologically incompetent lymphocytes[23, 42]. Advances in immunology in the ensuing two decades have led to the concept of CLL as a lymphoproliferative disorder involving a distinct subset of recirculating B-cells[12, 43], which may be found at the edges of normal germinal centres and not in normal bone marrow[15]. CLL has for many years been considered a model for the study of lymphoid malignancies and the pathogenesis of some manifestations such as hypogamma-globulinaemia and autoimmunity[23]. A transplantable leukaemia (KSL) of guinea-pigs has been described as a good model for human B-CLL[62]. KSL develops, as B-CLL, in spleen, lymph nodes and blood whereas another experimental B-cell leukaemia, BCL1 of BALB/c mice, develops mainly in the spleen[65], and can be considered as a model for B-PLL. This chapter will summarize and update the literature on human B-CLL with particular emphasis on the clinical and laboratory features with which the authors have greater experience.

Familial incidence

The best evidence for genetic susceptibility in leukaemia has resulted from family studies. The risk for familial leukaemia is greater in CLL than in any of the other leukaemias[51]; the evidence for familial incidence is almost non-existent in chronic granulocytic leukaemia. With modern immunological, serological and molecular biology methods it may be possible to study the factors responsible for the genetic susceptibility in some families. Findings of similar membrane immunoglobulins, such as the same class of light chain, has been a feature of the reported cases[93]. Although some of the studies in CLL and hairy cell leukaemia (HCL) suggested a linkage to HLA[18] this was absent in the family reported by Neuland et al.[93] where the father and four of five of his offspring were affected

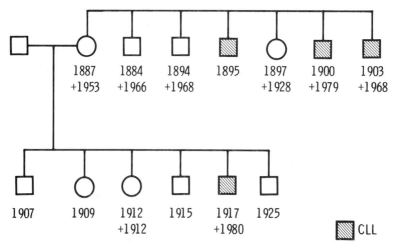

Figure 3.2 Pedigree of a family where the propositus (date of birth 1917) and three maternal uncles suffered from CLL. Dates of birth and of death (+) are given for family members

by CLL. Figure 3.2 illustrates the family tree of a patient whose three maternal uncles have also suffered from CLL. Future studies should include the analysis of the Ig idiotypes and of the configuration of the Ig genes, as well as the karyotype of the neoplastic cells, in order to obtain more precise clues about the genetic factors involved in the pathogenesis of familial CLL.

Clinical findings

A significant proportion (close to 20%) of CLL patients are asymptomatic and the diagnosis is made by chance following a blood examination. These patients usually have stage 0 disease in the Rai staging system[103]. Other patients present with symptoms of anaemia or notice lymph node enlargement; rarely splenomegaly comes to the attention of the patient as a result of symptoms of abdominal fullness or discomfort referred to the left hypochondrium. Constitutional 'B' symptoms (as in malignant lymphomas), e.g. pyrexia, sweating, malaise, weight loss, not related to an infectious complication, are rare as a presenting symptom. They are seen, however, as one of the manifestations of transformation of CLL: Richter's syndrome (see below)[2, 32, 41, 74, 105]. Lymph node enlargement is one of the cardinal features of B-CLL. These are usually bilateral (symmetrical) and involve the neck (anterior and posterior triangles and supraclavicular areas), the axillae and the inguinal regions including superficial femorals, and are found in two-thirds of cases. When palpable lymph nodes are often greater than 1 cm in diameter, are mobile and non-tender. The presence of lymphadenopathy in these three areas is important for staging purposes (see below).

Hepatomegaly and, more frequently, splenomegaly are also characteristic physical signs in half of the cases. Enlargement of these organs is also considered important for staging purposes. In the International Workshop system[56] both are considered as areas of organ enlargement. In Rai staging they define stage II, irrespective of the presence of lymphadenopathy. Splenomegaly without lymphadenopathy is rare (<5% of cases) and constitutes the 'splenic' form of the disease[26] which has been reported as being associated with good prognosis.

In addition to superficial organ enlargement, abdominal (retroperitoneal) or mediastinal and hilar region lymph nodes can be documented by means of special investigations: chest X-ray, abdominal ultrasound and/or computerized tomography scanning procedures. Lymphangiograms are rarely performed nowadays to demonstrate para-aortic lymphadenopathy in CLL. Although the presence of abdominal and/or mediastinal involvement does not seem to add to the prognostic features used in the staging of the disease the information may be important, in individual patients, to document either further progression of the disease or to assess the response to a particular treatment.

Laboratory investigations

The diagnosis of B-CLL is based on laboratory studies which currently include a full blood count with careful attention to the morphology of the lymphocytes, a bone marrow aspirate and trephine biopsy, and a minimum of cell markers to establish the B-cell nature of the lymphocytes and to show the characteristic phenotype of B-CLL (see Table 1.8, Chapter 1). Other tests may be necessary to assess the clinical status of patients and to make a precise diagnosis in borderline cases.

Blood counts

Lymphocytosis

Persistent lymphocytosis over $10 \times 10^9/l$ without apparent cause, may be sufficient for a diagnosis of CLL. Careful examination of the blood film should show the predominance of small lymphocytes with scanty cytoplasm, clumped nuclear chromatin, inconspicuous nucleolus and absence of azurophil granules in the cytoplasm. Lymphocyte counts range from 10 to $100 \times 10^9/l$; counts over $100 \times 10^9/l$ are not common at presentation; average values are $30–50 \times 10^9/l$. In addition to the lymphocyte morphology, the presence of smear cells, which correlates with the WBC count, is often diagnostic of B-CLL. A proportion of larger nucleolated lymphocytes (prolymphocytes) can be seen in blood films at presentation. In typical B-CLLs the proportion of prolymphocytes is, as a rule, less than 10% [84]. A group of patients with features intermediate between those of CLL and PLL has been recognized [84]. The proportion of these cells may remain stable or may progress, usually when associated with disease progression in what has been described as 'prolymphocytoid transformation' [27, 28]. Careful examination of blood films should exclude other causes of lymphocytosis, such as those associated with viral infections, and may suggest an alternative pathology, e.g. the presence of small cleaved (notched nuclei) cells with almost no cytoplasm may suggest follicular lymphoma, and the presence of lymphoplasmacytic cells may indicate a plasma cell disorder. In a minority of B-CLL cases the cells show crystalline inclusions, which correspond to Ig molecules, usually IgMλ, which are seen as unstained long inclusions in the cytoplasm. In addition to the CLL cells it is possible to recognize, in well-stained blood films, lymphocytes with more abundant cytoplasm and numerous azurophilic granules. These cells are more easily noted when the WBC count is low (and the relative proportion of T-cells higher) and correspond to Tγ-lymphocytes whose proportion is increased within the normal T-cell subsets in B-CLL [19, 69, 82]. The existence of a lymphopenic phase preceding the development of CLL has been suggested [10].

Anaemia

The investigation of anaemia has important diagnostic and prognostic implications in B-CLL. Haemoglobin less than 10 g/dl is an important prognostic feature and constitutes one of the components of the staging system (Rai stage III or stage C in the International system). However, the prognostic implication is valid only when anaemia results from advanced disease with bone marrow infiltration, with or without splenic enlargement. Secondary causes of anaemia, iron, folate or vitamin B_{12} deficiency, not uncommon in the CLL age group, should be identified and corrected appropriately before staging of the disease. Immune haemolytic anaemia may be suspected by the presence of reticulocytosis, spherocytes and proven by a positive direct antiglobulin (Coombs') test. The prognosis of immune haemolytic anaemia in B-CLL is more favourable than when the anaemia is caused by bone marrow failure.

Thrombocytopenia

Platelets counts below $100 \times 10^9/l$ are also considered a feature of poor prognosis (Rai stage IV or stage C in the International system) unless it is the result of immune phenomena, which could be corrected by corticosteroid therapy, or of splenic pooling, which improves with splenectomy.

Bone marrow

Aspirate

Increased lymphocyte infiltration ($\geq 40\%$ of the nucleated cells) is characteristic of CLL. The cells have the same morphology as those seen in the peripheral blood. The aspirate, stained with Romanovsky dyes, may show preservation of normal haemopoiesis, and therefore help to clarify the mechanism of anaemia or thrombocytopenia. A relative increase in erythroid precursors and/or megakary-ocytes in the bone marrow is a feature of hypersplenism, even in the presence of lymphocytic infiltration.

Trephine biopsy

This is more important than the aspirate and it is essential when adequate material is not obtained in the latter. A bone marrow core biopsy is required for:

1. Confirmation of the diagnosis and exclusion of other lymphoproliferative disorders (e.g. follicular lymphoma, hairy cell leukaemia), according to the pattern of infiltration.
2. To assess the bone marrow haemopoietic capacity in relation to the peripheral blood findings (anaemia or thrombocytopenia).
3. To define the patterns of bone marrow infiltration which have been shown to correlate with clinical stages and also to have independent prognostic value [5, 41a, 109].

Four histological patterns of infiltration have been described: interstitial, nodular, mixed (a combination of the interstitial and nodular pattern) and diffuse. The latter represents the most advanced degree of infiltration with complete replacement of the bone marrow spaces by diffuse lymphocytic infiltration, absence of normal haemopoiesis and of fat spaces [109]. The best preparations are those obtained with plastic embedding procedures followed by semi-thin sections which allow good preservation of the cell morphology. Furthermore, transformation of CLL to an immunoblastic lymphoma can also be documented in good trephine biopsies (Figure 3.3).

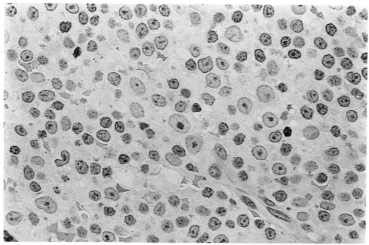

Figure 3.3 Bone marrow trephine biopsy of a CLL undergoing change to an immunoblastic lymphoma. Note the increased number of large cells with prominent nucleolus coexisting with a diffuse infiltration by small lymphocytes. $\times$ 200, reduced to 68% on reproduction

Lymph node biopsy

This is not a routine investigation for the diagnosis of CLL but is desirable for cases with low lymphocyte counts ($<10 \times 10^9/l$), when the morphology of the lymphocytes in blood films is equivocal and/or when the membrane phenotype of these cells is not typical. The lymph node histology of CLL shows diffuse lymphocytic infiltration with variable degrees of immaturity and a pseudonodular appearance [25]. The relationship of CLL with well-differentiated lymphocytic lymphoma (WDLL) is still the subject of debate. Histologically it is not possible to distinguish these conditions. The development of unilateral lymphadenopathy or the presence of systemic symptoms during the evolution of CLL is also an indication for lymph node biopsy to document large cell (immunoblastic) lymphoma, or Richter's syndrome [2, 4, 74]. Occasionally evidence of prolymph-ocytoid transformation can be obtained from a lymph node biopsy before the appearance of the typical peripheral blood changes.

Biochemical tests

A raised uric acid is frequent in CLL and tends to correlate with the degree of lymphocytosis and/or overall tumour mass. This should be appropriately treated with allopurinol if specific treatment for the disease will be given. Hypercalcaemia is a rare complication and will be discussed below. Liver function tests are usually normal. Significant proteinuria is not found even in cases with free light chains. Rarely heavy proteinuria suggests a nephrotic syndrome, a complication that will be discussed separately.

Serum immunoglobulins
Two types of change can be seen in B-CLL. A progressive reduction of the Ig levels is the rule, usually starting with low concentrations of IgA, followed later (Rai stages III–IV) by decrease in IgM and IgG [7, 33]. Even with good responses to treatment it is rare to see a return to normal of the serum Ig levels. The subnormal synthesis of Ig may have a complex pathogenesis and this will be discussed later in relation to the abnormal T-cell function in B-CLL.

Small monoclonal bands, usually IgM, can be demonstrated in the serum of 5–10% of cases by conventional protein electrophoresis. The appearance of such a band during the evolution of the disease may precede or be associated with the 'prolymphocytoid' or the immunoblastic transformations [18]. With more sensitive methods, such as high agarose gel electrophoresis combined with immunofixation or immunoisolectric focusing, it is possible to demonstrate small monoclonal bands (IgM, IgG or just light chains) in the serum and/or urine of a high proportion of B-CLL cases [24]. The presence of free light chains in the urine (κ or λ) can be shown by concentrating the sample 100-fold. With these methods monoclonal proteins can be found at the same time in the serum and urine in 25% of cases [24, 117]. The light chain of the 'M' band is always of the same type as the light chain expressed on the membrane of the B-CLL cells. Nevertheless, the serum or urine protein does not result from the turnover of SmIg but from the active secretion of more differentiated cells. These cells can be found in the blood, bone marrow or other tissues and express Ig in the cytoplasm (CyIg).

Membrane markers

Early studies on CLL cells were instrumental in demonstrating the existence in human blood of B- and T-lymphocytes[125]. The clonality of the B-cell proliferation in B-CLL is strongly suggested by evidence of a single light chain on the membrane of the peripheral blood lymphocytes[12]. More definitive proof came from studies with the enzyme glucose-6-phosphate dehydrogenase (G6PD) in CLL patients who were heterozygous at the G6PD locus. These studies also showed that the leukaemic clone derives from a committed B-progenitor cell[31, 116]. This contrasts with findings in myeloproliferative disorders, chiefly chronic granulocytic leukaemia, which involve pluripotent haemopoietic precursor cells. B-cell clonality can now be demonstrated elegantly by the analysis of DNA showing the rearrangement of the heavy and light chain Ig genes (see Chapter 2). The lymphocytes in a minority of B-CLL cases (about 5%) also show a clonal rearrangement of the T-cell receptor β-chain gene (see Chapter 8) but, in contrast to findings in normal and malignant T-cells, the gene for the γ-chain of the T-cell receptor is not found in a rearranged configuration[40b, 93a].

Advances in immunological methods in the last decade have facilitated the characterization of the cells in B-CLL and helped to define the distinguishing features from other B-cell disorders (see Table 1.8, Chapter 1). Before the advent of monoclonal antibodies, the circulating cells of B-CLL were identified by the binding of red blood cells (M-rosettes) (Figure 3.4) to an undefined receptor on the cell membrane, and by the weak expression of SmIg[12]. The mean percentage of M-rosettes in B-CLL, in studies of over 1000 cases in our laboratory, is 65% when the lymphocytes are pre-treated with neuraminidase[18]. Only rarely the percentage of M-rosettes reaches that value in other B-cell disorders which may also express receptors for mouse RBCs, such as follicular lymphoma centrocytes or

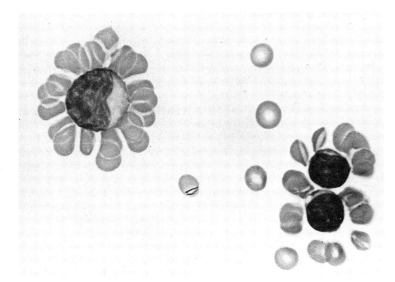

Figure 3.4 Cytospin preparation of M-rosettes obtained from peripheral blood lymphocytes from a case of CLL; note that both the small and large lymphocytes bind mouse RBCs. × 1200, reduced to 76% on reproduction

hairy cells. The high binding of mouse RBCs is a feature of peripheral blood lymphocytes in CLL; in the bone marrow the percentage of M-rosettes is often lower than in the blood.

The expression of membrane Ig (SmIg), IgM alone or IgM and IgD in most cases[12, 119], is weak and this may give rise to difficulties when the anti-human Ig reagents or the fluorescence microscope are not optimal. The density of SmIg on CLL cells is significantly lower than in normal B-lymphocytes and than in cells from other B-cell leukaemias, in particular B-PLL. Staining of fixed cells by immunoperoxidase[80] is more sensitive for demonstration of monoclonal Ig but this method does not distinguish between SmIg and CyIg and does not permit the accurate assessment of the intensity of Ig staining (see Chapter 1).

The B-cell nature of CLL can now be shown by specific monoclonal antibodies, e.g. CD19 (B4), CD20 (B1), CD24 (BA1), anti-Ia etc. (see Chapter 1); on the other hand B2 (CD21) is only expressed in 50% of cases. These reagents, whilst useful in demonstrating B-lineage, except for late B-cells and plasma cells, do not distinguish B-CLL from other B-cell malignancies. A characteristic feature, unique for its consistency in CLL, is the presence on its cells of the p67 antigen (CD5), also expressed in mature and immature T-lymphocytes[107, 122]. This antigen is also present on the prolymphocytes seen in typical CLLs, in half of the cases of B-PLLs, some centrocytes, but not on hairy cells. Other monoclonal antibodies of value in the characterization of B-CLL are FMC7 and mCD22 which are negative in most cases or expressed in a minority of cells whilst being always positive in B-PLL, hairy cell leukaemia and over half of the cases of follicular lymphoma (see Table 1.3, Chapter 1). The combination of weak SmIg, high M-rosettes, expression of p67 (CD5) and negative FMC7 is unique to B-CLL and has not been found by the authors in any other B-cell disorder. The activation antigen detected by antibodies of the CD23 group is also almost always expressed on B-CLL lymphocytes.

During the process of transformation of B-CLL to a disease resembling PLL[28] or to a large cell lymphoma, some changes on the membrane markers can occasionally be observed, namely an increase in the density of SmIg and, rarely, a decrease in the affinity for mouse RBCs. Strong CyIg staining is a feature of the immunoblastic or large cell lymphoma transformation.

E-rosettes provide one of the most specific tests for mature T-lymphocytes. A low percentage of E-rosettes in CLLs reflects the residual T-cell population which is often increased in absolute numbers[33] and has functional abnormalities (see below). In rare cases (<1%) the B-lymphocytes form spurious E-rosettes due to an anti-sheep RBC antibody activity by the monoclonal SmIg[90]. Such cases have the typical membrane phenotype of B-CLL except for a high percentage of E-rosettes; monoclonal antibodies against specific T-cell antigens including T11 (CD2) against the E-rosette receptor are negative. Incubation of the lymphocytes with monospecific antibodies will inhibit the formation of E-rosettes and this will confirm the non-specificity of the finding[90]. As other B-cells, CLL lymphocytes have receptors for the Fc fragments of IgG and IgM[110], demonstrable respectively by aggregated IgG and IgM, and for complement. Since the development of specific anti-B-cell monoclonal antibodies these tests are not used routinely in CLL.

Two groups have recently shown, directly and indirectly, that B-CLL lymphocytes express, albeit weakly, receptors for interleukin-2 (IL-2)[35, 118]. In only 25% of cases the percentage of CLL lymphocytes reactive with the monoclonal antibody anti-Tac (CD25) is 50% or greater (see Table 1.7, Chapter 1).

The percentage of Tac+ cells increases significantly after stimulation with the phorbol ester 12-*O*-tetradecanoylphorbol-13-acetate (TPA) in some cases[16]. As there is a major difference in the reactivity with anti-Tac compared with cells of hairy cell leukaemia, this reagent can still be used for the differential diagnosis of these two conditions (see Table 1.8, Chapter 1).

Maturation of B-CLL lymphocytes

Studies with monoclonal antibodies and receptors for IgM have suggested that although the B-cells have a consistent phenotype, they often represent discrete stages of B-cell maturation which can be documented with the appropriate combination of reagents[47, 48]. Thus, there are cases in which the cells are more immature, lack SmIg, express weakly B1 and the Fc receptor for IgM, and others in which the cells are more mature[48], often express CyIg and receptors for IL-2 and secrete 'M' components in the serum. Some of the latter cases are referred to as immunocytoma in the Swedish literature[59], although the authors prefer to reserve this term for disorders other than CLL where lymphoplasmacytic differentiation is the main feature (see Chapter 7).

A number of polyclonal B-cell activators (pokeweed mitogen, lipopolysaccharide, Epstein–Barr virus) and the phorbol ester TPA can stimulate B-CLL cells in vitro to acquire features suggestive of plasmacytoid differentiation. This drive towards immunological maturation can be shown by: the increase in the proportion of cells with CyIg and a concomitant increase in IgM secretion, the loss of the receptor for mouse RBCs, the switch from IgM to IgG in some experiments and the expression of FMC7 and Tac antigens with a corresponding reduction in the expression of B1 (CD29) and B2 (CD21)[16, 47, 48]. These maturation changes may be seen in vivo during the process of immunoblastic and, to a lesser degree, prolymphocytoid transformation, or in the rare transformation to plasmacytoma[99]. It has also been suggested[16] that the changes induced by TPA on CLL cells after 3 days of culture resemble, by a number of criteria, those of hairy cells, in particular the positivity with the monoclonal antibody LeuM5 (CD11c) against hairy cell antigens. As discussed in Chapters 1 and 6, the current concept of hairy cells as representing an activated B-cell is consistent with these findings, in as much as B-CLL cells are used as a model for B-lymphocytes. The evidence that hairy cells derive more specifically from a B-CLL-like cell is, however, far from proven.

Cell volume measurements

Precise estimation of the cell size of lymphocytes may be subjected to variation when these cells are examined in blood or bone marrow films of uneven thickness. As CLL is defined as a proliferation of small lymphocytes, the differential diagnosis from other lymphoproliferative disorders may depend, among many other features, on the evaluation of the cell size. A more accurate assessment of this feature can be obtained by volume measurements with a Coulter model ZBI or equivalent flow–cytometry equipment. Analysis of volume histograms on CLL samples in the authors' laboratory has confirmed that B-CLL consists of a uniform population of small cells (median volume 211.5 femtolitres or fl) which is significantly smaller than the larger cells which predominated in B-PLL (median volume of 281.8 fl in two-thirds of cases and 353.5 fl in one-third)[87]. Examination of CLL cases with an increased proportion of prolymphocytes always revealed two cell volume curves; in 80% of such cases the main cell population had, surprisingly, a volume larger than the small CLL cells (median 257.9 fl); in the remaining cases the major cell component was represented by cells of large volume, as in PLLs (median 349 fl)[87]. When the cell morphology was compared systematically with the volume measurements, the former always underestimated the cell size in PLL and in CLL with an increase in prolymphocytes in more than half of the cases. Volume estimations are also useful for identifying cells with an even larger size than prolymphocytes. The modal volume of these cells, which often correspond to immunoblasts, is over 500 fl[87]. When cell volume measurements are part of an FACS analyser the membrane phenotype of the distinct cell populations separated by size can be tested with more precision as in the case of hairy cell leukaemia (see Figure 1.4, Chapter 1).

Electron microscopy

Ultrastructural studies are not routinely performed for the diagnosis of B-CLL. In rare cases they may clarify the nature of cytoplasmic inclusions. Characteristically the B-CLL lymphocyte has a condensed nuclear chromatin and scanty cytoplasm with almost no organelles; a small nucleolus is sometimes seen (Figure 3.5a). In contrast to this typical cell, a prolymphocyte, as seen in B-PLL or in the CLL cases with increased number of prolymphocytes[84, 85], has more abundant cytoplasm, often with small electron-lucent granules, a nucleus with peripheral chromatin condensation, and a prominent nucleolus (Figure 3.5b). The distinction between these two cell types is further illustrated in Figure 3.6.

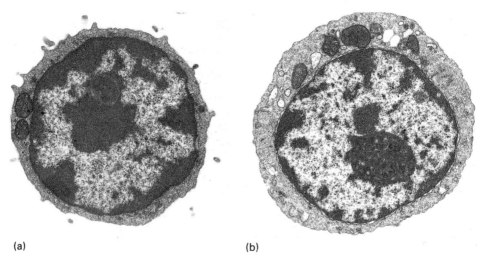

(a)   (b)

Figure 3.5 Electron microscopy of leukaemic lymphocytes. (a) Typical small lymphocyte of B-CLL; (b) prolymphocyte from a B-CLL case with an increased proportion of these cells. × 8000, reduced to 68% on reproduction

Prognostic factors

There have been numerous studies on prognostic factors in CLL, but few had utilized the modern methodology of the Cox multivariate regression analysis[8,

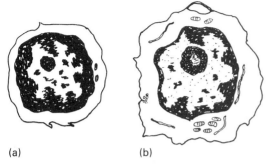

(a)   (b)

Figure 3.6 Diagram illustrating the main differences between (a) CLL lymphocytes and (b) B-PLL prolymphocytes: cell size, amount of cytoplasm and organelles, distribution of the nuclear chromatin and size of the nucleolus

18a, 86, 109]. In a disease with such variable patterns of survival it is important to define the factors which affect the outcome of patients. The studies by Dameshek[23], Boggs[9] and Galton[42] provided the basis for subsequent clinical staging systems[8, 45, 103]. These, in essence, compound the most significant features that influence survival and are, overall, the best indicators of prognosis. The staging evolves from the need to determine which cases may require treatment and to distinguish them from those which may have a long survival without the need of therapeutic intervention.

In addition to the factors included in the design of the staging systems, chiefly lymphadenopathy, hepatosplenomegaly, anaemia and thrombocytopenia, others have been shown to have independent prognostic value and to add to the prediction of survival within certain stages, namely, lymphocyte count[3, 108] and doubling time[92], bone marrow histology[5, 41a, 46, 53, 109], absolute number of prolymphocytes[86] and karyotype[54, 100].

A list of prognostic factors with key references is given in Table 3.1. Details of the two main staging systems will be discussed below; both have been shown in

Table 3.1 Prognostic factors in B-CLL[a]

Feature	Bad prognosis	References
Staging system		
International	Stage C[b]	[8, 18a, 45, 56]
Rai	Stage III–IV[b]	[8, 18a, 45, 53, 103]
Lymph node areas involved	$\geqslant 3$	[8, 97]
Splenomegaly	$\geqslant 10\,cm$	[8, 18a, 97]
Bone marrow histology	Diffuse involvement	[5, 41a, 46, 109]
Prolymphocyte count	$>15 \times 10^9/l$	[27, 86]
Lymphocyte count	$>50 \times 10^9/l$	[3, 108]
Lymphocyte doubling time	<12 months	[92]
Age	>70 years	[9, 18a, 103, 115]
Sex	Male	[18a, 103, 115]
Response to treatment	Poor or lack of response	[18a, 113]
Karyotype	14q+	[53, 54, 59, 95a]

a Listed in order of importance. Key references in brackets.
b Hb $<10\,g/dl$ and/or platelets $<100 \times 10^9/l$. In MRC CLL 1 trial [18a], low Hb was significant for prognnosis but not thrombocytopenia. In other studies too, anaemia was of greater prognostic value

many series to correlate with prognosis. The simplified prognostic grouping, A,B,C[56], based on the analysis of two series by Binet et al.[8] has probably greater power of prediction[18a]. Several of the factors listed in Table 3.1 have already been included in the design of staging systems, e.g. the number of lymph node areas involved and splenomegaly, both reflecting the tumour mass, or have been shown to be independent features in other studies[97]. The diameter of the largest lymph node and the spleen size (both in centimetres) are included, together with the square root of the lymphocyte count, in the elaborate 'total tumour mass' score proposed by Jaksic and Vitale[57] and recently applied in an Italian series[13]. Although anaemia and thrombocytopenia are used to define Rai stages III and IV and stage C in the Binet system, several studies[108, 109] including the analysis of the large MRC CLL 1 trial[18a], showed that haemoglobin (Hb) of less than 10 g/dl was stronger than platelets less than $100 \times 10^9/l$ as a prognostic factor.

The degree of bone marrow infiltration, particularly diffuse involvement, was shown by several groups to correlate with advanced disease and to have independent prognostic value[5, 41a]. In Rozman's study[109] each of the three stages, A,B,C, can be separated according to whether the bone marrow infiltration is diffuse or non-diffuse with the worse prognosis always corresponding to the diffuse groups. In Geisler's series this subclassification was shown to be useful in stage A patients[46]. A similar analysis by Han et al.[53] failed to show that the degree of bone marrow infiltration was an additional prognostic value over Rai's clinical staging. It should be noted here that the study of Rozman et al.[109] did not include clinical stage in the multivariate regression analysis. Assessment of bone marrow histology presupposes that all patients should have a trephine biopsy and that this should be uniformally reported by an experienced haematopathologist. It needs to be tested whether, although highly desirable, it would be possible to obtain this information easily in most patients.

Careful analysis of peripheral blood films in CLL discloses an increased proportion of prolymphocytes in some patients[84]. The prognostic value of the presence of prolymphocytes was analysed in a series from Hammersmith Hospital which included cases of CLL, PLL and intermediate CLL/PL, i.e. CLL cases with more than 10% prolymphocytes[84]. In that series the absolute number of prolymphocytes ($> 15 \times 10^9/l$) was the strongest predictor of survival, particularly for patients in the intermediate CLL/PL group[86]. The presence of large cells assessed by flow cytometry[66, 87] also seems to indicate a worse prognosis and to correlate with disease progression.

The height of the lymphocyte counts (> 40 or $> 50 \times 10^9/l$) was also shown to add additional prognostic information to the staging systems in two series[3, 108], particularly for patients with Rai stages I and II. Similarly, the lymphocyte doubling time, although shown to correlate partially with stage and bone marrow histology, seems to retain an independent prognostic value when analysed in relation to the interval of disease-free treatment[92]. Of the other factors listed in Table 3.1, age and sex, although available in most series, have not always been analysed systematically. Nevertheless, data from the authors' MRC CLL 1 trial[18a] as well as the large retrospective study from Skinnider et al.[115] suggest that males and individuals aged over 70 years have a worse prognosis than females and younger individuals. Age (> 60 years) did not enter the regression models in Rozman's series[109]. Analysis of survival by age and sex also requires careful analysis of causes of death[18a]. It is our impression that younger patients may present with a more advanced stage but may nevertheless survive longer than older patients in whom factors unrelated to CLL may operate. For example the series of Paolino et al.[97] showed that when CLL was complicated by 'chronic disorders', e.g. heart failure, diabetes, chronic lung problems etc., the survival was as short as that of patients with anaemia or thrombocytopenia.

The prognostic significance of karyotype abnormalities, shown in some studies[53, 59, 109], still needs a careful prospective analysis, because good chromosome preparations are not obtained in all cases. Furthermore, patients with more advanced disease usually have higher counts, and there is a trend for the cells of these cases to respond more readily in vitro to polyclonal B-cell mitogens[58]. The possible influence of the membrane phenotype, particularly the class of Ig heavy and light chains[4, 33, 52] has not been proven conclusively and awaits larger and more comprehensive studies. Overall patients with κ-bearing cells fare better than those with λ-bearing lymphocytes[18a].

Finally, the degree of response to the initial treatment is also a powerful indicator of subsequent prognosis[18a]. The authors' impression is that responses are better in early stages of the disease and that fewer good responses are seen in Rai stages III and IV. But, although it correlates with stage, response to treatment has been shown to have independent prognostic power by the Cox multivariate regression analysis[18a]. This is only possible in the context of multicentre therapy trials where this clinical parameter can be systematically recorded.

Staging systems

The development of staging systems stems from the concept of CLL as a slowly accumulative disease[23] which progresses in a predictable fashion from the blood and bone marrow, to lymph nodes and spleen, and finally to diffuse involvement of the bone marrow causing failure of normal haemopoiesis[42]. Evidence that this is the pattern of evolution derives from the observation that the probability of survival for a patient with CLL is the same whether he reaches a certain stage after progression from a lower stage or whether he presents in that particular stage[103]. Similarly, when good treatment responses are obtained the disease regresses to a lower stage and the subsequent patient survival will then be that of the new stage and not of the original one (E. Montserrat, personal communication).

The first staging system for CLL, proposed by Rai et al.[103], set the scene for clinical trials in this disease and has been used successfully for many years. This system consists of five stages which have been shown to correlate well with prognosis: 0, blood and bone marrow involvement only; I, as 0 plus lymphadenopathy; II, as 0 or I plus splenomegaly and/or hepatomegaly; III, as 0, I

Table 3.2 International staging system for CLL

Group	(Rai)	Areas involved[a]	Hb (g/dl)	Platelets ($\times 10^9$/l)
A	(0), (I), (II)	<3	>10	>100
B	(I) or (II)	≥3	>10	>100
C	(III) or (IV)	<3 or >3	<10	<100

[a] Each of the following counts as one area: palpable lymph nodes in the neck, axillae and groin, spleen and liver (clinically enlarged).

or II plus anaemia (< 11 g/dl); and IV, as 0, I, II or III plus thrombocytopenia (< 100 g/dl). Subsequent studies by Binet et al.[8], based on multivariate analysis of prognostic features, suggested a modification of the Rai staging which was later adopted by an International Workshop[56]. The new system which incorporates the Rai staging is shown in Table 3.2. The main reasons for the change, in addition to simplifying the prognostic groups from five to three, was based on evidence that patients with splenomegaly alone fare better than those with splenomegaly and/or extensive lymphadenopathy, and the need to adopt lower levels of haemoglobin for stage III (or C). The prognostic value of this staging system has been shown in several series[18a, 45, 108]. The analysis of the MRC CLL trial 1 shows that stage A(II) patients fare better than stage B(I) patients, confirming that with three or more areas of involved lymph nodes the prognosis is worse than with only splenomegaly.

Whether a subdivision of group A into A(0), A(I) and A(II) is justified at the present time is not clear, but it was considered important to retain Rai's stage 0 for future studies as this represents the minimal expression of CLL[56]. In the analysis of Binet the inclusion of patients with lymphadenopathy and/or splenomegaly in stage A did not suggest a worse survival for the whole group A. In the analysis of survival of patients entered into the MRC CLL 1 trial there was a distinct trend for worse prognosis in groups A(I) and A(II) compared with A(0). The distribution of cases in the various published series according to the two staging systems is shown in Tables 3.3 (Rai staging) and 3.4 (International staging) and the respective median survivals are shown in Tables 3.5 and 3.6. Overall, the proportion of cases in the Rai stages is not very different in these series. The slightly higher incidence of stage C patients in the MRC CLL 1 trial and in the series of Rozman et al.[109] (Table 3.4) may relate to the possible preferential entry of patients with more advanced disease in therapeutic trials in which no treatment is considered for those in early stages. Analysis of survival according to either staging system shows clearly major differences between the early and late stages of the disease.

Complications

There are several types of complication and clinical problems directly or indirectly related to the disease process that could affect patients with B-CLL. The most common and most important ones are infections and autoimmune phenomena. Other problems such as erythroaplasia, nephrotic syndrome and osteolytic lesions, although less common, are nevertheless well documented in the literature.

Infections

These are, as a rule, due to bacteria and relate to the degree of hypogammaglobulinaemia. In late stages of the disease they may also be caused by neutropenia resulting from marrow failure and/or cytotoxic therapy and often result in terminal pneumonia. Overwhelming pneumococcal infection may occur following splenectomy but this can be prevented by long-term prophylaxis with oral penicillin. There is a well-established concept that CLL patients do not respond to vaccines by raising appropriate levels of antibodies. This humoral immunodeficiency is more marked in the late stages of the disease. A rise in antibody titres to pneumococcal vaccine was observed in 5 of 18 CLL patients, mainly with early disease, studied in Boston (A. Zimelman, personal communication). Viral

Table 3.3 Distribution of cases in various series according to the Rai staging

Series	No. of cases	Stage (% of cases)					
		0	*I*	*II*	*III*	*IV*	*(III+IV)*
Rai et al. [103]	125	18	23	31	17	11	(28)
Geisler and Hansen [45]	102	20	36	19	17	8	(25)
Baccarani et al. [3]	188	26.5	26.5	21	9	17	(26)
Skinnider et al. [115]	745	19	21	31	16	13	(29)
MRC CLL 1[a] [18a]	660	28	18	29	10	15	(25.5)

[a] The haemoglobin level for stage III in this study was <10 g/dl; in the other series <11 g/dl.

Table 3.4 Distribution of cases in various series according to the International (Binet) system

Series	No. of cases	Stages (% of cases)		
		A	*B*	*C*
Binet et al. [8]	295	55	30	15
Geisler and Hansen [45]	102	44	41	15
Rozman et al. [109][a]	329	43	28	29
MRC CLL 1 [18a]	660	46	29	25

[a] Spanish Cooperative Group for the study of CLL.

Table 3.5 Median survival (in months) according to Rai staging system

Series	No. of cases	Rai stage				
		0	*I*	*II*	*III*	*IV*
Rai et al. [103]	125	>150	101	71	19	19
Boggs et al. [9]	84	–	130	108	9	42
Geisler and Hansen [45]	102	>78	50	36	30	6
Skinnider et al. [115]	745	>200	91	56	30	34

Table 3.6 Median survival (in months) according to the International Workshop staging system

Series	No. of cases	Stage		
		A	*B*	*C*
Binet et al. [8]	295	>120	84	24
Geisler and Hansen [45]	102	>60	36	15
Rozman et al. [109]	329	>80	52	19

infections, resulting from a deficient cell-mediated immunity, may prove difficult to document because specific antibodies are not a reliable indicator of infection in CLL. Herpes zoster is common and can occasionally result in disseminated varicella-zoster. A haemophagocytic syndrome resembling histiocytic medullary reticulosis has been documented in CLL patients and is probably due to intercurrent infections caused by DNA viruses[78]. Patients deteriorate rapidly with fever and jaundice and show large numbers of macrophages in the bone marrow exhibiting active haemophagocytosis. It was intriguing to observe, in the authors' own series, that this complication was more often documented in cases developing immunoblastic transformation[78].

Unusually large urticarial reactions as a result of insect bites are well known to occur in CLL patients. The exact nature of this allergic manifestation is not clear; some of these lesions can become secondarily infected.

Autoimmune phenomena

There are two well-known manifestations of autoimmunity in CLL: immune haemolytic anaemia (IHA) and immune thrombocytopenic purpura (ITP)[17], both resulting from the formation of autoantibodies, warm antibodies with anti-D specificity in IHA[106] and against platelet antigens in ITP.

A positive direct antiglobulin (Coombs') test is found in 10–20% of cases. However, overt IHA is documented only in half of those patients. The demonstration of haemolysis as a cause of anaemia in CLL may not be easy as the degree of reticulocytosis is lower than in idiopathic IHA, due to the bone marrow infiltration by lymphocytes. The presence of spherocytes in the blood films and a rise in bilirubin levels may facilitate the diagnosis which is proven by a positive Coombs' test. The demonstration of platelet-associated IgG[55] in CLL may also be more frequent than the incidence of ITP; overall thrombocytopenia due to autoantibodies is seen in 1–2% of cases. The diagnosis should be suspected when platelet counts are very low, e.g. less than $20 \times 10^9/l$, and megakaryocytes can be found in normal or increased numbers in the bone marrow. In patients with massive splenomegaly and resulting hypersplenism, pooling of RBCs and/or platelets in the spleen may mimic IHA or ITP, but the specific tests for antibodies are always negative. ITP and IHA can occur simultaneously; this is known as Evans' syndrome.

The propensity of CLL patients for autoantibody formation may relate to the T-cell abnormalities observed in this disease (see below). The antibodies are polyclonal, mostly of IgG class (as in idiopathic IHA or ITP), and thus bear no relation to the Ig class present on the membrane of the leukaemic B-lymphocytes. The T-cell imbalance, or some other mechanism, may be triggered by alkylating agents or radiotherapy as described for the first time by Lewis et al.[73]. This sequence of events has been confirmed by the authors in several patients. This relation to treatment may explain the higher incidence of IHA or ITP in more advanced stages of the disease. It should be noted that the nature of the T-cell abnormalities seen in hairy cell leukaemia and its autoimmune manifestations, e.g. systemic lupus erythematosus, vasculitis, caused by antibodies against tissue components[123] are different from those of CLL where the antibodies are directed against blood elements.

Anaemia or thrombocytopenia when due to autoantibodies does not carry the same bad prognosis as when resulting from bone marrow failure. For this reason it has been suggested that the subscript 'i' for immune should be used, to designate the CLL stages, e.g. III_i, IV_i or C_i. The current MRC CLL 2 trial recommends the randomization of these patients once the autoimmune cytopenia has responded to treatment. IHA and ITP respond to corticosteroid therapy and often benefit from splenectomy, which is indicated when immunosuppressive drugs fail to control the process. A period of treatment with cyclophosphamide is often necessary in our experience to induce a remission or a definitive cure of the autoimmune complication.

Red cell aplasia

Acquired pure red cell aplasia is a relatively uncommon complication ($< 1\%$ of cases) of CLL, but which has lately been recognized in several cases[77, 127]. Erythroaplasia has been associated with other forms of malignancy, chiefly with thymoma. In CLL this complication may develop spontaneously or may follow treatment with alkylating agents. Considering the many possible mechanisms for anaemia in this disease, the diagnosis of erythroaplasia may not be easy. It should be suspected when profound anaemia ($\leqslant 7\,g/dl$), with macrocytosis and reticulocytopenia ($\leqslant 0.1\%$) develop in a patient known to have had CLL for some years, especially after the initiation of therapy. The Coombs' test is negative and the bone marrow aspirate shows an almost complete absence of erythroid precursurs. This complication may be due to autoantibodies against erythroid precursors, as suggested by some studies, or to a direct effect by suppressor T-cells.

Nephrotic syndrome

Another rare but well-known complication (12 cases reported in the literature) is the nephrotic syndrome which, in the majority of cases, is due to a membranous glomerulopathy with deposition of IgG and C3[29]. The diagnosis is suspected when oedema and heavy proteinuria are detected at the time of diagnosis (half of the cases) or during the evolution of the disease; a renal biopsy is required to document the pathogenic mechanism. The authors have treated two CLL patients with nephrotic syndrome by means of corticosteroids and cyclophosphamide in one, and diuretics and chlorambucil in the other, and achieved a complete remission in both. Similar results have been reported[49]. Of interest is the observation in one of the authors' patients, in whom the CLL was in a quiescent phase not requiring therapy, that the additional treatment with chlorambucil reduced the lymphocyte counts to very low levels and induced, in addition, a complete haematological remission.

Hypercalcaemia and osteolytic lesions

These features, characteristic of multiple myeloma, are rare, in CLL[22, 67, 76, 104]. Patients either present with hypercalcaemia[76] or develop this complication after many years of evolution[22, 104]. All the reported cases had generalized osteolytic lesions and some also had pathological fractures; occasionally these features were associated with free light chains in the urine[104]. In general, it is thought that the lesions reflect the production of an 'osteoclast activating factor' by the neoplastic cells, as in myelomatosis. This is supported by the histology of the bone lesions which show numerous osteoclasts[76, 104]. In one case the hypercalcaemia was thought to result from increased serum concentrations of parathyroid hormone[67].

The even rarer association of CLL with multiple myeloma[11, 30] could also be responsible for clinical manifestations of osteolysis. According to studies by Brouet et al.[11] the two B-cell neoplasms usually have a different cell of origin. However, CLL could also transform into plasmacytoma as a result of the plasma cell maturation of the CLL clone[99]. Because of these various possibilities it is important to thoroughly document the immunopathology of the bone lesions and ascertain, whenever possible, whether the new clone represents the malignant evolution of the CLL clone or a new, possibly related, event.

Transformation of B-CLL

Two types of transformation have been recognized in CLL: 'prolymphocytoid'[28, 63, 85] and 'immunoblastic'. Both of them represent a profound biological change within the leukaemic B-cell clone with different morphological expressions. This development is analogous to the well-known transformation of chronic granulocytic leukaemia (CGL), but an acute blast crisis is only rarely seen in CLL whilst it is the rule in CGL. The changes seen in CLL are more subtle, particularly when an increased proportion of prolymphocyte-like cells is observed. In fact this phenomenon may not always indicate a progressive transformation. For this reason it may be more accurate to designate the cases with increased prolymphocytes as CLL/PL, also because it raises the question of the relationship between CLL and PLL[84–87]. Observations in a number of patients lead the authors to believe that the transformation of CLL is a process which occurs in stages, each one more aggressive and less responsive to the conventional therapy for the disease.

The rare but well-documented evolution to acute myeloid leukaemia (AML), observed either at diagnosis or later in the evolution of the disease, before any cytotoxic therapy or after treatment with alkylating agents, should not be regarded as a true transformation of CLL. It has probably the same pathogenesis as other cases of secondary or de novo AML[128]. Secondary AML following chlorambucil therapy is less common in CLL than in myelomatosis treated by melphalan.

B-CLL with an increased proportion of prolymphocytes

A detailed clinical and laboratory analysis of 300 cases defined the cut-off points in the percentage of peripheral blood prolymphocytes characteristic of typical CLL ($<10\%$ prolymphocytes), the intermediate CLL/PL group (11–55% prolymphocytes) and typical B-PLL ($>55\%$ prolymphocytes)[84]. The CLL/PL group (Figure 3.7a,b) is heterogeneous and includes the cases formerly described as 'prolymphocytoid' transformation of CLL[28]. The clinical features of this group are intermediate between those of CLL and PLL, namely the degree of splenomegaly is greater than in CLL and the number of cases with lymphadenopathy are significantly higher than in PLL. The immunological profile of the cells in CLL/PL is closer to that of CLL but with more cases with strong SmIg than in CLL and less than in PLL[84]. The proportion of M-rosettes and of FMC7+ cells is very similar in CLL and CLL/PL although a minority of the latter (18%) has a similar phenotype to PLL (e.g. two of the following: low M-rosettes, high FMC7 or strong SmIg).

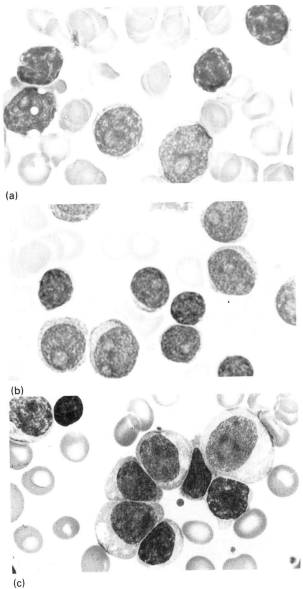

(a)

(b)

(c)

Figure 3.7 Peripheral blood morphology of CLL in transformation. (a,b) Examples from cases with CLL/PL showing the coexistence of small lymphocytes with large nucleolated prolymphocytes. Some of the small cells in (b) also have a distinct nucleolus. (c) The rare immunoblastic transformation affecting the peripheral blood. The large immunoblasts have an abundant, deeply basophilic cytoplasm. × 1400, reduced to 59% on reproduction

Sequential morphological studies in 55 patients over long periods of time showed that one-third of typical CLL cases experience, after diagnosis, a steady rise in the proportion of prolymphocytes (>10%, but <55%)[85]. One such patient presented with 4% prolymphocytes and reached 40% more than 2 years later. Of the patients presenting as CLL/PL (11–55% prolymphocytes), 20% may develop a blood picture resembling PLL. One patient, for example, presented with 16% prolymphocytes and reached 80% prolymphocytes within a 4-year period. In rare cases the morphological changes are associated with changes on the cell membrane (decrease in M-rosettes, increase in FMC7 and stronger SmIg staining).

Overall, good responses to treatment, partial and complete, in CLL/PL are lower (42%) than in CLL (53%). However, the response rate is much lower in the CLL and CLL/PL patients who experience the progressive prolymphocytoid transformation[27]. The latter definition can be used in cases where sequential changes take place, associated sometimes with phenotypic changes, disproportionate splenic enlargement and poor response to conventional treatment.

The most important prognostic feature in the CLL/PL group is the absolute number of prolymphocytes. Patients with more than $15 \times 10^9/l$ prolymphocytes have a median survival of 3.5 years which is similar to that of B-PLL[86]. The response to treatment also correlates inversely with the absolute prolymphocyte count. When CLL and CLL/PL cases were analysed as a single group by means of a multivariate regression model, the absolute number of peripheral blood prolymphocytes was the strongest factor to predict survival. This suggests that the dynamic changes that result in a high WBC count and an increased proportion of prolymphocytes reflect the process of transformation well and predict the clinical outcome.

Immunoblastic transformation

The development of a large cell lymphoma (or Richter's syndrome) during the evolution of CLL is a well-recognized form of malignant transformation in this disease[2, 105]. This change can occur in a single lymph node or, more often, in a group of them and is associated with characteristic clinical features, namely fever, weight loss and/or abdominal symptoms, simultaneous to asymmetrical enlargement of lymph nodes in the neck, mediastinal or para-aortic regions.

The lymph node histology shows a large cell 'immunoblastic' lymphoma, often with pleomorphic multinucleated cells which, not infrequently, have been confused with Reed–Sternberg cells[74]. Evidence that immunoblasts arise from the original CLL clone has been obtained by specific Ig staining in many cases[6, 41]. However, in some instances the presence of a different rearrangement of the Ig heavy and light chain genes[120] suggests that a new independent malignancy has developed. In fact, in about half of the cases of Richter's syndrome the disease appears to arise from a different B-cell clone. As a rule the amount of Ig in the transformed cells is considerably greater than in the peripheral blood lymphocytes, shown by strong CyIg staining associated with Ig and the appearance of an 'M' band in the serum and/or free light chains in the urine[74].

The diagnosis of Richter's syndrome should always be suspected when typical symptoms develop in a patient showing evidence of resistance to treatment. The incidence of this transformation is at least 3–5%, but it may be higher if lymph node biopsies are systematically carried out whenever there is a clinical suspicion. The interval from the diagnosis of CLL to this complication is variable; it can occur simultaneously as in Richter's original case[32, 105] or as long as 23 years after the original diagnosis[120]. Blood changes do not necessarily accompany this syndrome, although lymphopenia has been recorded in some cases.

Richter's syndrome is always associated with bad prognosis, less than 1-year survival in most series. Recently some remissions have been obtained with combination chemotherapy. Bauman et al.[6] reported a case who achieved a complete remission following three courses of CHOP (cyclophosphamide, hydroxydaunorubicin, oncovin and prednisolone) and returned to a relatively stable chronic phase. We have observed transient responses to CHOP in some patients.

Rarely the immunoblastic transformation resembles an acute leukaemia and involves mainly the blood and bone marrow (Figure 3.7c and Figure 3.8a,b), contrasting with Richter's syndrome which affects primarily lymph nodes (Figure 3.8c). The cells in these cases are large blasts with a deep basophilic cytoplasm and can be recognized by cell volume measurements which delineate both the immunoblasts and the small CLL lymphocytes[87]. The cells in some cases resemble those of ALL (Figure 3.8b) but marker studies will show a mature B-cell

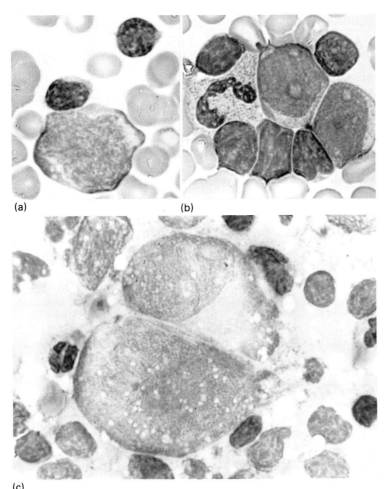

(a)   (b)

(c)

Figure 3.8 Immunoblastic transformation of CLL. (a,b) Large blast cells on blood films of two patients; (c) an imprint preparation from a lymph node with large cell lymphoma (Richter's syndrome) showing two very large immunoblasts contrasting with residual small CLL cells. × 1400, reduced to 62% on reproduction

phenotype. The diagnosis of the underlying CLL may be difficult if the 'immunoblastic leukaemia' develops very early in the evolution of the disease. It can nevertheless be suspected by the presence of a residual population of small lymphocytes in blood and/or bone marrow films.

Association of CLL with other malignancies

There are strong indications that the incidence of second neoplasms in CLL is higher than would have been expected by chance alone[50], even when corrected for age and sex, although this last point has been contested[75]. Some studies have suggested that this incidence is three-fold higher in CLL than in the normal population, and eight-fold greater when skin tumours are considered[79]. It is important in these types of survey to consider more precisely the type of cancer concerned. Skin cancer may not be a reliable indicator because CLL patients are under more regular surveillance than normal individuals and thus may have these changes detected more readily. In the MRC CLL trial 1, the incidence of epithelial cancers as a cause of death in CLL was 13.4%, which is comparable to the frequency of 15% observed in other European studies. An American survey indicates that an excess of cancers of lung, prostate and kidney, and cutaneous melanoma, observed in a population of leukaemic patients, was derived mainly from CLL patients, which constituted 28% of the total cohort and 47% of the total person-years of observation due to their longer survival[50].

Although the association of CLL with other haemopoietic malignancies has been recognized, there should be caution about reports of the association with Hodgkin's disease[128], unless there is good evidence that this does not refer to the development of Richter's syndrome (see above) and that both neoplasms arise from separate cell lineages.

Treatment

Although the treatment of CLL is largely palliative, good responses are, as a rule, correlated with prolonged survival[18a, 113]. It is clear that with a disease of such variable evolution the indications for treatment will depend on the clinical stage and symptomatology. The use of haematology charts to assess the response to treatment and/or observe the progress of the disease without therapy is essential for the management of patients (Figure 3.9). In this way it is possible to predict the time when a particular patient may become symptomatic and require treatment.

Accepted indications for treatment are stage C, stage B with evidence of progression and/or symptomatic lymphadenopathy or splenomegaly, and stage A (substage I or II) with progressive disease. Disease progression in this context is defined as a persistent downward trend in the haemoglobin concentrations or platelet counts with an increase in physical signs or a consistent upward trend in the lymphocyte count or constitutional symptoms such as unexplained fever, sweating, malaise, weight loss etc. When anaemia is an indication for treatment it is important to exclude secondary causes, e.g. iron or folate deficiency etc.

The treatment of patients with stage A (substage 0) or stage A (I and II) with stable disease is not normally indicated. However, a number of studies are now considering whether treatment at this early stage could improve patients' response and overall survival. Part of the argument relates to the evidence that response to

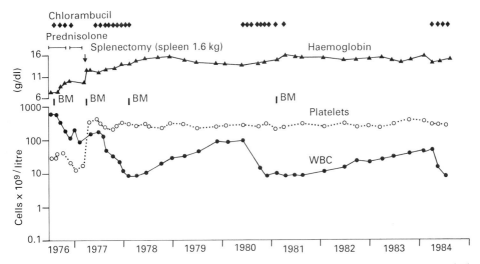

Figure 3.9 Haematology chart of a CLL patient presenting with massive splenomegaly and stage C (IV) disease whose hypersplenism corrected by splenectomy. Further courses of therapy given at 3-year intervals, kept the disease in good control thereafter. The patient was alive and well in 1989

treatment correlates with clinical staging, better responses always being recorded in early disease. Recent analysis of several trials at the International Workshop on CLL, in London 1989[56a], showed no evidence for an advantage in treating early (stage A) disease.

To assess the effect of treatment some standard definitions of response are necessary[113]. *Complete response* indicates the resolution of all physical signs, normalization of blood counts including the lymphocyte count ($< 3.5 \times 10^9$/l), and normalization of the bone marrow ($< 30\%$ lymphocytes). More stringent definitions of complete response can be based on membrane markers (e.g. with anti-light chain reagents) or even molecular biology methods, but they are probably of little practical value for general use. *Partial response* is defined by the regression by at least 50% of the abnormal physical signs, normalization of blood count (haemoglobin, platelets and neutrophils) and lymphocyte counts to less than 15×10^9/l; the bone marrow will still show lymphocyte infiltration ($> 30\%$ lymphocytes). Responses less than partial and complete are often called improvement, although their significance is not very different from a lack of response. Some authors use the change (downwards) of the clinical stage as an indication of a good response, e.g. the return from stage B to A or from C to A or B. Similarly, the semi-quantitation of the 'total tumour mass' index has also been proposed[13, 57].

The kinetics of the leukaemic cells, namely the proportion of cells in a particular stage of the cell cycle, is not currently used for the design of treatment in CLL. However, as the methodology for DNA staining and cell cycle analysis by flow cytometry are more widely used, it may be possible in the near future to define kinetic parameters which indicate the need for particular treatment modalities.

There are two main forms of treatment in CLL: chemotherapy, with alkylating agents and corticosteroids, and radiation therapy. Supportive measures are also important and splenectomy has clear indications which will be discussed below.

Chemotherapy

This is the most frequent treatment modality and consists mainly of alkylating agents used alone or in combination with prednisolone. Three-, four- or five-drug combinations are sometimes employed. The most common of them, COP (cyclophosphamide, oncovin and prednisolone), has been tried based on the relatively good responses seen in lymphocytic lymphomas. There is, however, no good evidence that COP is superior to chlorambucil or to its combination with prednisolone, in CLL. The MRC CLL 1 trial failed to show any advantage for COP vs monthly chlorambucil and similar results were obtained in the Spanish Pethema Cooperative trial[91] and in the American ECOG trial (J. Bennett, personal communication). This suggests that the addition of a vinca alkaloid, such as oncovin, has no appreciable effect in a disease with a low proliferating rate. It is possible that such an effect could be demonstrated in cases with more active disease and short doubling times. A recently completed French multicentre trial has shown that CHOP (COP plus hydroxydaunorubicin given at $25 \, mg/m^2$) was superior to COP for the treatment of stage C disease. The differences in favour of CHOP were a higher percentage of good responses and a better survival $(P < 0.002)$[7a]; CHOP is now being tested in stage B patients. The benefits of CHOP are probably due to the anthracycline doxorubicin. A new MRC trial, CLL3, will test this hypothesis directly by comparing chlorambucil alone vs chlorambucil + a new anthracycline epirubicin, in stage B and C CLL. The Memorial Sloan Kettering group has used a five-drug combination (carmustine, cyclophosphamide, melphalan, oncovin and prednisolone), the M2 protocol, in newly diagnosed and previously treated CLL patients[61]. Although the response rate was high it is difficult to appreciate the real value of this intensive form of chemotherapy in CLL as no randomized comparison was tested at the same time.

Alkylating agents
These are also known as radiomimetic agents because of the similarity of their cytolytic effect on lymphoid cells to that of ionizing radiation. Chlorambucil has been used for over 25 years[44] and still remains the drug of choice in CLL. Cyclophosphamide has probably a similar effect but has been used less as a single agent and almost always in combination, e.g. COP, CHOP or the M2 protocol.

Chlorambucil can be given orally at a low dose continuously, e.g. $0.1 \, mg/kg$ daily, adjusted according to haematological toxicity. A higher dose given intermittently in pulses, e.g. $0.5 \, mg/kg$ or $20 \, mg/m^2$ daily for 3 days every 4 weeks, is now more popular and may be advantageous to the low daily dose regimen because a similar good response can be obtained with a smaller total amount of drug[113], thus reducing the risk of leukaemia or myelodysplasia. The intermittent high dose therapy also has the theoretical advantage of sparing the normal bone marrow, and consequently allowing a faster haemopoietic recovery between courses.

Overall, 50% of previously untreated CLL patients are expected to experience good responses (partial or complete remission) with chlorambucil. This response rate may be as high as 70% in Rai stages I and II and usually low, about 30%, in advanced disease. When used in stage C patients with a severely compromised bone marrow by diffuse lymphocytic infiltration, the initial treatment with alkylating agents should be given with caution as haemopoiesis is likely to deteriorate first, before an improvement can be observed. Therefore it has been the authors' practice for many years to give prednisolone first in order to allow the improvement of the blood counts and then give chlorambucil. It would appear that the better survival of patients with Rai stages III and IV entered into the MRC CLL 1 trial, compared with other published series, could have resulted from the recommendation to use corticosteroids as the initial form of therapy.

It is advisable to continue treatment with alkylating agents until the best possible response can be obtained and then stop to observe how long the remission can be maintained. This period will be longer in patients achieving a complete remission. There is little benefit in continuing treatment when no objective response is observed, but it is preferable to continue therapy whilst a response is still being recorded aiming at achieving a complete remission. Some patients who experience incomplete responses and tend to relapse shortly when therapy is discontinued may require long-term maintenance to keep the disease under control. Once treatment is indicated in a particular patient it is likely that it will continue to be needed in the foreseeable future. Chlorambucil has few side effects and this is one of the reasons for its popularity. Nausea may be a problem when using the higher doses but this can be overcome by halving the daily dose and prolonging the duration of the course, e.g. from 3 to 6 days. Rarely, hypersensitivity reactions such as urticaria or other allergic skin manifestations may require a change from chlorambucil to cyclophosphamide. For patients on cyclophosphamide, it is important always to recommend adequate hydration and to monitor the urine regularly for evidence of blood because haemorrhagic cystitis is one of the severe long-term complications of this agent.

Corticosteroids

The effect of these agents in CLL has been known for many years[44]. Prednisone or prednisolone, when given alone as initial treatment, causes a characteristic rise in the WBC count during the first 4–6 weeks which gradually declines to below the initial level by 8–12 weeks. This typical curve of the WBC count, which can be observed in haematological charts, is usually associated with a decrease in size of lymph nodes and spleen and a concomitant improvement in the levels of haemoglobin and platelets. This lympholytic action of corticosteroids is extremely useful in the early stages of treatment. It is not clear whether this redistribution of lymphocytes is due to a change in the membrane of these cells affecting their pattern of recirculation, or whether it is the result of changes at the level of the post-capillary venules which prevent the normal traffic of lymphocytes. However, prednisolone used as single agent is not effective for the long-term management of this disease as the proportion of good responses obtained with this agent is lower than when used in combination with chlorambucil[113]. Prolonged use of this drug is associated with complications and side effects which constitute obvious disadvantages. In addition to the initial beneficial effect in patients with bone marrow failure, there have been suggestions that the addition of prednisolone to chlorambucil, both given in pulses, may potentiate the effect of the latter and increase the response rates. This proposition has not been previously tested in a randomized trial and it is for this reason that it is being examined in the MRC CLL 2 trial. This study includes stage B and C patients and compares chlorambucil alone vs chlorambucil plus prednisolone, both regimens given intermittently at 4-week intervals. Preliminary analysis shows no differences with respect to survival.

Another indication for corticosteroids in CLL is the treatment of autoimmune complications, chiefly immune haemolytic anaemia (IHA) and immune thrombocytopenic purpura (ITP). In this situation, treatment is given at a relatively high dose, e.g. 60 mg a day, until a response is recorded and then continues with gradually decreasing doses. Some patients require being maintained on low doses, e.g. 10–20 mg a day, and others achieve prolonged remissions without the need of further therapy. Non-responders may benefit from splenectomy. To prevent the relapse of the autoimmune complication it is often necessary also to administer an alkylating agent (for this, daily cyclophosphamide may be more useful than chlorambucil), or to continue with corticosteroids for prolonged periods of time.

Patients on steroids experience an increase in well being but, if treatment is prolonged, they will gain weight, and have many side effects such as abdominal discomfort, flatulence, heartburn, cramps etc. It is important to prevent some of the complications by appropriate measures, for example the H_2-receptor antagonists (cimetidine or ranitidine) to prevent gastric bleeding or duodenal ulcers, and oral antifungals (amphotericin, nystatin or ketoconazole) to prevent candidiasis.

Radiation

Lymphocytes are highly susceptible to the effects of ionizing irradiation both in vitro and in vivo. CLL lymphocytes are as radiosensitive as, or more so than, normal lymphocytes and this may be due to a failure in DNA repair mechanisms. The lympholytic effect of irradiation is independent of the cell cycle phase. Two forms of delivering X-ray therapy have been used in CLL: total body and splenic irradiation. Low dose total body irradiation given at a rate of 5–10 cGy, two or three times a week up to a total dose of 100–150 cGy, was shown to be effective in patients without bone marrow failure but also to be highly toxic in stage C patients. Overall this modality has no advantages over more conventional methods. Splenic irradiation has been used on and off for a number of years[14, 44]. One remarkable, although still poorly explained phenomenon following irradiation of the spleen, is the regression of lymph nodes distant from the irradiated field, which often occurs at the same time as the reduction in spleen size and WBC count. This effect can also be obtained by the irradiation of other sites, for example the mediastinum, although the latter modality has proven too toxic.

The benefits of splenic irradiation are seen equally in patients with small or large spleens, including those with B-PLL (see also Chapter 5). Splenic irradiation was shown not to be inferior to chlorambucil or COP in the MRC CLL 1 trial and is being re-examined in the MRC CLL 2 trial. The modality of irradiation adopted in these studies is a technique used in Padova by Dr M. Fiorentino (personal communication) which consists of weekly doses of 100 cGy given for 10 weeks (total dose 1000 cGy). The radiation field should relate to the spleen size, usually starting off with a field of 10 × 15 cm with the option of reducing it as the spleen becomes smaller during treatment. Anterior and posterior irradiation fields should preferably be used and the specified dose calculated at the centre of the spleen. Treatment may be delayed for an extra week if the platelet count is below $50 \times 10^9/l$ and the neutrophils are less than $1 \times 10^9/l$. In responding cases it is advisable to complete the 10-week treatment in order to achieve the best response. After a suitable interval (at least 6 months) a further course can be given. In general, no more than two courses of splenic irradiation are recommended to avoid damage to the left kidney or to cause a functional hyposplenism with respect to the antibacterial activity of the spleen (see below). Prolonged periods of remission have been recorded in some patients receiving only splenic irradiation. A significant reduction in spleen size ($>25\%$) and relief of symptoms relating to a large spleen can be obtained in 80% of patients[14]. Partial responses are possible in close to 50% of cases – again better in those with less advanced CLL. Good responses are nevertheless rare in patients shown to be resistant to chemotherapy, thus confirming that both modalities may act upon the cells by a similar cytotoxic mechanism. Possible advantages of a weekly over a daily dose of irradiation, in addition to considerations of convenience, are: less bone marrow toxicity (as when using chemotherapy in pulses) and greater effectivity due to the irradiation of a different fraction of lymphocytes circulating through, or pooled in, the spleen.

Splenectomy

There have been few reports analysing the indications for splenectomy in CLL[1, 21, 41b, 88, 116a, 126]. The following considerations derive from the authors' experience with splenectomy in CLL patients presenting with a large spleen. An analysis of 20 splenectomies for stage C showed that these patients fared significantly better ($P < 0.01$) than a control group (non-splenectomized) matched for age, sex and stage[41b]. The clinical evolution of one such patient is illustrated in Figure 3.9.

Splenectomy should be considered in CLL in three situations:

1. Refractory IHA or ITP, non-responding to or requiring high doses of prednisolone.
2. Hypersplenism, i.e. splenomegaly with anaemia or thrombocytopenia due to splenic pooling.
3. Poor response, with a residual large spleen despite an adequate trial of therapy: often, but not always, this is associated with hypersplenism.

The indications for splenectomy in the authors' series of 20 cases were mainly (2) and (3). It should be noted that a strict criterion for hypersplenism is not always applicable in CLL because the bone marrow is often heavily infiltrated[1]. After splenectomy blood counts improve in over 50% of cases, even in cases without evidence of splenic sequestration of ^{51}Cr-labelled RBCs[1, 21]. Trephine biopsies of the bone marrow are better than aspirates for assessing residual haemopoietic activity, particularly identifying megakaryocytes in cases with thrombocytopenia.

New treatment modalities

2′-Deoxycoformycin (DCF), a drug of value in the treatment of hairy cell leukaemia (see Chapter 6), has also shown useful therapeutic activity in CLL. The authors have used DCF to treat 17 patients with refractory advanced disease and documented partial responses in 47%. Ten of the treated patients eventually died of disease progression but only 4 out of the 10 were responders to DCF. One patient with high WBC count and anaemia had prolonged responses to two series of treatments with DCF, starting in January 1987 and continuing through October 1989.

Another promising agent, fludarabine monophosphate, a fluorinated analogue of adenine, has been reported to induce complete and partial remissions in 50% of previously treated CLL patients[60a]. Major toxicities are myelosuppression, mainly neutropenia, and infections, but this may reflect that mainly patients with advanced disease have been treated. There is little doubt that this agent will have a role in the management of CLL and this is likely to be defined better in current treatment trials. Neither DCF nor fludarabine are yet widely available for clinical use but are being carefully monitored for efficacy and toxicity in phase II studies.

α-Interferon, another agent useful in the treatment of hairy cell leukaemia (see Chapter 6), has recently been shown also to have activity in patients with early B-CLL[109a, 129]. Although the need to treat such patients can be questioned, there is no doubt that interferon has a favourable effect on several disease features. It could therefore be considered, in future studies, to try to prolong the duration of remissions in patients with stages B and C once they have responded to chemotherapy or in combination with cytotoxic agents.

Supportive therapy

In addition to the occasional requirements for blood products, there are some other measures to take into account when treating CLL. When initiating therapy in patients with a high WBC count ($> 50 \times 10^9$/l) and/or in patients with raised uric acid levels, it is important to add allopurinol together with the courses of therapy.

The prevention and treatment of infections constitute an important aspect of management, more specifically in patients with recurrent upper respiratory tract infections. It is helpful to have a low threshold for giving appropriate antibiotics. Our practice is to supply the patient with antibiotics, e.g. amoxycillin, which are taken immediately after starting a febrile illness or a respiratory complaint. Patients with advanced disease and profound hypogammaglobulinaemia benefit from γ-globulin replacement therapy given intramuscularly or intravenously. This is indicated in patients with repeated infections, particularly if some of them are severe. Long-term oral phenoxymethylpenicillin (penicillin V 250 mg two or three times a day) is essential in splenectomized patients in order to prevent sudden overwhelming infections due to pneumococci, meningococci, *Haemophilus influenzae* or similar organisms. The risk is greater in the first 2 years, but serious infections have been seen with those micro-organisms many years after splenectomy, often following dental manipulations. It is thus important to recommend antibiotic cover before and after any dental surgery and/or possibly to continue penicillin prophylaxis for many years. Although immunization with polyvalent pneumococcal polysaccharide vaccines (e.g. the pneumococcal vaccine Pneumovax) is now possible, the antibody response of B-CLL patients is likely to be suboptimal (see above).

Viral complications are less common in CLL but the risk of disseminated herpes simplex or herpes zoster infections is always present following localized lesions. Nowadays, early prophylaxis with oral or topical acyclovir should be considered according to the circumstances. Intravenous infusions with acyclovir are indicated for the treatment of such complications.

Patients with high WBC counts which are resistant to therapy may have their symptoms palliated by leucapheresis procedures. This has not been shown to be highly beneficial in CLL, but it may be successful, both in B-CLL and B-PLL, after removal of a large spleen.

T-cell phenotype and function in B-cell leukaemias

The interest in the role played by T-lymphocytes in the chronic B-cell disorders has increased over the last few years in conjunction with a greater knowledge of the close interaction between T- and B-lymphocytes. The demonstration that

T-lymphocytes have a primary role in the process of B-cell maturation suggests that a balance between T- and B-lymphocytes is essential for normal immunosurveillance. In turn, T-cell abnormalities may be relevant to the pathogenesis and/or influence the clinical course of some B-cell leukaemias.

The possibility of identifying T-cell subsets with specific regulatory functions, first by the presence of Fc receptors for IgG (Tγ) and IgM (Tμ) and more recently by monoclonal antibodies (see Chapter 1), has provided the necessary laboratory tools for the characterization of these cells. The membrane phenotype analysis, coupled with various functional assays, has permitted, in the last few years, a better understanding of the function of T-cells in most B-cell disorders. In this respect B-CLL has been more extensively studied than the other lymphoproliferative disorders. The findings in this disease will be compared with those obtained in other chronic B-cell leukaemias and in multiple myeloma.

Chronic lymphocytic leukaemia

The interest in the role of the T-cells in B-CLL is underlined by the known discrepancy between the low proportion of circulating T-lymphocytes and their high absolute number, which suggests that these cells may have some pathogenic relevance to the subsequent clinical course of the disease.

Although early results of the responses in vitro of the T-cells of B-CLL to phytohaemagglutinin (PHA) have been conflicting[36, 68], most studies have since reported a decreased and delayed response to PHA compared with that of normal T-lymphocytes, particularly in patients with advanced disease. The first suggestion of a defect within the T-cell population was made by Kay[60], and thereafter by other groups[69], which demonstrated a significant increase in the proportion of Tγ-cells and a decrease in Tμ-cells which was found to correlate with the clinical stages of the disease[19].

Results obtained with monoclonal antibodies have confirmed the abnormal T-cell subset distribution in B-CLL showing a significant increase in the proportion of CD8+ cells and a decrease in CD4+ cells[81, 102, 114], which is more accentuated in patients with advanced disease. In a recent study of 70 B-CLL patients a reduced CD4/CD8 ratio has been observed in all stages of the disease, although without major differences between Rai stages 0–I and II. Despite these changes in the proportion of CD4 and CD8 cells, the absolute number of both these lymphocyte subsets in the peripheral blood was higher than normal. The increase in the number of CD8+ cells was several times greater than the increase of the CD4+ cells. Studies with the immunoperoxidase technique without the need for isolating the E-rosette population have confirmed the reduction of the CD4/CD8 ratio and the absolute increase in CD8+ cells[80].

Pizzolo et al.[101] have shown that the proportion of T-cells in the bone marrow of B-CLL is also greater than in normal. Immunohistochemical analysis with monoclonal antibodies showed, in addition, that CD4+ cells were the predominant subset, with CD4/CD8 ratios ranging from 2 to 10. This finding suggests that the preferential homing of CD4+ lymphocytes to the bone marrow may contribute to the T-subset imbalance which is observed in the peripheral blood.

Studies in vitro corroborate the T-cell subset imbalance in B-CLL, namely a reduced T-colony-forming capacity[36], a reduced mixed lymphocyte reaction[68] and a reduced helper activity, in a pokeweed mitogen (PWM) driven system[20, 72]. Studies in the authors' laboratory have shown that the low T-colony growth and defective helper function are mainly due to an intrinsic defect of the T-helper (CD4+) population and is not just a reflection of the T-cell imbalance[36, 72]. Further evidence of an abnormality within the T-helper subset in B-CLL is provided by studies with the monoclonal antibody 5.9. This reagent recognizes a subset of T-cells (about 20%) in normal blood which contains the cells with helper activity[68]. In B-CLL the proportion of 5.9+ T-cells is reduced compared with normal blood and isolated 5.9+ T-cells also show a reduced T-colony-forming capacity as well as a decreased response to PHA.

B-CLL T-cells also have defective natural killer (NK) and killer (K)[38, 102] cytotoxic functions. Incubation with human γ-interferon and interleukin-2 (IL-2) can induce NK activity in these cells, but still at below normal levels. Other studies point to a discrepancy between the low NK activity assessed in vitro and the relative high proportion of cells positive with the monoclonal antibody Leu7. Studies by two-colour immunofluorescence show that the expression of the Leu7 (CD57)[38] antigen is observed mainly in CD8+ cells which were shown by cytochemical stains to correspond mainly to granular lymphocytes. These cells co-expressing CD8 and CD57 are rare in normal blood[121]. The use of monoclonal antibodies (e.g. CD16) which correlate more strictly with cytotoxic functions (see Chapter 1) has confirmed the low numbers of NK cells in B-CLL[34].

Abnormalities in the T-lymphocytes of B-CLL have also been observed at ultrastructural level by means of the immunogold technique and monoclonal antibodies[82]. These morphological studies have confirmed that the membrane phenotype in T-cells from B-CLL is abnormal (shown by the weak expression of CD3) and have demonstrated the increase in the population of large granular lymphocyte Tγ-cells.

Unlike the phenotypic and functional abnormalities, the production of soluble factors by the T-cell population in B-CLL appears to be normal[35]. Both the release of γ-interferon and of IL-2 from mitogen-stimulated cells is similar to that of normal T-cells. It is of interest that the leukaemic B-cells, which weakly express the receptor for IL-2[35, 118], can absorb the IL-2 produced by the T-cells[35]; this in turn may affect indirectly the normal function of this lymphokine on the T-cells in this disease.

The significance of the T-cell defects described in B-CLL is not yet fully understood; for example, it is not clear whether they are primary or secondary to the leukaemic process, whether they play a part in the onset of the disease itself and its progression, and to what extent they are implicated in the hypogammaglobulin-aemia which so frequently affects the patients. Because many of the abnormalities are spared in early stages and deteriorate with disease progression the current view is that they represent a secondary rather than a primary event. It cannot be ruled out, however, that the abnormalities may contribute to the gradual accumulation of immature B-cells which occurs as the disease progresses. The correlation between the T-cell defects and the levels of serum immunoglobulins, both of which progressively deteriorate in advanced stages, suggest that defective T-cells may reduce even further the subnormal antibody production in B-CLL and thus, implicitly, influence the clinical course of the disease.

Prolymphocytic leukaemia

There is little information on the distribution and functional behaviour of T-lymphocytes in B-PLL. Such studies have been hampered by the high WBC count and the very low proportion of T-cells in the peripheral blood. In a study of six cases[37], a significant increase in Tγ-cells and a decrease in Tμ-cells, compared with findings in the equivalent E-rosette positive fraction of normal blood, was observed in five and four cases respectively.

Functional studies have shown a marked reduction in colony growth in four out of five cases studied[37]. Despite the small number of cases evaluated so far the findings in B-PLL appear to be similar to those of B-CLL.

Hairy cell leukaemia

Contradictory results have been reported regarding the T-cell function in hairy cell leukaemia (HCL) and this may have been due in part to the presence of hairy cells in the samples tested. Studies carried out with enriched T-lymphocytes point to a weak response to the mitogens concanavalin A (ConA) and pokeweed mitogen (PWM), whilst the response to phytohaemagglutinin (PHA) appears normal[111]. The reduced activation with ConA and PWM may be restored following the addition of allogeneic monocytes[111].

Analysis of the distribution of T-cell subsets has revealed an overall increase in Tγ-cells accompanied by a reduction in Tμ-cells[111]. These observations have partly been confirmed using monoclonal antibodies. Lauria et al.[71] observed a marked increase in CD8+ cells and a decrease in CD4+ cells in half of the cases studied. When the T-cell subset distribution was analysed according to the clinical state of the disease, it appeared that the abnormality was present only in patients with active disease[71].

In contrast to B-CLL, T-colony growth is normal in most HCL cases and the helper function in vitro is preserved[40]. Both these functions are maintained regardless of whether the T-cell phenotype is normal or not. Studies on the NK function point to a frequent defective cytotoxic function in some individuals with a reduced response to interferon in vitro[39]. As in B-CLL[34] an increased proportion of CD57+ cells was found in HCL, but not with Leu11c (CD16) and AB8.28 monoclonal antibodies, which correlated better with NK function[39].

Myelomatosis

The possibility that T-lymphocytes may be implicated in the pathogenesis of myeloma has been suggested by Oken and Kay[95] who demonstrated a significant increase in Tγ-cells and a reduction in Tμ-cells in patients in whom the disease was under control; these findings have been confirmed by other groups. Patients with progressive disease showed, however, a normal proportion of Tγ-cells and a reduction of Tμ-cells[95]. In addition, an increased suppressor activity has been reported[96] together with an enhanced sensitivity of myeloma B-cells to Tγ-cell suppression[98]. These observations have led to the suggestion that the increase in suppressor Tγ-cells may play a part in controlling the proliferation of the neoplastic clone and also in the progressive depletion of the residual normal serum immunoglobulins.

Studies using monoclonal antibodies have confirmed the abnormality of the T-cell subset distribution showing a decrease of CD4+ cells in absolute and relative values[112]. When these findings are analysed according to the clinical stages of the disease the low absolute numbers of CD4+ cells are more evident in advanced stages of the disease[70, 89]. An increase in CD8+ cells was found only in stage I patients although the inversion of the CD4/CD8 ratio is more pronounced in stage III. Changes similar to those found in myeloma have been reported in Waldenström's macroglobulinaemia whilst findings in benign monoclonal gammopathy are close to normal[83, 112].

Functional studies have shown that the helper capacity of T-lymphocytes from myeloma is depressed irrespective of clinical stage[70] and that the T-colony-forming capacity is reduced in the majority of cases. These findings are consistent with the suggestion of an increased suppressor activity in peripheral blood lymphocytes in this disease which is associated with a quantitative reduction in T-helper cells. This reduced helper capacity indicates that this abnormality may be involved in the progressive hypogammaglobulinaemia which accompanies this disease.

Conclusions

It is now apparent that a range of T-cell abnormalities can be found in chronic B-cell disorders. These abnormalities tend to be specific for a particular disease, as illustrated in Table 3.7. Close monitoring of the changes within the T-cell

Table 3.7 T-cell functional activity in chronic B-cell leukaemias

Disease	PHA TI	T-colony growth	Help[a]	NK/K	CD4/CD8 ratio
B-CLL	Low	Low[b]	Low	Low	Reversed
B-PLL	Low	Low	Low	Low	Reversed
HCL	Normal	Normal	Normal	Normal or low	Reversed in active disease
Myeloma	Variable	Variable	Low[c]	Normal	Reversed[d]

TI, transformation index; NK/K, natural killer and killer function in vitro; NT, not tested.
[a] Suppressor function is not included in the table because there are few data with isolated CD8+ cells in these disorders.
[b] Partially spared in stage 0 patients.
[c] Probably due to excessive suppressor function; isolated (CD4+) cells function normally.
[d] More evident in patients with advanced disease.

population in individual patients throughout the course of the disease and in relation to treatment, will help to define better the role of these cells and to answer the question as to whether the abnormalities are a primary or a secondary phenomenon. This type of information gains particular relevance also in view of the possibility of using immunomodulatory agents in association with conventional chemo- and radiotherapy in the management of these disorders.

Chromosome abnormalities in B-CLL

The use of polyclonal B-cell activators (Table 3.8) has facilitated the demonstration of chromosome aberrations in CLL and other B-cell leukaemias. Analysable metaphases can now be obtained in over 50% of cases. Early work with PHA, a T-cell mitogen, rendered few mitoses, and as a rule these were normal.

The most common abnormalities are trisomy 12 (+12) and a 14q+ marker with breakpoint at 14q32 coinciding with the localization of the Ig heavy chain gene.

Table 3.8 Chromosomal abnormalities in B-CLL

Authors	No. of cases[a]	Mitogens used	Abnormalities (%)		Normal karyotype (%)
			+12	14q+	
Han et al. [54]	53	EBV, PWM, protein A	24.5	5.6	60
Pittman and Catovsky [100]	33	PWM[b], LPS	21	51	0
Juliusson et al. [59]	43	EBV, LPS, TPA	37	14	26
Nowell et al. [94]	40	PWM, TPA	10[c]	12.5[c]	65

[a] With analysable metaphases; the number of successful preparations ranged in the various series between 52% and 78%.
[b] Pre-treatment of the cells with neuraminidase and galactose oxidase.
[c] If considering only cases with abnormal karyotype these figures are 28.5% and 36%, close to those observed by the author [100].

Abbreviations: EBV, Epstein–Barr virus; PWM, pokeweed mitogen; LPS, lipopolysaccharide from *E. coli*; TPA, 12-*O*-tetradecanoylphorbol-13-acetate.

Table 3.8 summarizes the incidence of these abnormalities in four series. Differences in the incidence, particularly of 14q+, related to:

1. The number of cases with successful metaphases, and this depends on culture techniques and mitogens used.
2. The proportion of normal metaphases (Table 3.8) which may in turn depend on the mitogen used (e.g. higher with TPA which also stimulates T-cells) and on the proportion of normal T-cells.
3. The stage of the disease, the WBC count and the percentage of prolymphocytes.

It is our impression that mitoses are more easy to obtain in cases of CLL/PLL with high WBC counts and this is corroborated by the demonstration of abnormalities in nearly all cases of B-PLL (see Chapter 5). Juliusson et al.[58] noted that a high [^{3}H]thymidine uptake in 4-day cultures with B-cell mitogens correlates with shorter periods free of treatment, thus indirectly relating the response to mitogens to disease activity.

Other abnormalities seen in B-CLL, but with lower frequency than +12 and 14q+, are: 6q−, trisomy 3, del(12)(p13), del(2)(p13), abnormal 13q etc.[59, 95a, 100]. Trisomy 12 was considered initially to be a primary event with the other changes occurring mainly during clonal evolution. In some cases, however, +12 is not present in all the abnormal metaphases and is thus considered to be a secondary change. The marker 14q+ seems to be associated with a worse form of CLL either from presentation or secondary, in association with changes suggestive of clinical progression or transformation[100]. Available data suggest that abnormal karyotypes are more frequent in advance stages of CLL and are thus associated with a short survival and diffuse patterns of bone marrow infiltration[53]. In this respect, the presence of 14q+, or of numerous abnormalities and/or complex translocations, carry the worst prognosis[95a, 100]. Trisomy 12 by itself does not appear to be associated with worse prognosis[53, 95a]. However, a Swedish study suggested that patients with +12 more often require active therapy than those without[59]. It has been noted too that +12 and 14q+ tend to occur in different patients suggesting that each may relate to a different form of the disease. Alternatively the acquisition of either abnormality may influence the clinical outcome. Clearly the best prognosis is in patients with a normal karyotype and the worst in those with 14q+; trisomy 12 has an intermediate prognostic significance.

It is not clear at the present time whether the presence of normal metaphases reflects the residual normal T-cell population or may be compatible with a benign CLL clone. When normal metaphases coexist with abnormal ones it has been our experience that the former correlate with the proportion of E-rosettes in the sample. However, when all the mitoses have a normal karyotype, as seen in over 50% of cases in some series (Table 3.8), the answer is not so simple. It should be noted however, that when these 'normal' cases are excluded from the analysis, the incidence of +12 and 14q+ tends to be the same in most series (Table 3.8), thus suggesting that normal karyotypes, particularly if TPA is used as mitogen, may not necessarily reflect the 'leukaemic clone'. Recently, Knuutila et al.[64] demonstrated, by an elegant method that allows the simultaneous analysis of karyotype and immunological phenotype in cultures stimulated by PWM and TPA, that all mitoses with monoclonal κ- or λ-chain had trisomy 12, whereas the Ig− cells or those positive with T-markers had normal karyotypes. This, and the observations mentioned above, suggest strongly that normal metaphases in CLL may reflect only the normal T-cells. Nevertheless, further studies are necessary to ascertain whether this is also true for the cases in which all the metaphases obtained are normal.

Tumour necrosis factor alpha (TNF) in B-CLL

Recent data indicate that detectable levels of TNF may be found in most B-CLL sera and that purified B-CLL cells may release, particularly in the early stages of the disease, high quantities of TNF[40a]. These findings, together with the demonstration that in the presence of an anti-TNF antibody the proliferation of B-CLL cells can be significantly enhanced, suggest that TNF may play a regulatory role on the progression of B-CLL cells[40a], and thus be implicated in the characteristic accumulative status of this disease.

References

1. Adler, S., Stutzman, L., Sokal, J. E. and Mittelman, A. (1975) Splenectomy for hematologic depression in lymphocytic lymphoma and leukaemia. *Cancer*, **35**, 521–528
2. Armitage, J. O., Dick, F. R. and Corder, M. P. (1978) Diffuse histiocytic lymphoma complicating chronic lymphocytic leukemia. *Cancer*, **41**, 422–427
3. Baccarani, M., Cavo, M., Gobbi, M., Lauria, F. and Tura, S. (1982) Staging of chronic lymphocytic leukemia. *Blood*, **59**, 1191–1196
4. Baldini, L., Mozzana, R., Cortelezzi, A. et al. (1985) Prognostic significance of immunoglobulin phenotype in B cell chronic lymphocytic leukemia. *Blood*, **65**, 340–344
5. Bartl, R., Frisch, B., Burkhardt, R., Hoffmann-Fezer, G., Demmler, K. and Sund, M. (1982) Assessment of marrow trephine in relation to staging chronic lymphocytic leukaemia. *British Journal of Haematology*, **51**, 1–15
6. Baumann, M. A., Libnoch, J. A., Patrick, C. W., Choi, H. and Keller, R. H. (1985) Prolonged survival in Richter syndrome with subsequent reemergence of CLL: A case report including serial cell surface phenotypic analysis. *American Journal of Hematology*, **20**, 67–72
7. Ben-Bassat, I., Many, A., Modan, M., Peretz, C. and Ramot, B. (1979) Serum immunoglobulins in chronic lymphocytic leukemia. *American Journal of Medical Sciences*, **278**, 4–9
7a. Binet, J-L. (1988) Clinical classifications and treatment of chronic lymphocytic leukemia: the experience of the French Co-operative Group Trials. In *Chronic Lymphocytic Leukaemia*, edited by A. Polliack and D. Catovsky, pp. 123–138. New York: Harwood Academic Publishers
8. Binet, J. L., Auquier, A., Dighiero, G. et al. (1981) A new prognostic classification of chronic lymphocytic leukemia derived from a multivariate survival analysis. *Cancer*, **48**, 198–206
9. Boggs, D. R., Sofferman, S. A., Wintrobe, M. M. and Cartwright, G. E. (1966) Factors influencing the duration of survival of patients with chronic lymphocytic leukaemia. *American Journal of Medicine*, **40**, 243–254

10. Brandt, L. and Nilsson, P. G. (1980) Lymphocytopenia preceding chronic lymphocytic leukemia. *Acta Medica Scandinavica,* **208,** 13–16

11. Brouet, J. C., Fermand, J. P., Laurent, G. et al. (1985) The association of chronic lymphocytic leukaemia and multiple myeloma: a study of eleven patients. *British Journal of Haematology,* **59,** 55–66

12. Brouet, J-C. and Seligmann, M. (1977) Chronic lymphocytic leukaemia as an immunoproliferative disorder. *Clinics in Haematology,* **6,** 169–184

13. Brugiatelli, M., Morabito, F., Restifo, D. and Neri, A. (1985) Staging of chronic lymphocytic leukemia by total tumor mass (TTM) score. Evaluation of 121 patients. *Haematologica,* **70,** 405–413

14. Byhardt, R. W., Brace, K. C. and Wiernik, P. H. (1975) The role of splenic irradiation in chronic lymphocytic leukemia. *Cancer,* **35,** 1621–1625

15. Caligaris-Cappio, F., Gobbi, M., Bofill, M. and Janossy, G. (1982) Infrequent normal B lymphocytes express features of B-chronic lymphocytic leukemia. *Journal of Experimental Medicine,* **155,** 623–628

16. Caligaris-Cappio, F., Pizzolo, G., Chilosi, M. et al. (1985) Phorbol ester induces abnormal chronic lymphocytic leukemia cells to express features of hairy cell leukemia. *Blood,* **66,** 1035–1042

17. Carey, R. W., McGinnis, A., Jacobson, B. M. and Carvalho, A. (1976) Idiopathic thrombocytopenic purpura complicating chronic lymphocytic leukemia. *Archives of Internal Medicine,* **136,** 62–66

18. Catovsky, D. (1984) Chronic lymphocytic, prolymphocytic and hairy cell leukaemias. In *The Leukaemias,* edited by J. M. Goldman and H. D. Preisler, pp. 266–298. London: Butterworths

18a. Catovsky, D., Fooks, J. and Richards, S. (1989) Prognostic factors in chronic lymphocytic leukaemia: the importance of age, sex and response to treatment in survival. *British Journal of Haematology,* **72,** 141–149

19. Catovsky, D., Lauria, F., Matutes, E. et al. (1981) Increase in Tγ lymphocytes in B-cell chronic lymphocytic leukaemia. II. Correlation with clinical stage and findings in B-prolymphocytic leukaemia. *British Journal of Haematology,* **47,** 539–544

20. Chiorazzi, N., Fu, S., Ghodrat, M., Kunkel, H. G., Rai, K. and Gee, T. (1979) T cell helper defect in patients with chronic lymphocytic leukemia. *Journal of Immunology,* **122,** 1087–1090

21. Christensen, B. E., Hansen, M. M. and Videbaek, A. A. (1977) Splenectomy in chronic lymphocytic leukaemia. *Scandinavian Journal of Haematology,* **18,** 279–287

22. Clinicopathological Conference (1970) A case of chronic lymphocytic leukaemia. Presented at the Royal Postgraduate Medical School. *British Medical Journal,* **i,** 546–551

23. Dameshek, W. (1967) Chronic lymphocytic leukemia – an accumulative disease of immunologically incompetent lymphocytes. *Blood,* **29,** 556–584

24. Deegan, M. J., Abraham, J. P., Sawdyk, M. and Van Slyck, E. J. (1984) High incidence of monoclonal proteins in the serum and urine of chronic lymphocytic leukemia patients. *Blood,* **64,** 1207–1211

25. Dick, F. R. and Maca, R. D. (1978) The lymph node in chronic lymphocytic leukemia. *Cancer,* **41,** 283–292

26. Dighiero, G., Charron, D., Debre, P. et al. (1979) Identification of a pure splenic form of chronic lymphocytic leukaemia. *British Journal of Haematology,* **41,** 169–176

27. Economopoulos, T., Fotopoulos, S., Hatzioannou, J. and Gardikas, C. (1982) 'Prolymphocytoid' cells in chronic lymphocytic leukaemia and their prognostic significance. *Scandinavian Journal of Haematology,* **28,** 238–242

28. Enno, A., Catovsky, D., O'Brien, M., Cherchi, M., Kumaran, T. O. and Galton, D. A. G. (1979) 'Prolymphocytoid' transformation of chronic lymphocytic leukaemia. *British Journal of Haematology,* **41,** 9–18

29. Feehally, J., Hutchinson, R. M. and Mackay, E. H. (1981) Recurrent proteinuria in chronic lymphatic leukaemia. *Clinical Nephrology,* **16,** 51–54

30. Fermand, J. P., James, J. M., Herait, P. and Brouet, J. C. (1985) Association chronic lymphocytic leukemia and multiple myeloma: Origin from a single clone. *Blood,* **66,** 291–293

31. Fialkow, P. J., Najfeld, V., Reddy, A. L., Singer, J. and Steinmann, L. (1978) Chronic lymphocytic leukaemia: clonal origin in a committed B-lymphocyte progenitor. *Lancet,* **ii,** 444–446

32. Fialon, P., Hoerni, B., Mascarel, A. de, Hoerni-Simon, G. and Eghbali, M. H. (1979) Le syndrome de Richter. A propos de 7 observations. *Bordeaux Medical*, **12**, 367–374

33. Foa, R., Catovsky, D., Brozovic, M. et al. (1979) Clinical staging and immunological findings in chronic lymphocytic leukemia. *Cancer*, **44**, 483–487

34. Foa, R., Fierro, M. T., Lusso, P. et al. (1986) Reduced natural killer T-cells in B-cell chronic lymphocytic leukaemia identified by three monoclonal antibodies: Leu-11, A10, AB8.28. *British Journal of Haematology*, **62**, 151–154

35. Foa, R., Giovarelli, M., Jemma, C. et al. (1985) Interleukin 2 (IL2) and Interferon-γ production by T lymphocytes from patients with B-chronic lymphocytic leukemia: evidence that normally released IL2 is absorbed by the neoplastic B cell population. *Blood*, **66**, 614–619

36. Foa, R. and Lauria, F. (1982) Reduced T lymphocyte colonies in B chronic lymphocytic leukaemia. III. Evidence of a proliferative abnormality of the T helper cell population. *Clinical and Experimental Immunology*, **50**, 336–340

37. Foa, R., Lauria, F., Catovsky, D. and Galton, D. A. G. (1982) Reduced T-colony forming capacity in B-chronic lymphocytic leukaemia. II. Correlation with clinical stage and findings in B-prolymphocytic leukaemia. *Leukemia Research*, **6**, 329–333

38. Foa, R., Lauria, F., Lusso, P. et al. (1984) Discrepancy between phenotypic and functional features of natural killer T-lymphocytes in B-cell chronic lymphocytic leukaemia. *British Journal of Haematology*, **58**, 509–516

39. Foa, R., Lauria, F., Lusso, P. et al. (1986) Phenotypic and functional characterization of the circulating NK compartment in hairy cell leukaemia. *Clinical and Experimental Immunology*, **64**, 392–398

40. Foa, R., Lauria, F., Raspadori, D. et al. (1983) Normal helper T-cell function in hairy-cell leukaemia. *Scandinavian Journal of Haematology*, **31**, 322–328

40a. Foa, R., Massaia, M., Cardona, S. et al. (1990) Production of tumor necrosis factor alpha (TNF) by B-cell chronic lymphocytic leukemia cells. A possible role for TNF in the progression of the disease. *Blood*, in press

40b. Foroni, L., Foldi, J., Matutes, E. et al. (1987) α, β and γ T-cell receptor genes: rearrangements correlate with haematological phenotype in T cell leukaemias. *British Journal of Haematology*, **67**, 307–318

41. Foucar, K. and Rydell, R. E. (1980) Richter's syndrome in chronic lymphocytic leukemia. *Cancer*, **46**, 118–134

41a. Frisch, B. and Bartl, R. (1988) Histologic classification and staging of chronic lymphocytic leukemia. A retrospective and prospective study of 503 cases. *Acta Haematologica*, **79**, 140–152

41b. Gallhofer, G., Melo, J. V., Spencer, J. and Catovsky, D. (1987) Splenectomy in advanced chronic lymphocytic leukaemia. *Acta Haematologica*, **77**, 78–82

42. Galton, D. A. G. (1966) The pathogenesis of chronic lymphocytic leukemia. *Canadian Medical Association Journal*, **94**, 1005–1010

43. Galton, D. A. G. and MacLennan, I. C. M. (1982) Clinical patterns in B lymphoid malignancy. *Clinics in Haematology*, **11**, 561–587

44. Galton, D. A. G., Wiltshaw, E., Szur, L. and Dacie, J. V. (1961) The use of chlorambucil and steroids in the treatment of chronic lymphocytic leukaemia. *British Journal of Haematology*, **7**, 73–98

45. Geisler, C. and Hansen, M. M. (1981) Chronic lymphocytic leukaemia: a test of a proposed new clinical staging system. *Scandinavian Journal of Haematology*, **27**, 279–286

46. Geisler, C., Ralfkiaer, E., Mork Hansen, M., Hou-Jensen, K. and Olesen Larsen, S. (1986) The bone marrow histological pattern has independent prognostic value in early stage chronic lymphocytic leukaemia. *British Journal of Haematology*, **62**, 47–54

47. Gordon, J., Mellstedt, H., Aman, P., Biberfeld, P., Bjorkholm, M. and Klein, G. (1983) Phenotypes in chronic B-lymphocytic leukemia probed by monoclonal antibodies and immunoglobulin secretion studies: Identification of stages of maturation arrest and the relation to clinical findings. *Blood*, **62**, 910–917

48. Gordon, J., Mellstedt, H., Aman, P., Biberfeld, P. and Klein, G. (1984) Phenotypic modulation of chronic lymphocytic leukemia cells by phorbol ester: induction of IgM secretion and changes in the expression of B cell-associated surface antigens. *Journal of Immunology*, **132**, 541–547

49. Gouet, D., Marechand, R., Touchard, G., Abadie, J. C., Pourat, O. and Sudre, Y. (1982) Syndrome nephrotique associé a une leucemie lymphoide chronique. *Nouvelle Presse Medicale*, **11**, 3047–3049

50. Greene, M. H. and Wilson, J. (1985) Second cancer following lymphatic and hematopoietic cancers in Connecticut, 1935–82. *National Cancer Institute Monograph*, **68**, 191–217

51. Gunz, F. M. (1977) The epidemiology and genetics of the chronic leukaemias. *Clinics in Haematology*, **6**, 3–20

52. Hamblin, T. and Hough, D. (1977) Chronic lymphocytic leukaemia: correlation of immuno-fluorescent characteristics and clinical features. *British Journal of Haematology*, **36**, 359–365

53. Han, T., Barcos, M., Emrich, L. et al. (1984) Bone marrow infiltration patterns and their prognostic significance in chronic lymphocytic leukemia: corelations with clinical, immunologic, phenotypic and cytogenetic data. *Journal of Clinical Oncology*, **2**, 562–570

54. Han, T., Ozer, H., Sadamori, N. et al. (1984) Prognostic importance of cytogenetic abnormalities in patients with chronic lymphocytic leukemia. *New England Journal of Medicine*, **310**, 288–292

55. Hegde, U. M., Williams, K., Devereux, S., Bowes, A., Powell, D. and Fisher, D. (1983) Platelet associated IgG and immune thrombocytopenia in lymphoproliferative and autoimmune disorders. *Clinical and Laboratory Haematology*, **5**, 9–15

56. International Workshop on CLL (1981) Chronic lymphocytic leukaemia: proposals for a revised prognostic staging system. *British Journal of Haematology*, **48**, 365–367

56a. International Workshop on CLL (1989) *Lancet*, **ii**, 986–969

57. Jaksic, B. and Vitale, B. (1981) Total tumour mass score (TTM): a new parameter in chronic lymphocytic leukaemia. *British Journal of Haematology*, **49**, 405–413

58. Juliusson, G., Robert, K-H., Nilsson, B. and Gahrton, G. (1985) Prognostic value of B-cell mitogen-induced and spontaneous thymidine uptake *in vitro* in chronic B-lymphocytic leukaemia cells. *British Journal of Haematology*, **60**, 429–436

59. Juliusson, G., Robert, K-H., Öst, Å. et al. (1985) Prognostic information from cytogenetic analysis in chronic B-lymphocytic leukemia and leukemic immunocytoma. *Blood*, **65**, 134–141

60. Kay, N. E. (1981) Abnormal T-cell subpopulation function in CLL: excessive suppressor (Tγ) and deficient helper (Tμ) activity with respect to B-cell proliferation. *Blood*, **57**, 418–420

60a. Keating, M. J., Kantarjian, H., Talpaz, M. et al. (1989) Fludarabine: a new agent with major activity against chronic lymphocytic leukemia. *Blood*, **74**, 19–25

61. Kempin, S., Lee III, B. J., Thalen, H. T. et al. (1982) Combination chemotherapy of advanced chronic lymphocytic leukemia: The M-2 protocol (vincristine, BCNU, cyclophosphamide, melphalan and prednisone). *Blood*, **60**, 1110–1121

62. Key, M. E., Brandhorst, J. S., Bucana, C. D. and Hanna, M. G. Jr (1983) Development of a model of chronic lymphocytic leukemia in inbred strain 2 guinea pigs. *Journal of the National Cancer Institute*, **70**, 1139–1149

63. Kjeldsberg, C. R. and Marty, J. (1981) Prolymphocytic transformation of chronic lymphocytic leukemia. *Cancer*, **48**, 2447–2457

64. Knuutila, S., Elonen, E., Teerenhovi, L. et al. (1986) Trisomy 12 in B cells of patients with B-cell chronic lymphocytic leukemia. *New England Journal of Medicine*, **314**, 865–869

65. Krolick, K. A., Isakson, P. C., Uhr, J. W. and Vitetta, E. S. (1979) BCL1, a murine model for chronic lymphocytic leukemia. Use of the surface immunoglobulin idiotype for the detection and treatment of the tumor. *Immunological Reviews*, **48**, 81–106

66. Lanza, F., Scapoli, G. L., Spanedda, R., Franze, D. and Castoldi, G. L. (1985) Automated assessment of lymphoid cells in chronic lymphocytic leukemia: Correlation with prognostic features. *Haematologica*, **70**, 212–220

67. Laugen, R. H., Carey, R. M., Wills, M. R. and Hess, C. E. (1979) Hypercalcemia associated with chronic lymphocytic leukemia. *Archives of Internal Medicine*, **139**, 1307–1309

68. Lauria, F. and Foa, R. (1985) T-lymphocytes in B-cell chronic lymphocytic leukaemia. *Haematologica*, **70**, 445–450

69. Lauria, F., Foa, R. and Catovsky, D. (1980) Increase in Tγ lymphocytes in B-cell chronic lymphocytic leukaemia. *Scandinavian Journal of Haematology*, **24**, 187–190

70. Lauria, F., Foa, R., Cavo, M. et al. (1984) Membrane phenotype and functional behaviour of T lymphocytes in multiple myeloma: correlation with clinical stages of the disease. *Clinical and Experimental Immunology*, **56**, 653–658

71. Lauria, F., Foa, R., Gobbi, M. et al. (1982) Characterization of T-lymphocyte subsets in hairy-cell leukaemia (HCL) by monoclonal antibodies: comparison with Fcγ, Fcμ receptors and correlation with disease activity. *British Journal of Haematology*, **52**, 657–662

72. Lauria, F., Foa, R., Mantovani, V., Fierro, M. T., Catovsky, D. and Tura, S. (1983) T-cell functional abnormality in B-chronic lymphocytic leukaemia: evidence of a defect of the T-helper subset. *British Journal of Haematology*, **54**, 277–283

73. Lewis, F. B., Schwartz, R. S. and Dameshek, W. (1966) X-radiation and alkylating agents as possible 'trigger' mechanisms in the autoimmune complications of malignant lymphoproliferative disease. *Clinical and Experimental Immunology*, **1**, 3–11

74. Long, J. C. and Aisenberg, A. C. (1975) Richter's syndrome: A terminal complication of chronic lymphocytic leukemia with distinct clinicopathologic features. *American Journal of Clinical Pathology*, **63**, 786–795

75. Lopaciuk, H. Z., Wieczorek, A. J., Romejko, M. et al. (1977) Occurrence of malignant neoplasms in patients with chronic lymphatic leukaemia. *Haematologica*, **11**, 279–287

76. McMillan, P., Mundy, G. and Mayer, P. (1980) Hypercalcaemia and osteolytic bone lesions in chronic lymphocytic leukaemia. *British Medical Journal*, **281**, 1107

77. Mangan, K. F. and D'Alessandro, L. (1985) Hypoplastic anemia in B cell chronic lymphocytic leukemia: Evolution of T cell-mediated suppression of erythropoiesis in early-stage and late-stage disease. *Blood*, **66**, 533–541

78. Manoharan, A., Catovsky, D., Lampert, I. A., Al-Mashadani, Gordon-Smith, E. C. and Galton, D. A. G. (1981) Histiocytic medullary reticulosis complicating chronic lymphocytic leukaemia: malignant or reactive? *Scandinavian Journal of Haematology*, **26**, 5–13

79. Manusow, D. and Weinerman, B. H. (1975) Subsequent neoplasia in chronic lymphocytic leukemia. *Journal of the American Medical Association*, **232**, 267–269

80. Markey, G. M., Alexander, H. D., Agnew, A. N. D. et al. (1986) Enumeration of absolute numbers of T lymphocyte subsets in B-chronic lymphocytic leukaemia using an immunoperoxidase technique: relation to clinical stage. *British Journal of Haematology*, **62**, 257–273

81. Matutes, E., Wechsler, A., Gomez, R., Cherchi, M. and Catovsky, D. (1981) Unusual T-cell phenotype in advanced B-chronic lymphocytic leukaemia. *British Journal of Haematology*, **49**, 635–642

82. Matutes, E., Crockard, A. D. and Catovsky, D. (1983) The ultrastructural morphology of T-lymphocytes in B-chronic lymphocytic leukaemia: a study with monoclonal antibodies and the immunogold technique. *British Journal of Haematology*, **55**, 273–283

83. Mellstedt, H., Holm, G., Pettersson, D. et al. (1982) T cells in monoclonal gammopathies. *Scandinavian Journal of Haematology*, **29**, 57–64

84. Melo, J. V., Catovsky, D. and Galton, D. A. G. (1986) The relationship between chronic lymphocytic leukaemia and prolymphocytic leukaemia. I. Clinical and laboratory features of 300 patients and characterisation of an intermediate group. *British Journal of Haematology*, **63**, 377–387

85. Melo, J. V., Catovsky, D. and Galton, D. A. G. (1986) The relationship between chronic lymphocytic leukaemia and prolymphocytic leukaemia. II. Patterns of evolution of 'prolymphocytoid' transformation. *British Journal of Haematology*, **64**, 77–86

86. Melo, J. V., Catovsky, D., Gregory, W. M. and Galton, D. A. G. (1987) The relationship between chronic lymphocytic leukaemia and prolymphocytic leukaemia. IV. Analysis of survival and prognostic features. *British Journal of Haematology*, **65**, 23–29

87. Melo, J. V., Wardle, J., Chetty, M. et al. (1986) The relationship between chronic lymphocytic leukaemia and prolymphocytic leukaemia. III. Evaluation of cell size by morphology and volume measurements. *British Journal of Haematology*, **64**, 469–478

88. Merl, S. A., Theodorakis, M. E., Goldberg, J. and Gottlieb, A. J. (1983) Splenectomy for thrombocytopenia in chronic lymphocytic leukemia. *American Journal of Hematology*, **15**, 253–259

89. Mills, K. H. G. and Cawley, J. C. (1983) Abnormal monoclonal antibody-defined helper/suppressor T-cell subpopulations in multiple myeloma: relationship to treatment and clinical stage. *British Journal of Haematology*, **53**, 271–275

90. Mills, L. E., O'Donnell, J. F., Guyre, P. M., LeMarbre, P. J., Miller, I. D. and Bernier, G. M.

(1985) Spurious E rosette formation in B cell chronic lymphocytic leukemia due to monoclonal anti-sheep RBC antibody. *Blood,* **65**, 270–274

91. Montserrat, E., Alcala, A., Parody, R. et al. (1986) Treatment of chronic lymphocytic leukemia in advanced stages: a randomized trial comparing chlorambucil plus prednisone *vs* cyclophosphamide, vincristine and prednisone. *Cancer,* **56**, 2369–2375

92. Montserrat, E., Sanchez-Bisono, J., Vinolas, N. and Rozman, C. (1986) Lymphocyte doubling time in chronic lymphocytic leukaemia: analysis of its prognostic significance. *British Journal of Haematology,* **62**, 567–575

93. Neuland, C. Y., Blattner, W. A., Mann, D. L., Fraser, M. C., Tsai, S. and Strong, D. M. (1983) Familial chronic lymphocytic leukemia. *Journal of the National Cancer Institute,* **71**, 1143–1150

93a. Norton, J. D., Pattinson, J., Hoffbrand, A. V., Jani, H., Yaxley, J. C. and Leber, B. F. (1988) Rearrangement and expression of T cell antigen receptor genes in B cell chronic lymphocytic leukemia. *Blood,* **71**, 178–185

94. Nowell, P. C., Vonderheid, E. C., Besa, E., Hoxie, J. A., Moreau, L. and Finan, J. B. (1986) The most common chromosome change in 86 chronic B cell or T cell tumors: A 14q32 translocation. *Cancer Genetics and Cytogenetics,* **19**, 219–227

95. Oken, M. M. and Kay, N. E. (1981) T-cell subpopulations in multiple myeloma: correlation with clinical disease status. *British Journal of Haematology,* **49**, 629–634

95a. Oscier, D. G., Fitchett, M. and Hamblin, T. J. (1988) Chromosomal abnormalities in B-CLL. *Nouvelle Revue Française d'Hematologie,* **30**, 397–398

96. Ozer, H., Han, T., Henderson, E. S., Nussbaum, A. and Sheedy, D. (1981) Immunoregulatory T cell function in multiple myeloma. *Journal of Clinical Investigation,* **67**, 779–789

97. Paolino, W., Infelise, V., Levis, A. et al. (1984) Adenosplenomegaly and prognosis in uncomplicated and complicated chronic lymphocytic leukemia. A study of 362 cases. *Cancer,* **54**, 339–346

98. Perri, R. T., Oken, M. M. and Kay, N. E. (1982) Enhanced T cell suppression is directed toward sensitive circulating B cells in multiple myeloma. *Journal of Clinical and Laboratory Medicine,* **99**, 512–519

99. Pines, A., Ben-Bassat, I., Selzer, G. and Ramot, B. (1984) Transformation of chronic lymphocytic leukemia to plasmacytoma. *Cancer,* **54**, 1904–1907

100. Pittman, S. and Catovsky, D. (1984) Prognostic significance of chromosome abnormalities in chronic lymphocytic leukaemia. *British Journal of Haematology,* **58**, 649–660

101. Pizzolo, G., Chilosi, M., Ambrosetti, A., Semenzato, G., Fiore-Donati, L. and Perona, G. (1983) Immunohistologic study of bone marrow involvement in B-chronic lymphocytic leukemia. *Blood,* **62**, 1289–1296

102. Platsoucas, C. D., Galinski, M., Kempin, S., Reich, L., Clarkson, B. and Good, R. A. (1982) Abnormal T lymphocyte subpopulations in patients with B-cell chronic lymphocytic leukaemia: an analysis by monoclonal antibodies. *Journal of Immunology,* **129**, 2305–2311

103. Rai, K. R., Sawitsky, A., Cronkite, E. P., Chanana, A. D., Levy, R. N. and Pasternack, B. S. (1975) Clinical staging of chronic lymphocytic leukemia. *Blood,* **46**, 219–234

104. Redmond III, J., Stites, D. P., Beckstead, J. H., George, C. B., Casavant, C. H. and Gandara, D. R. (1983) Chronic lymphocytic leukemia with osteolytic bone lesions, hypercalcemia and monoclonal protein. *American Journal of Clinical Pathology,* **79**, 616–620

105. Richter, M. N. (1928) Generalized reticular cell sarcoma of the lymph nodes associated with lymphatic leukemia. *American Journal of Pathology,* **4**, 285–292

106. Rosse, W. F. (1981) The acquired haemolytic anaemias. In *Postgraduate Haematology*, 2nd edn, edited by A. V. Hoffbrand and S. M. Lewis, pp. 229–268. London: W. Heineman Medical Books Ltd.

107. Royston, I., Majda, J. A., Baird, S. M., Meserve, B. L. and Griffiths, J. C. (1980) Human T-cell antigens defined by monoclonal antibodies: the 65,000 Dalton antigen of T-cells (T65) is also found on chronic lymphocytic leukemia cells bearing surface immunoglobulin. *Journal of Immunology,* **125**, 725–731

108. Rozman, C., Montserrat, E., Feliu, E. et al. (1982) Prognosis of chronic lymphocytic leukemia: a multivariate survival analysis of 150 cases. *Blood,* **59**, 1001–1005

109. Rozman, C., Montserrat, E., Rodriguez-Fernandez, J. M. et al. (1984) Bone marrow histologic

pattern – the best single prognostic parameter in chronic lymphocytic leukemia: A multivariate survival analysis of 329 cases. *Blood,* **64**, 642–648

109a. Rozman, C., Montserrat, E., Vinolas, N. et al. (1988) Recombinant α_2-Interferon in the treatment of B chronic lymphocytic leukemia in early stages. *Blood,* **71**, 1295–1298

110. Rudders, R. A. and Poldre, P. A. (1984) The B cell IgM Fc receptor: further evidence for the B cell origin of 'null' chronic lymphocytic leukemia. *Blood,* **64**, 375–379

111. Sabbe, L. J. M., Meijer, C. J. L. M. and Jansen, J. (1980) T lymphocyte function in hairy cell leukaemia. *Clinical and Experimental Immunology,* **42**, 336–344

112. San Miguel, J. F., Caballero, M. D. and Gonzalez, M. (1985) T-cell subpopulations in patients with monoclonal gammopathies: Essential monoclonal gammopathy, multiple myeloma, and Waldenström macroglobulinemia. *American Journal of Hematology,* **20**, 267–273

113. Sawitsky, A., Rai, K. R., Glidewell, O., Silver, R. T. and participating members of CALGB (Cancer and Leukemia Group B) (1977) Comparison of daily versus intermittent chlorambucil and prednisone therapy in the treatment of patients with chronic lymphocytic leukemia. *Blood,* **50**, 1049–1059

114. Semenzato, G., Pezzutto, A., Foa, R., Lauria, F. and Raimondi, R. (1983) T lymphocytes in B-cell lymphocytic leukemia: Characterization by monoclonal antibodies and correlation with Fc receptors. *Clinical Immunology and Immunopathology,* **26**, 155–161

115. Skinnider, L. F., Tan, L., Schmidt, J. and Armitage, G. (1982) Chronic lymphocytic leukemia. A review of 745 cases and assessment of clinical staging. *Cancer,* **50**, 2951–2955

116. Solanki, D. L., McCurdy, P. R. and MacDermott, R. P. (1982) Chronic lymphocytic leukemia: a monoclonal disease. *American Journal of Hematology,* **13**, 159–162

116a. Stein, R. S., Weikert, D., Reynolds, V., Greer, J. P. and Flexner, J. M. (1989) Splenectomy for end-stage chronic lymphocytic leukemia. *Cancer,* **59**, 1815–1818

117. Stevenson, F. K., Spellerberg, M. and Smith, J. L. (1983) Monoclonal immunoglobulin light chain in urine or patients with B lymphocytic disease: Its source and use as a diagnostic aid. *British Journal of Cancer,* **47**, 607–612

118. Touw, I. and Lowenberg, B. (1985) Interleukin 2 stimulates chronic lymphocytic leukemia colony formation in vitro. *Blood,* **66**, 237–240

119. van der Reijden, H. J., van der Gaag, R., Pinkster, J. et al. (1982) Chronic lymphocytic leukemia. Immunologic markers and functional properties of the leukemic cells. *Cancer,* **50**, 2826–2833

120. van Dongen, J. J. M., Hooijkass, H., Michiels, J. J. et al. (1984) Richter's syndrome with different immunoglobulin light chains and different heavy chain gene rearrangements. *Blood,* **64**, 571–575

121. Velardi, A., Prchal, J. T., Prasthofer, E. F. and Grossi, C. E. (1985) Expression of NK-lineage markers on peripheral blood lymphocytes with T-helper (Leu3$^+$/T4$^+$) phenotype in B cell chronic lymphocytic leukemia. *Blood,* **65**, 149–155

122. Wang, C. Y., Good, R. A., Ammirati, P., Dymbort, G. and Evans, R. L. (1980) Identification of a p69,71 complex expressed on human T-cells sharing determinants with B-type chronic lymphatic leukemic cells. *Journal of Experimental Medicine,* **151**, 1539–1544

123. Westbrook, C. A. and Golde, D. W. (1985) Autoimmune disease in hairy-cell leukaemia: clinical syndromes and treatment. *British Journal of Haematology,* **61**, 349–356

124. Williams, C. K. O., Essien, E. M. and Bamgboye, E. A. (1984) Trends in leukemia incidence in Ibadan, Nigeria. In *Pathogenesis of Leukemias and Lymphomas: Environmental influences,* edited by I. T. Magrath, G. T. O'Conor and B. Ramot, pp. 17–27. New York: Raven Press

125. Wilson, J. D. and Nossal, G. J. V. (1971) Identification of human T and B lymphocytes in normal peripheral blood and in chronic lymphatic leukaemia. *Lancet,* **ii**, 788–791

126. Yam, L. T. and Crosby, W. H. (1974) Early splenectomy in lymphoproliferative disorders. *Archives of Internal Medicine,* **133**, 270–274

127. Yoo, D., Pierce, L. E. and Lessin, L. S. (1983) Acquired pure red cell aplasia associated with chronic lymphocytic leukemia. *Cancer,* **51**, 844–850

128. Zarrabi, M. H., Grunwald, H. W. and Rosner, F. (1977) Chronic lymphocytic leukemia terminating in acute leukemia. *Archives of Internal Medicine,* **137**, 1059–1064

129. Ziegler-Heitbrock, H. W. L., Schlag, R., Flieger, D. and Thiel, E. (1989) Favorable response of early stage B CLL patients to treatment with IFN-α_2. *Blood,* **73**, 1426–1430

T-cell chronic lymphocytic leukaemia/T-cell lymphocytosis

Introduction

Considerable confusion has surrounded the definition of T-cell chronic lymphocytic leukaemia (T-CLL). This has originated mainly from the wide use of the term 'T-CLL' to define various T-cell lymphoproliferative disorders as one disease when in fact they have different morphological, cytochemical, immunological and clinical characteristics. In classifying these diseases at least four major subgroups should be taken into account considering the clinical and laboratory findings: T-CLL, T-prolymphocytic leukaemia (T-PLL), Sézary syndrome, as the leukaemic manifestation of cutaneous T-cell lymphoma (CTCL), and adult T-cell leukaemia/ lymphoma (ATLL). A common denominator of these T-cell leukaemias is the mature (post-thymic) phenotype of the cells, i.e. they are TdT− and CD1a−(T6−) (see Table 1.10, Chapter 1).

In the authors' view the term 'T-CLL' should encompass only cases characterized by the proliferation of mature-looking T-lymphocytes, whilst those with larger or more pleomorphic cells can be referred to the other diagnostic entities. Typical T-CLL cells are represented by lymphocytes with azurophil granules (see below) and it is of interest that an animal model for this disease is a leukaemia of large granular lymphocytes described in F344 rats[70]. Based on the morphology of the expanded population, the term 'large granular lymphocyte leukaemia' can also be used to describe T-CLL[42a, 56].

The reason for using the term 'T-cell lymphocytosis' in addition to T-CLL, implies that in a proportion of patients the neoplastic nature of the T-cell proliferation has not been proven; some authors believe that most cases are in fact non-neoplastic[2, 62].

Some cases reported in earlier series do not appear to fulfil this morphological definition of T-CLL as they also included patients with T-PLL and ATLL as well as T-cell lymphomas in leukaemic phase[9, 54, 59, 68]. The first series of T-CLL reported by Brouet et al. in 1975[12] included nine cases with the morphological criteria used in this chapter, and two in which the cells were described as prolymphocytes and the clinical features clearly identified them as having T-PLL.

The different forms of chronic T-cell leukaemia other than T-CLL will be described in Chapters 5, 8 and 9.

Clinical and laboratory features

Immunological markers carried out in 1000 samples from patients with a diagnosis of CLL studied at the MRC Leukaemia Unit showed that only 20 cases (2%) had T-cell markers. This series did not include cases diagnosed as PLL, ATLL or CTCL.

The age distribution of T-CLL patients is wide ranging from the paediatric to the older age group; the mean age at presentation is 50 years. This feature distinguishes this disorder from B-CLL, which is seen more frequently in older people and only rarely occurs below the age of 40 years.

Symptoms at presentation may be variable and include fatigue, weight loss and infections; often the disease is discovered only through routine blood counts in patients who are otherwise asymptomatic. The main clinical and laboratory features of T-CLL are shown in Table 4.1. Splenomegaly is the most frequent

Table 4.1 Clinical and laboratory features of T-CLL

Features	Incidence[a] (%)
Splenomegaly	80
Hepatomegaly	30
Skin rash	25
Lymphadenopathy	10
Neutropenia	80
Anaemia	50
Thrombocytopenia	30
WBC count ($\times\ 10^9$/l)[b]	
<10	55
10–20	30
>20	15

[a] Based on cases diagnosed with the criteria described in this chapter [12, 44, 50].
[b] 70–95% of the cells are large granular lymphocytes (LGLs) with azurophil granules; a persistent T-lymphocytosis, with LGLs of $\geqslant 5 \times 10^9$/l for at least 3 months without obvious cause, is a good criterion to consider a diagnosis of T-CLL, and is helpful to exclude secondary or reactive causes.

finding on physical examination; in the majority of patients, however, the spleen is only moderately enlarged. Significant hepatic enlargement occurs only in a minority, and lymphadenopathy is even more rare. Skin lesions may be present in 25% of patients. These consist of non-specific erythematous rashes which only occasionally are papular. If biopsied they show lymphocytic infiltration in the deep dermis[12].

The blood picture described in the literature reflects the heterogeneity of cases reported as T-CLL. However, when the assessment is confined to patients who fulfil the criteria used here the white blood cell (WBC) count shows only a moderate increase (Table 4.1). In most cases the WBC count is below 20×10^9/l; rare cases with high WBC counts has been reported[61].

One of the striking laboratory features of T-CLL is the presence of cytopenia which is, as a rule, unrelated to the degree of bone marrow infiltration. The cytopenia usually affects only one of the three bone marrow lineages; rarely, bicytopenia or pancytopenia is seen. Neutropenia is the most frequent finding, whilst both thrombocytopenia and anaemia, the latter resulting from red cell hypoplasia, may also occur. It is likely that the haematological manifestations seen in T-CLL result from a specific inhibitory effect of the proliferating T-lymphocytes rather than from a significant degree of bone marrow involvement by these cells. The findings also point to the proliferation of a T-cell subset with a specific functional capability. Similarly, the predominance of suppressor T-cells may result in the progressive hypogammaglobulinaemia seen in some patients[49, 67]; more commonly polyclonal hypergammaglobulinaemia accompanies T-CLL[12, 50].

It is of interest that a proportion of cases (about 20%) has been shown to have serological evidence of rheumatoid arthritis. When analysed in a series of 21 patients, 7 were found to have a past history and laboratory findings consistent with rheumatoid arthritis[50]. The reason for this association is not clear, but it is possible that rheumatoid arthritis, which affects the T-cell compartment, may in some cases lead to a progressive T-lymphocyte derangement and, ultimately, to a lymphoproliferative disorder.

Diagnostic criteria

Morphology

Although the recognition of T-CLL has only been possible since the advent of immunological markers, it is apparent nevertheless that this disease has typical morphological features that can help distinguish it from other T-cell leukaemias and from B-CLL. An alert observer may suspect the diagnosis of T-CLL from the examination of blood films stained with May–Grünwald–Giemsa. Typical T-CLL lymphocytes are mature looking with relatively abundant cytoplasm, a low nuclear cytoplasmic ratio and prominent azurophilic granules (Figure 4.1). In most cases the nuclear outline is round or indented. They resemble the so-called large granular lymphocytes (LGLs) and justify the designation of LGL-leukaemia[42a, 44].

Electron microscopy (Figure 4.2) confirms the maturity and slight irregularity of the nucleus and the relatively abundant cytoplasm[18]. The nuclear chromatin is

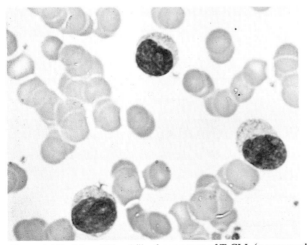

Figure 4.1 Peripheral blood film from a case of T-CLL (common phenotype). The lymphocytes have a slightly eccentric nucleus and a moderately abundant cytoplasm with fine azurophil granules. × 1200, reduced to 60% on reproduction

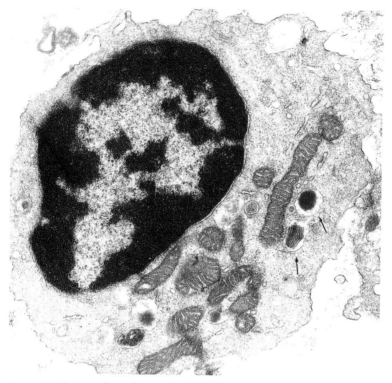

Figure 4.2 Electron photomicrograph of a T-CLL lymphocyte showing abundant cytoplasm with long mitochondria, several parallel tubular arrays (arrows) and membrane-bound electron dense granules. × 10 000, reduced to 74% on reproduction

well condensed and a small nucleolus may be found in a proportion of cells. Scattered electron-dense granules 0.1–0.7 μm in diameter are usually visible in the cytoplasm. Structures defined as parallel tubular arrays (PTAs) which consist of bundles of microtubules (Figure 4.2) are seen in most cases[18]. The function of these PTAs, which have been described in several other conditions, including rheumatoid arthritis[35], sarcoidosis[5], infectious mononucleosis[47], as well as in a minority of normal lymphocytes[14], is uncertain. A study of normal T-lymphocytes with the immunogold method has shown that PTAs are found in cells which are CD8+(T8+) and/or CD11b+(OKM1+) and correspond to Tγ− lymphocytes[44a].

Bone marrow

The bone marrow of these patients is always less heavily infiltrated than in B-CLL. The degree of infiltration is often moderate, ranging from 30% to 50% of lymphocytes; in some cases the proportion of bone marrow lymphocytes may be near normal[12]. The morphology of the bone marrow lymphocytes resembles that of the circulating T-cells. Bone marrow trephine biopsies show moderately diffuse or nodular infiltration.

Cytochemistry

The content of acid hydrolases in the cytoplasm of these cells is usually high. The acid phosphatase reaction is strongly positive and ultrastructural cytochemistry has shown that this enzyme is localized in the cytoplasmic granules and in the PTAs[18, 45]. β-Glucuronidase and β-glucosaminidase are also positive. In contrast, the α-naphthylacetate esterase (ANAE) reaction is often weak or negative[19]. Another enzyme, dipeptidylaminopeptidase IV (DAP IV), which has a more restricted distribution than the other acid hydrolases reacting mainly with CD4+(T4+) (helper) T-lymphocytes[23], also tends to be negative or is only weakly positive in the common type of T-CLL with a CD8+(T8+) membrane phenotype[20].

The cytochemistry of T-CLL is discussed further in the context of the other T-cell leukaemias in Chapter 5.

Membrane markers

All cases of T-CLL so far reported express a mature post-thymic phenotype (see Chapter 1). Prior to the advent of monoclonal antibodies the T-cell origin of the proliferating cells was demonstrated by the capacity to form E-rosettes and the mature origin of the circulating cells by the absence of terminal deoxynucleotidyl transferase (TdT) activity. In the majority of cases the cells express the receptor for the Fc portion of IgG (Tγ-cells)[8, 16, 47]; only one series[12] reported Fcμ receptors in a minority of T-CLL patients.

The use of monoclonal antibodies in the characterization of T-CLL cases can help to identify 'clones' of cells which express similar, and sometimes rare, phenotypes (Table 4.2). In reactive cases[62] or in postsplenectomy subjects[50] there appears to be a 'polyclonal' expansion of T-lymphocytes (i.e. of different subsets), sometimes including large granular cells.

Table 4.2 Phenotypic expression of T-CLL lymphocytes (all CD2+, CD1a−, TdT−)

Phenotype	No. of cases	Reactivity with monoclonal antibodies						References
		CD3	CD4	CD8	CD11b	CD57	CD16[b]	
Common	38	+	−	+	−	+/−	−	[2, 16, 17, 33, 42a, 44, 50, 53, 54, 60, 63, 67][a]
Uncommon and/or unusual	4	+	−	+	+	−	(+)	[31, 61][a]
	3	−	−	−	+	−		[60, 66][a]
	2	−	−	−	−		+	[55]
	1	+	−	−	−		+	[36]
	4[c]	+	+	−	−			[54]
	1	+	+	−	−	+	−	a
	1	+	+	−	+	−	+	[48]
	2	+	+	+	−	+		[27][a]
	1	+	+	+	+	+	−	a
	2	+	−	−	−		−	a

[a] Cases observed by the authors.
[b] The monoclonal antibody Leu11 (CD16) has not been tested in many of the cases reported early on; (+) indicated that it was positive in two cases studied by the authors.
[c] Three of these cases may correspond to T-PLL.

All cases referred to in Table 4.2 appear to represent the expansion of a single population of cells. In the great majority the cells are T-lymphocytes which are E-rosette+, CD3+(T3+), CD1a−(T6−), and CD2+(T11+). In the majority of T-CLLs the cells express the T8(CD8) antigen (common phenotype) (Table 4.2), whilst the T4 (CD4) antigen is either absent or present only on a minority or cells[44]. These cases may or may not express the Leu7(CD57) antigen[1]. OKM1 (CD11b) is expressed only on very few CD8+ T-CLLs and therefore CD8+, CD11b+ cases (Table 4.2) may be considered as uncommon. Other reported cases which are morphologically indistinguishable from CD8+ T-CLL have a more unusual membrane phenotype (Table 4.2). The cells have been found to lack the CD3, CD4 and CD8 antigens[42a] despite the high percentage of E-rosettes or CD2+ cells and to have a variable expression of the CD11b antigen. A variant of this CD4− and CD8− group was described as CD3+ and Leu7+[36]. Finally, in a group of patients the large granular cells express the CD4 antigen with or without the expression of CD8, CD11b and CD57 (Table 4.2).

Surprisingly, other monoclonal antibodies which react against T-lymphocyte antigens such as T1 (CD5), which is characteristically positive in B-CLL (see Chapter 3), and 3A1 (CD7) are negative in most cases of T-CLL; in other cases the reactivity may be weak. At present it is still uncertain whether this unexpected finding relates to an aberrant antigenic expression of a pathological cell or rather to the expansion of a T-cell subset also present in normal peripheral blood as suggested by Callard et al.[15]. On the other hand another anti-T monoclonal antibody, OKT17, is positive in all T-CLL cases[46]. In a few cases HLA-DR+ T-cells may also be found[16, 65]. The monoclonal antibody anti-Tac (CD25), which reacts with the receptor for interleukin-2 (IL-2) and which is expressed on activated T-cells, is negative in T-CLL cells even after mitogenic stimulation.

T-CLL, as described here, represents a good model to study the phenotypic expression of large granular lymphocytes in humans, particularly in view of the important role that these cells play in the host reactions to infection and tumour formation[30]. It is likely, therefore, that cases of T-CLL will help to recognize the existence of hitherto unrecognized T-cell subsets because they probably represent monoclonal expansions of both common and rare populations or T-cells. The frequency of the common and rare phenotypes in T-CLL reflects well the relative frequency of the equivalent T-cell subsets as represented in normal peripheral blood.

Differential diagnosis

On the basis of clinical, morphological, cytochemical and immunological features the recognition of T-CLL and its differential diagnosis from other related conditions have become easier. The distinction between T-CLL and B-CLL, which could be suspected on morphological grounds by the appearance of the lymphocytes on slides well stained with May–Grünwald–Giemsa and on clinical features by the absence of lymphadenopathy in most T-CLL cases, can be established by cytochemical reactions and surface marker analysis.

When a T-cell proliferation has been documented, the differential diagnosis between T-CLL and the other T-cell disorders should be considered. As illustrated in Table 4.3 each type of chronic T-cell leukaemia shows distinct clinical and laboratory features. If the definition of T-CLL is confined to cases with a

Table 4.3 Summary of clinical and laboratory features of the chronic T-cell leukaemias

Disease	Cell morphology	Cytochemistry	Phenotype[a]	WBC count ($\times 10^9$/l)	Clinical course
T-CLL	Lymphocytes with abundant cytoplasm, azurophil granules and no visible nucleolus	AP++ ANAE−	CD8+ CD4− CD8+	Low(<20)	Benign, slowly progressive Aggressive in some cases
T-PLL	Cells with basophilic cytoplasm and prominent nucleolus	AP++ ANAE+++	CD4+ CD8−	High(>100)	Progressive, often rapidly
CTCL	Cerebriform nucleus (small and large Sézary cells)	AP++ ANAE++	CD4+ CD8−	Low (about 20)	Usually progressive
ATLL	Variable size, irregular, often multilobed nucleus	AP++ ANAE++	CD4+ CD8−	Intermediate (about 40)	Progressive, rapidly fatal

[a] Findings in the majority of cases with respect to the two major lymphocyte subsets: CD4 and CD8. All cases have a mature T-cell membrane phenotype: CD1a−, TdT−; most cases are E+/CD2+, CD3+, CD7− (except T-PLL); most ATLLs are CD25+.

AP: acid phosphatase; ANAE: α-naphthylacetate esterase.

moderately raised WBC count ($\geq 5 \times 10^9$/l) and the presence of large granular lymphocytes, mature looking with azurophil granules in the cytoplasm, the diagnosis of this disorder should not be difficult. Furthermore, the cells of all types of chronic T-cell leukaemia other than common T-CLL consistently display the T4 (CD4) antigen with only the rare expression of T8 (CD8) in T-PLL (Table 4.3).

T-PLL can be distinguished from T-CLL by its characteristic high WBC count, marked splenomegaly and aggressive clinical course. Furthermore, the neoplastic cells clearly differ from those of T-CLL by their basophilic cytoplasm without azurophil granules and by the presence of a prominent nucleolus. A few localized electron-dense granules may be seen by electron microscope analysis. The cells in the majority of T-PLL are CD4+, CD8−, whilst CD4−, CD8+ and CD4+, CD8+ cases are less common (see Chapter 5). T-PLL cells show as a rule a very strong positivity with the cytochemical reactions for all acid hydrolases; this contrasts with the pattern in T-CLL cells in which the ANAE reaction is generally negative or weak (see Table 5.5, Chapter 5).

A few T-PLL cases in which the cells are CD4+ and appear to be more mature than typical prolymphocytes, showing some degree of nuclear chromatin condensation and a small nucleolus but no azurophil granules in the cytoplasm, have sometimes a lower WBC count and a less aggressive clinical course than typical T-PLL[39]. These rare cases, which may represent a variant form of T-PLL, could have been considered as T-CLL in some reports.

Cases of CTCL can be distinguished on morphological grounds particularly by electron microscopic examination where the cells reveal the characteristic cerebriform aspect of the nucleus. Skin lesions, usually erythroderma due to infiltration by CD4+ lymphocytes with typical epidermotropism, are the rule. As in the skin, the pathological cells in the blood display the phenotypic and functional features of CD4+ lymphocytes (see Chapter 9).

ATLL represents a more recently identified condition frequent in some areas of

Japan and the Caribbean (see Chapter 8). This disorder is clearly different from T-CLL because of its relatively high WBC count and aggressive clinical course. Furthermore, unlike T-CLL the morphology of ATLL cells is pleomorphic ranging in size from small lymphocytes to large blast cells. The nucleus is characteristically irregular, polylobed and often markedly convoluted. The membrane phenotype is usually CD4+, but the cells display suppressor activity in vitro (see Chapter 8).

Natural history and prognosis

Unlike other chronic T-lymphoproliferative disorders, e.g. T-PLL or ATLL, the clinical course of T-CLL is often benign. This had led some authors to question whether it is in fact a true malignant disorder or rather a reactive proliferation of a given lymphocyte subset (see below). A survey of the literature shows that, even within typical T-CLL, the clinical course may be heterogeneous. Thus, together with cases with a benign, asymptomatic disease which may not require any form of treatment for many years, some others have a progressive illness with a frank leukaemic evolution. Most often the disease remains static without significant clinical and haematological changes for many years. In these cases a slowly progressive increase in the size of the spleen, which may be impalpable or only mildly enlarged at diagnosis, is often observed after some years, sometimes accompanied by a moderate rise in the lymphocyte count. Repeated bone marrow aspirates also reveal a progressive lymphocyte infiltration in these cases (Figure 4.3).

Some patients are asymptomatic except for complaints related to infections with no skin involvement or lymph node enlargement. In others a more aggressive clinical picture is observed. These patients tend to have more pronounced

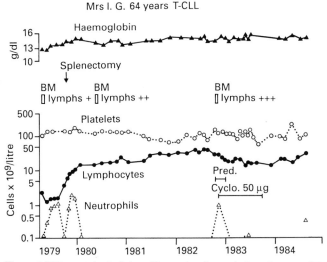

Figure 4.3 Haematological chart illustrating the evolution of a case of T-CLL (CD8+) with marked neutropenia. The graph illustrates the rise in lymphocyte count and progressive bone marrow (BM) infiltration following splenectomy and the reduction in the lymphocyte count with cyclophosphamide which did not correct the neutropenia

splenomegaly, skin rashes, liver function abnormalities and often show progressive cytopenias. This particular evolution of T-CLL may be seen from diagnosis or, very rarely, as a terminal event with a Richter-type of transformation[13, 51]. Some of these patients may respond successfully to chemotherapy and achieve prolonged remissions. Others, however, do not respond and progress to frank leukaemia with a rapidly fatal outcome. The latter course characterized by systemic symptoms and marked organ infiltration is more frequent in young patients. Rare patients may present with a clinicohaematological picture of overt leukaemia[61].

At the present time it is not clear whether patients with a more aggressive disease are part of the same spectrum as the more benign cases or whether they represent distinct clinical entities. Some of the differences in the clinical evolution correlate with the various membrane phenotypes expressed by the T-CLL cells (see Table 4.2). There is some evidence to suggest that the common form of T-CLL (CD3+, CD8+, CD11b−) is more benign, whilst a more aggressive disease has been associated with some of the uncommon phenotypes[44, 61]. This was the case ein three patients treated by one of the authors (DC), one with CD4+, CD11b+, CD16+ cells and two with CD8+, CD11b+ cells, the latter being similar to the case reported by Schlimok et al.[61]. It is also possible that the different clinical pictures may reflect the timing of the diagnosis and that the benign cases with low WBC count and very slowly progressive disease may have been diagnosed earlier. In this respect it should be recalled that the latter evolution is not rare in B-CLL where some stage 0 patients have a mild disease with low lymphocyte counts and often do not require treatment for long periods[28]. In the series of 21 T-CLL patients reported by Newland et al.[50] the median survival was 4 years but with many patients still alive and well at the time of reporting. Five patients of that series had died; two of them were from unrelated causes while the other three showed an aggressive clinical picture and had required chemotherapy.

Management

Patients fulfilling the diagnostic criteria for T-CLL should not necessarily be treated at presentation and should instead be observed for some time to assess the rate of progression of the disease. This rule does not apply to cases with a frank leukaemic picture. The main reason for an expectant approach is the possibility that some patients may not have a true malignancy and that, in these circumstances, chemotherapy may be harmful.

In patients with T-CLL treatment is indicated in two situations: (1) in an attempt to correct the cytopenia(s) and (2) to treat progressive lymphocytoses with organomegaly. Alkylating agents, chlorambucil or cyclophosphamide, alone or in combination with prednisolone have been reported to be effective in reducing the lymphocyte count[49, 50]. This is illustrated by graphs of patients treated by the authors (Figures 4.3–4.5). With regard to the cytopenias, alkylating agents may easily improve the anaemia (Figure 4.4) whilst the neutropenia is generally difficult to correct (see Figure 4.3).

More intensive chemotherapy regimens (COP–CHOP; C = cyclophosphamide, H = hydroxydaunorubicin, O = oncovin and P = prednisolone) have been used in patients who showed more aggressive clinical evolution following an initial response to single agent treatment[50] and in those with a frank leukaemic picture[53].

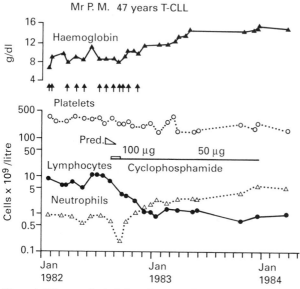

Figure 4.4 Haematological chart from a T-CLL (CD8+) patient who presented with neutropenia and anaemia and required numerous blood transfusions (arrows) through 1982. Treatment with cyclophosphamide resulted in a complete normalization of the blood counts; this improvement persisted until 1988 when he relapsed and had a splenectomy

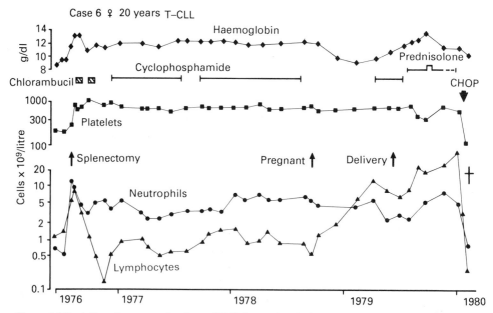

Figure 4.5 Evolution of an aggressive from of T-CLL associated with lymphocyte infiltration in the liver. Splenectomy resulted in a rising lymphocyte count that promptly fell with chlorambucil. The treatment maintained a precarious control of the disease until it was stopped during pregnancy. This was followed by a rising lymphocyte count and septic complications which eventually lead to her death

Splenectomy has often been performed in patients with T-CLL in order to reduce transfusion requirements and to correct the cytopenia. Neutropenia does not appear to be influenced by splenectomy, thus suggesting that hypersplenism is unlikely to play an important role in the pathogenesis of this complication. In most cases splenectomy is followed by marked postoperative lymphocytosis (Figures 4.3 and 4.5)[50, 53] which is often associated with increased bone marrow infiltration by lymphocytes. The peripheral blood lymphocytes in these cases maintain the morphological and phenotypic characteristics of the original cells, thus excluding a reactive lymphocytosis postsplenectomy. This has been confirmed by marker studies in subjects with a circulating T-lymphocytosis following splenectomy for non-neoplastic diseases[50]. In these cases, unlike splenectomized patients with T-CLL, the lymphocytosis is characterized by a 'polyclonal' increase of both CD4+ and CD8+ T-lymphocytes with a normal or near-normal CD4/CD8 ratio.

A new therapeutic approach has been attempted by means of the pan-T monoclonal antibody UCHT1 (CD3)[40, 41]. Although this produced a fall in the peripheral blood WBC count and a reduction in the bone marrow infiltration, the development of anti-mouse antibodies prevented further treatment.

The adenosine deaminase inhibitor, 2'-deoxycyformycin (DCF), has also been used with some success in the treatment of T-CLL and other T-cell disorders[64]. A dramatic response to this treatment was observed by the authors in a patient with an unusual phenotype – CD4+, CD11b+ (see Table 4.2). Following a short course of intravenous 2'-deoxycoformycin, the WBC count dropped from 70×10^9/l to 3×10^9/l, the abnormal liver function tests improved markedly and the enlarged spleen (6 cm) became impalpable. This complete response lasted almost 2 years. Following a relapse, this patient has responded again to DCF. Experience at the MRC Leukaemia Unit has shown that good responses with DCF are seen only in cases of T-CLL and other T-cell leukaemias with CD4+, CD8− cells, but not with other phenotypes[21a].

At the present time the best approach for the management of T-CLL patients appears to be a close clinicohaematological follow-up. This is particularly relevant in patients with a static clinical picture and no systemic symptoms. In such patients cytotoxic agents may indeed be harmful. Only cases with signs of progression or marked cytopenia will require treatment, which may initially be confined to a single alkylating agent and later to a more intensive multiple drug regimen. Splenectomy does not appear to be beneficial in the management of T-CLL, although removal of a large spleen may facilitate additional therapy. Further trials of 2'-deoxycoformycin are warranted as this agent given in low doses (i.e. $4 \, mg/m^2$ per week) is not toxic and has a marked lympholytic effect[21a].

T-cell functional studies

The functional behaviour of T-CLL lymphocytes has been extensively investigated in order to give a better definition of the properties of the proliferating cells and to correlate them with the membrane antigenic expression. As there is no complete concordance between phenotype and function (see Figure 1.5, Chapter 1) these studies may be relevant for identifying the specific T-cell subset involved in the disease. Furthermore, in the absence of other markers the demonstration of a specific function behaviour by the T-CLL cells may be taken as an indicator of clonality.

Another aspect that has been explored with studies in vitro is the possible correlation between the nature of the T-cell proliferation and the pathogenesis of the cytopenias.

Correlation between T-cell phenotype and function

As summarized in Table 4.4, the lymphocytes in the common form of T-CLL (CD3+, CD8+) often have killer (K) function with or without concomitant natural killer (NK) activity. Only in a few cases has the expression of the CD8 antigen been associated with suppressor capacity. The latter, when present, may contribute to the marked hypogammaglobulinaemia observed in some of these patients[49, 67]. It is of interest too that cells in two cases have been shown to display helper activity despite expressing the CD8 antigen (Table 4.4). The possibility that this may be

Table 4.4 T-cell lymphocyte function in T-CLL

Membrane phenotype	No. of cases	PHA TI	Helper	Suppressor	Natural killer (NK)	ADCC or killer (K)	References
CD8+, CD3+							
CD11b− { 8	8	−	−	−	−	+	[2, 17, 60]
2	2	−	−	+	−	−	[56, 67]
3	3	−/+	+	−	−	+	[63]
1	1	−	−	+	+		[53]
CD11b+ { 1	1		−	−	+	+	[61]
1	1		−	+	+		[31]
CD8−, CD11b+							
CD3− { 2	2	+			+		[55]
CD4− { 1	1	−	−	−	+	+	[60]
1	1	−	+	−	+		
CD3+ { 1	1	−	−	−	−	+	[48]
CD4+							

PHA TI: phytohaemagglutinin transformation index; ADCC: antibody-dependent cell-mediated cytotoxicity or killer (K) function.

due to residual CD4+ cells was ruled out in one study[63] by purification experiments and was highly unlikely in the other because of the very low proportion of CD4+ cells present in the sample tested[39].

As described above, a group of T-CLL with unusual membrane phenotypes has been identified (see Table 4.3); cases which lack the CD3, CD4 and CD8 antigens but express OKM1 (CD11b) and Leu11b (CD16) consistently show high NK activity (Table 4.4). These patients are characterized by the expansion of a CD2+, CD8− subset of large granular lymphocytes which lack other T-cell markers and which is also represented, albeit in a small proportion, in normal peripheral blood[7]. The functional properties of this rare subset are identical to those of the T-CLL cells with a similar phenotype. The existence in normal blood of this subset has been confirmed by the establishment of a cell line with similar functional characteristics[38]. Little information is presently available on the functional behaviour of the rare cases which express the CD4 antigen. One of them (CD4+, CD11b+, CD16+) studied by the authors had only K function[48].

Although the cells in most T-CLL cases show K and/or NK activity, the expression of the Leu7 (CD57) antigen, which has been reported to react primarily with human cytotoxic cells encompassing both NK and K functions[1], is variable and does not always correlate with the functional behaviour of the cells. It would appear that other monoclonal antibodies, such as CD16, may correlate better with NK activity than any of the other monoclonal antibodies (see Figure 1.2).

A consistent feature of T-CLL lymphocytes, regardless of the membrane phenotype, appears to be the significantly depressed response to mitogens or to recall antigens (Table 4.4) along with a decreased T-colony-forming capacity[25]. This is largely due to the reduced or absent proportion of CD4+ cells in the majority of cases.

The evaluation of the T-cell functional properties has confirmed the heterogeneity of T-CLL and shown that different T-cell functions can be found in individual patients. The continued use of phenotypic and functional analyses is therefore essential for a better characterization of this disease and also for a better understanding of the various properties of the T-cell subsets in humans. T-CLL in fact represents a good model for studying the phenotype and function of normal subsets, which may be present only in very small numbers in the peripheral blood and are thus difficult to recognize and analyse.

Release of soluble factors

γ-Interferon and IL-2 are released by normal T-lymphocytes upon mitogenic stimulation. This function is not confined to a given T-cell subset as both CD4+ and CD8+ cells can release these two lymphokines[37]. In T-CLL the capacity to produce soluble factors following different stimuli has been investigated in a few cases. Two reports have shown that in T-CLL, unlike normal peripheral blood, a spontaneous release of interferon may occur[34, 36]. In two cases studied by one of the authors (RF, unpublished data) no spontaneous release of γ-interferon or of IL-2 was observed but both lymphokines were detected in the cell supernatants after mitogenic stimulation. One case had the common membrane phenotype CD2+, CD3+, CD8+ and the other had a rare one CD2+, CD3−, CD4−, CD8−. Release of IL-2 following mitogens has also been reported in T-CLL by Friedman et al.[26]. These findings suggest that despite phenotypic and functional dissimilarities the release of soluble factors by T-CLL may be preserved.

Role of T-cells in the pathogenesis of cytopenias

Several studies have been carried out to ascertain whether the neutropenia and/or the anaemia (often resulting from pure red cell aplasia) could be mediated via the abnormally expanded T-cell population.

The capacity of bone marrow cells from T-CLL patients with neutropenia to give rise to myeloid colonies has been described as normal in some cases[16] and reduced in others[11]. Although it has been observed that in some of these patients bone marrow T-cells may induce suppression of myeloid colony growth[4, 22], it is uncertain whether the T-cell population of T-CLL is directly involved in the pathogenesis of the neutropenia. Removal of the T-cells does not induce enhancement of myeloid colony formation; these cells also do not suppress the growth of allogeneic bone marrow cells unless they are stimulated by mitogen[16]. The existence of a population of T-cells that suppress myelopoiesis following mitogenic activation has been described in studies with normal peripheral blood[3]. Furthermore, two reports have suggested that some leukaemic T-cell lines may produce factors capable of suppressing the in vitro growth of myeloid precursors[6, 69]. The authors have shown that conditioned medium derived from CD3+, CD4−, CD8+ cells from a T-CLL patient was markedly inhibitory to the in vitro growth of allogeneic myeloid precursors (RF, unpublished data).

With regards to the erythroid stem cell compartment there is good evidence that in T-CLL cases with pure red cell aplasia or with severe anaemia removal of bone marrow T-cells can enhance significantly BFU-E colony growth and also that the patient's T-cells are capable of suppressing allogeneic erythroid colony growth[32, 42, 49].

The possibility that the abnormal cell proliferation in T-CLL patients may be involved in the pathogenesis of the neutropenia, anaemia and/or hypogamma-globulinaemia (see above) awaits further studies particularly in view of the physiological role that large granular lymphocytes play in the growth regulation of the myeloid and erythroid compartments[29, 43, 57].

Cytogenetic studies

Whilst in other chronic T-cell leukaemias, such as T-PLL and ATLL, clonal chromosome abnormalities can always be demonstrated (see Chapters 5 and 8), the cytogenetic data in T-CLL have so far been more difficult to obtain. This has been largely due to the poor response of T-CLL cells to the mitogen phytohaemaggluti-nin (PHA) resulting in an inadequate number of mitotic figures. There is little published evidence of karyotypic abnormalities in CD8+ proliferations. For example trisomy 22[63] was described in an unusual case in which the CD8+ T-cells showed helper activity in vitro. Earlier cytogenetic studies were performed prior to the advent of monoclonal antibodies and thus without an adequate definition of the lymphoproliferative process[10, 52]. Two studies in CD8+ T-CLL cases have shown either non-consistent chromosome abnormalities or normal karyotypes[21, 58]. The structural clonal abnormalities found by Dallapiccola et al.[21] in two CD4+ cases with an aggressive clinical picture and a relatively high WBC count may in fact refer to T-PLL cases.

In a report by Zech et al.[71] four of five cases showed a consistent chromosome change in the form of an inversion of the long arm of chromosome 14 [inv(14)(q11;q32)] and trisomy 8 in three of five patients. Unfortunately, no haematological or immunological data on the nature of the cells were given in that study; the only case with an apparently normal karyotype had a relatively benign disease. The authors have recently demonstrated an inverted 14q and trisomy for 8q as characteristic abnormalities of T-PLL (see Chapter 5). The possibility that clonal cytogenetic changes may also occur in patients with typical CD8+ T-CLL with slowly progressive disease has recently been documented in several cases which showed, after 5 days' culture in the presence of PHA and IL-2, structural abnormalities, namely: t(11;15) (q13;q22–24), t(1;5) (q12;q35), t(4;17) (p15–16; q23), and int.del(14) (q22–24)[9a]. It is of interest that the latter abnormality was observed in the case described in Figure 4.3. These observations suggest that karyotypic analyses under adequate culture conditions may help to distinguish the clonal and thus possibly leukaemic conditions from the reactive processes. They also suggest that there are no characteristic chromosome abnormalities unique to T-CLL.

Reactive or neoplastic nature of the T-cell proliferation

The question of whether many cases classified as T-CLL have in fact a true clonal lymphoproliferative disease is now largely resolved[9a, 25a, 25b, 42a]. The clinical course of this disorder is rather heterogeneous because it includes patients with a progressive disease or frank leukaemic picture and others in whom the disease remains static with little evidence of progression. The nature of some of these cases remains uncertain and in this respect many different designations other than T-CLL have been suggested: chronic T-cell lymphocytosis[2], Tγ-cell proliferation[8] or abnormal expansion of large granular lymphocytes[56]. Until clear evidence of malignancy is demonstrated, it is probably also correct to designate some cases as chronic T-cell lymphocytosis.

However, it is becoming apparent that in most cases which fulfil the criteria for T-CLL, there is clear evidence of a monoclonal T-cell proliferation as shown by the rearrangement of the T-cell receptor (TCR) β- and/or γ-chain genes[25a, 25b, 42a]. For details and other references see Chapter 8. All the cases studied by the authors with uncommon and unusual phenotypes and the majority, but not all, with the common membrane phenotype (CD3+, CD8+) were shown to be monoclonal proliferations by DNA analysis. The past difficulties in defining the neoplastic origin of the non-progressive cases were mainly due to the absence of good markers for T-cell clonality. For example, one study suggested[62] that some patients have a reactive lymphocytosis rather than a lymphoproliferative disorder on the stability of the clinicohaematological picture, on the morphological and immunological heterogeneity of the expanded lymphocyte population, which was nevertheless consistent within individual patients, and on positive serology for chronic infections [Epstein–Barr virus titres, HBsAg (hepatitis B surface antigen) and/or the Widal reaction]. A T-cell lymphocytosis has also been reported in patients with solid tumours[24, 47].

The evidence, in addition to DNA analysis, in favour of the neoplastic nature of most T-CLL cases, not just of those presenting with a clearly leukaemic picture, is based on the presence of a persistent lymphocytosis which often is slowly but consistently progressive and includes the gradual enlargement of the spleen and the progressive infiltration of the bone marrow. Spontaneous regressions are extremely rare[17]. A further indication of the clonal origin of this process comes from surface marker analysis which shows a clear predominance of a single T-cell subset usually with a specific function. The evidence of clonal chromosome abnormalities, well documented in some cases[9a] and discussed above, supports the concept that this is a neoplastic disorder. An objective way to resolve this question is the use of the recently cloned probes for the β-, γ- and δ-chains of the human TCR. Data from several laboratories (see Chapter 8) support the view that T-CLL cells show a monoclonal rearrangement of the genes for the different chains of the T-cell receptor. If studied consistently in all cases of T-CLL these techniques with molecular probes may be invaluable to demonstrate the neoplastic or clonal nature of some cases or, by the same token, to recognize those cases with T-cell lymphocytosis resulting from reactive causes, as evidenced by a polyclonal configuration of the TCR genes[39].

In most T-CLLs both the TCR β- and γ-genes are clonally rearranged. However, rare cases may show a germ-line configuration of the TCR β-gene. This was the case in the CD3+, CD8+ T-CLL whose clinical course is shown in Figure 4.3. The granular lymphocytes of this case were germ-line for β and rearranged for γ and δ[25b]. It is likely that the leukaemia has arisen in this case from a rare normal T-cell bearing a γ/δ TCR rather than an α/β heterodimeric molecule. This observation is important because other patients with T-CLL have been reported with TCR β-genes in germ-line configuration. On the other hand, clonal proliferations of rare CD3− T-CLL cases (see Table 4.2), which may correspond to NK cells, will not show evidence for rearrangement or expression of TCR α-, β- or γ-chain genes[42a]. It is essential that analysis at DNA level of the TCR γ- and δ-genes should be carried out before concluding that the disease is non-clonal.

References

1. Abo, T. and Balch, C. M. (1981) A differentiation antigen of human NK and K cells identified by a monoclonal antibody (HNK-1). *Journal of Immunology,* **127**, 1024–1029
2. Aisenberg, A. C., Wilkes, B. M., Harris, N. L., Ault, K. A. and Carey, R. W. (1981) Chronic T-cell lymphocytosis with neutropenia: report of a case studied with monoclonal antibody. *Blood,* **58**, 818–822
3. Bacigalupo, A., Podesta, M., Mingari, M. C. et al. (1981) Generation of CFU-C/suppressor T cells in vitro: an experimental model for immune-mediated marrow failure. *Blood,* **57**, 491–496.
4. Bagby, G. C. Jr (1981) T lymphocytes involved in inhibition of granulopoiesis in two neutropenic patients are of the cytotoxic/suppressor (T3+ T8+) subset. *Journal of Clinical Investigation,* **68**, 1597–1600
5. Belcher, R. W., Czarnetzki, B. M. and Campbell, P. B. (1975) Ultrastructure of inclusions in peripheral blood mononuclear cells in sarcoidosis. *American Journal of Pathology,* **78**, 461–466
6. Bellone, G., Giovinazzo, B., Garbarino, G. et al. (1984) Suppression of myelopoiesis by a human leukemia T-cell line (PF-382). In *New Trends in Experimental Hematology,* edited by C. Peschle and C. Rizzoli, pp. 110–113. Ares Serono Symposia
7. Beverley, P. C. L. and Callard, R. E. (1981) Distinctive functional characteristics of human 'T' lymphocytes defined by E rosetting or a monoclonal anti-T cell antibody. *European Journal of Immunology,* **11**, 329–334
8. Bom-van Noorloos, A. A., Pegels, H. G., van Oers, R. H. J. et al. (1980) Proliferation of Tγ cells with killer-cell activity in two patients with neutropenia and recurrent infections. *New England Journal of Medicine,* **302**, 933–937
9. Boumsell, L., Bernard, A., Reinherz, E. L. et al. (1981) Surface antigens on malignant Sézary and T-CLL cells correspond to those of mature T cells. *Blood,* **57**, 526–530
9a. Brito-Babapulle, V., Matutes, E., Parreira, L. and Catovsky, D. (1986) Abnormalities of chromosome 7q and Tac expression in T cell leukemias. *Blood,* **67**, 516–521
10. Brody, J. I., Burningham, R. A., Nowell, P. C., Rowlands, D. T., Freiburg, P. and Daniele, R. P. (1975) Persistent lymphocytosis with chromosomal evidence of malignancy. *American Journal of Medicine,* **58**, 547–552
11. Brouet, J. C. (1980) Proliferation of Tγ cells with killer-cell activity in patients with neutropenia. *New England Journal of Medicine,* **303**, 882
12. Brouet, J. C., Flandrin, G., Sasportes, M., Preud'homme, J. L. and Seligmann, M. (1975) Chronic lymphocytic leukaemia of T-cell origin. Immunological and clinical evaluation in eleven patients. *Lancet,* **ii**, 890–893
13. Brouet, J-C. and Seligmann, M. (1981) T-derived chronic lymphocytic leukemia. *Pathology Research and Practice,* **171**, 262–267
14. Brunning, R. D. and Parkin, J. (1975) Ultrastructural studies of parallel tubular arrays in human lymphocytes. *American Journal of Pathology,* **78**, 59–64

15. Callard, R. E., Smith, C. M., Worman, C., Linch, D., Cawley, J. C. and Beverley, P. C. L. (1981) Unusual phenotype and function of an expanded subpopulation of T cells in patients with haemopoietic disorders. *Clinical Experimental Immunology,* **43**, 497–505

16. Catovsky, D., Linch, D. C. and Beverley, P. C. L. (1982) T cell disorders in haematological diseases. *Clinics in Haematology,* **11**, 661–695

17. Chan, W. C., Check, I., Schick, C., Brynes, R. K., Kateley, J. and Winton, E. F. (1984) A morphologic and immunologic study of the large granular lymphocyte in neutropenia with T lymphocytosis. *Blood,* **63**, 1133–1140

18. Costello, C., Catovsky, D., O'Brien, M., Morilla, R. and Varadi, S. (1980) Chronic T-cell leukemias. I. Morphology, cytochemistry and ultrastructure. *Leukemia Research,* **4**, 463–476

19. Crockard, A., Chalmers, D., Matutes, E. and Catovsky, D. (1982) Cytochemistry of acid hydrolases in chronic B- and T-cell leukemias. *American Journal of Clinical Pathology,* **78**, 437–444

20. Crockard, A. D., Macfarlane, E., Andrews, C., Bridges, J. M. and Catovsky, D. (1984) Dipeptidylaminopeptidase IV activity in normal and leukemic T cell subpopulations. *American Journal of Clinical Pathology,* **82**, 294–299

21. Dallapiccola, B., Alimena, G., Chessa, L. et al. (1984) Chromosome studies in patients with T-CLL chronic lymphocytic leukemia and expansions of granular lymphocytes. *International Journal of Cancer,* **34**, 171–176

21a. Dearden, C., Matutes, E., Brozovic, N. et al. (1987) Response to deoxycoformycin in mature T cell malignancies relates to membrane phenotype. *British Medical Journal,* **295**, 873–875

22. Delforge, A., Bron, D. and Stryckmans, P. (1981) Neutropenia associated with excess of T cell lymphocytes. *British Journal of Haematology,* **49**, 488–489

23. Feller, A. C., Heijnen, C. J., Ballieux, R. E. and Parwaresch, M. R. (1982) Enzyme histochemical staining of Tμ lymphocytes for glycylproline-4-methoxy-beta-naphthylamide-peptidase (DAP IV). *British Journal of Haematology,* **51**, 227–234

24. Ferrarini, M., Romagnani, S., Montesoro, E. et al. (1983) A lymphoproliferative disorder of the large granular lymphocytes with natural killer activity. *Journal of Clinical Immunology,* **3**, 30–41

25. Foa, R., Catovsky, D., Incarbone, E. et al. (1982) Chronic T-cell leukaemias. III. T-colonies, PHA response and correlation with membrane phenotype. *Leukemia Research,* **6**, 809–814

25a. Foa, R., Pelicci, P. G., Migone, N. et al. (1986) Analysis of T-cell receptor beta chain (Tβ) gene rearrangements demonstrates the monoclonal nature of T-cell chronic lymphoproliferative disorders. *Blood,* **67**, 247–250

25b. Foroni, L., Matutes, E., Foldi, J. et al. (1988) T-cell leukemias with rearrangement of the γ but not β T-cell receptor genes. *Blood,* **71**, 356–362

26. Friedman, S. M., Thompson, G., Halper, J. P. and Knowles, D. M. (1982) OT-CLL: a human T cell chronic lymphocytic leukemia that produces IL 2 in high titer. *Journal of Immunology,* **128**, 935–940

27. Gallart, T., Anegon, I., Woessner, S. et al. (1983) Clinically benign adult T-cell chronic lymphocytosis with unusual phenotype. *Lancet,* **i**, 769–770

28. Han, R., Ozer, H., Gaigan, M. et al. (1984) Benign monoclonal B cell lymphocytosis. A benign variant of CLL: clinical, immunologic, phenotypic, and cytogenetic studies in 20 patients. *Blood,* **64**, 244–252

29. Hansson, M., Beran, M., Andersson, B. and Kiessling, R. (1982) Inhibition of in vitro granulopoiesis by autologous allogeneic human NK cells. *Journal of Immunology,* **129**, 126–132

30. Herberman, R. B. and Ortaldo, J. R. (1981) Natural killer cells: their role in defenses against disease. *Science,* **214**, 24–30

31. Herrmann, F., Sieber, G., Enders, B., Bochert, G., Reim, J. and Ruehl, H. (1982) Chronic lymphocytic leukaemia of T-G cell type with NK and suppressor activity clinically presented as hypogammaglobulinaemia. Functional and surface markers characteristics of the proliferating cell clone. *Immunobiology,* **162**, 363–364

32. Hoffman, R., Kopel, S., Hsu, S. D., Dainiak, N. and Zanjani, E. D. (1978) T cell chronic lymphocytic leukaemia: Presence in bone marrow and peripheral blood of cells that suppress erythropoiesis in vitro. *Blood,* **52**, 255–260

33. Hofman, F. M., Smith, D. and Hocking, W. (1982) T cell chronic lymphocytic leukaemia with suppressor phenotype. *Clinical and Experimental Immunology,* **49**, 401–409

34. Hooks, J. J., Haynes, B. F., Detrick-Hooks, B., Diehl, L. F., Gerrard, T. L. and Fauci, A. S. (1982) Gamma (immune) interferon production by leukocytes from a patient with a T_G cell proliferative disease. *Blood*, **59**, 198–201

35. Hovig, T., Jeremic, M. and Stavem, P. (1968) A new type of inclusion bodies in lymphocytes. *Scandinavian Journal of Haematology*, **5**, 81–96

36. Itoh, K., Tsuchikawa, K., Awataguchi, T., Shiiba, K. and Kumagai, K. (1983) A case of chronic lymphocytic leukemia with properties characteristic of natural killer cells. *Blood*, **61**, 940–948.

37. Kasahara, T., Hooks, J. J., Dougherty, S. F. and Oppenheim, J. J. (1983) Interleukin 2-mediated immune interferon (IFN-γ) production by human T cells and T cell subsets. *Journal of Immunology*, **130**, 1784–1789

38. Kornbluth, J., Flomenberg, N. and Dupont, B. (1982) Cell surface phenotype of a cloned line of human natural killer cells. *Journal of Immunology*, **129**, 2831–2837

39. Lauria, F., Foa, R. and Giubellino, M. C. (1987) Heterogeneity of large granular lymphocyte proliferations: morphological, immunological molecular analysis in 7 patients. *British Journal of Haematology*, **66**, 187–191

40. Linch, D. C., Beverley, P. C. L., Newland, A. C. and Turnbull, A. L. (1981) Treatment of T cell proliferation with monoclonal antibody. *Lancet*, **ii**, 524

41. Linch, D. C., Beverley, P. C. L., Newland, A. C. and Turnbull, A. L. (1983) Treatment of a low grade T cell proliferation with monoclonal antibody. *Clinical and Experimental Immunology*, **51**, 133–140

42. Linch, D. C., Cawley, J. C., MacDonald, S. M. et al. (1981) Acquired pure red cell aplasia associated with an increase of T cells bearing receptors for the Fc of IgG. *Acta Haematologica*, **65**, 270–274

42a. Loughran, T. P., Starkebaum, G. and Aprile, J. A. (1988) Rearrangement and expression of T-cell receptor genes in large granular lymphocyte leukemia. *Blood*, **71**, 822–824

43. Mangan, K. F., Hartnett, M. E., Matis, S. A., Winkelstein, A. and Abo, T. (1984) Natural killer cells suppress human erythroid stem cell proliferation in vitro. *Blood*, **63**, 260–269

44. Matutes, E., Brito-Babapulle, V., Worner, I., Sainati, L., Foroni, L. and Catovsky, D. (1988) T-cell chronic lymphocytic leukaemia: the spectrum of mature T-cell disorders. *Nouvelle Revue Française d'Hematologie*, **30**, 347–351

44a. Matutes, E. and Catovsky, D. (1982) The fine structure of normal lymphocyte subpopulations – a study with monoclonal antibodies and the immunogold technique. *Clinical and Experimental Immunology*, **50**, 416–425

45. Matutes, E., Crockard, A. D., O'Brien, M. and Catovsky, D. (1983) Ultrastructural cytochemistry of chronic T-cell leukaemias. A study with four acid hydrolases. *Histochemical Journal*, **15**, 895–909

46. Matutes, E., Parreira, A., Foa, R. and Catovsky, D. (1985) Monoclonal antibody OKT17 recognises most cases of T-cell malignancy. *British Journal of Haematology*, **61**, 649–656

47. McKenna, R. W., Parkin, J., Kersey, J. H., Gajl-Peczalska, K. J., Peterson, L. and Brunning, R. D. (1977) Chronic lymphoproliferative disorder with unusual clinical, morphologic, ultrastructural and membrane surface marker characteristics. *American Journal of Medicine*, **62**, 588–596

48. Moss, V. E., Miedema, F., Matutes, E. et al. (1986) An unusual variant of T-CLL: evidence for the existence of a hitherto unrecognized T cell subset. *Clinical and Experimental Immunology*, **63**, 303–311

49. Nagasawa, T., Abe, T. and Nakagawa, T. (1981) Pure red cell aplasia and hypogammaglobulinemia associated with Tγ-cell chronic lymphocytic leukemia. *Blood*, **57**, 1025–1031

50. Newland, A. C., Catovsky, D., Linch, D. et al. (1984) Chronic T cell lymphocytosis: a review of 21 cases. *British Journal of Haematology*, **58**, 433–446

51. Nowell, P., Finan, J., Glover, D. and Guerry, D. (1981) Cytogenetic evidence for the clonal nature of Richter's syndrome. *Blood*, **58**, 183–186

52. Nowell, P., Jensen, J., Winger, L., Daniele, R. and Growney, P. (1976) T cell variant of chronic lymphocytic leukaemia with chromosome abnormality and defective responsive to mitogens. *British Journal of Haematology*, **33**, 459–468

53. Palutke, M., Eisenberg, L., Kaplan, J. et al. (1983) Natural killer and suppressor T-cell chronic lymphocytic leukemia. *Blood*, **62**, 627–634

54. Pandolfi, F., De Rossi, G., Semenzato, G. et al. (1982) Immunologic evaluation of T chronic lymphocytic leukemia cells: correlations among phenotype, functional activities, and morphology. *Blood*, **59**, 688–695

55. Pandolfi, F., Quinti, I., De Rossi, G. et al. (1982) A population of sheep rosetting cells lacking T and monocyte-specific antigens, as detected by monoclonal antibodies. *Clinical Immunology and Immunopathology*, **22**, 331–339

56. Pandolfi, F., Semenzato, G., De Rossi, G. et al. (1983) HNK-1 monoclonal antibody (Leu-7) in the identification of abnormal expansions of large granular lymphocytes. *Clinical and Experimental Immunology*, **52**, 641–647

57. Pistoia, V., Ghio, R., Nocera, A., Leprini, A., Perata, A. and Ferrarini, M. (1985) Large granular lymphocytes have a promoting activity on human peripheral blood erythroid burst-forming units. *Blood*, **65**, 464–472

58. Pittman, S., Morilla, R. and Catovsky, D. (1982) Chronic T cell leukemias. II Cytogenetic studies. *Leukemia Research*, **6**, 33–42

59. Reinherz, E. L., Nadler, L. M., Rosenthal, D. S., Moloney, W. C. and Schlossman, S. F. (1979) T-cell-subset characterization of human T-CLL. *Blood*, **53**, 1066–1075

60. Rümke, H. C., Miedema, F., Ten Berge, I. J. M. et al. (1982) Functional properties of T cells in patients with chronic Tγ lymphocytosis and chronic T cell neoplasia. *Journal of Immunology*, **129**, 419–426

61. Schlimok, G., Thiel, E., Rieber, E. P. et al. (1982) Chronic leukemia with a hybrid surface phenotype (T lymphocytic/myelomonocytic): leukemic cells displaying natural killer activity and antibody-dependent cellular cytotoxicity. *Blood*, **59**, 1157–1162

62. Semenzato, G., Pizzolo, G., Ranucci, A. et al. (1984) Abnormal expansion of polyclonal large to small size granular lymphocytes: reactive or neoplastic process? *Blood*, **63**, 1271–1277

63. Siegal, F. P., Rambotti, P., Siegal, M. et al. (1982) Helper cell function of leukemic Leu-2a+, histamine receptor+, Tγ lymphocytes. *Journal of Immunology*, **129**, 1775–1781

64. Spiers, A. S. D., Ruckdeschel, J. C. and Horton, J. (1984) Effectiveness of Pentostatin (2′-deoxycoformycin) in refractory lymphoid neoplasms. *Scandinavian Journal of Haematology*, **32**, 130–134

65. Strong, D. M., Pandolfi, F., Slease, R. B., Budd, J. E. and Woody, J. N. (1981) Antigenic characterization of a T-CLL with heteroantisera and monoclonal antibodies: evidence for the T cell lineage of an Ia-positive Fc-IgG-positive, suppressor-cell population. *Journal of Immunology*, **126**, 2205–2208

66. Tagawa, S., Konishi, I., Kuratune, H. et al. (1983) A case of T-cell chronic lymphocytic leukemia (T-CLL) expressing a peculiar phenotype (E+, OKM1+, Leu1+, OKT3− and IgG EA−). *Cancer*, **52**, 1378–1384

67. Thien, S. L., Catovsky, D., Oscier, D. et al. (1982) T-chronic lymphocytic leukaemia presenting as primary hypogammaglobulinaemia – evidence of a proliferation of T-suppressor cells. *Clinical and Experimental Immunology*, **47**, 670–676

68. Toben, H. R. and Smith, R. G. (1977) T lymphocytes bearing complement receptors in a patient with chronic lymphocytic leukaemia. *Clinical and Experimental Immunology*, **27**, 292–302

69. Trucco, M., Rovera, G. and Ferrero, D. (1984) A novel human lymphokine that inhibits hematopoietic progenitor cell proliferation. *Nature*, **309**, 166–168

70. Ward, J. M. and Reynolds, C. W. (1983) Large granular lymphocyte leukemia. A heterogeneous lymphocytic leukemia in F344 rats. *American Journal of Pathology*, **111**, 1–10

71. Zech, L., Gahrton, G., Hammarstrom, L. et al. (1984) Inversion of chromosome 14 marks human T-cell chronic lymphocytic leukaemia. *Nature*, **308**, 858–860

Chapter 5

Prolymphocytic leukaemia

Introduction

Prolymphocytic leukaemia (PLL) has been recognized as a clinicomorphological entity in the last 15 years. Galton et al.[21] published a series of 15 patients who had been seen over an 18-year period with characteristics different from classic chronic lymphocytic leukaemia (CLL). PLL was initially described as a rare variant of CLL[21] but it has since become apparent that the only link with the latter is provided by patients with intermediate features, i.e. CLL with more than 10% prolymphocytes or CLL/PL[32], discussed in Chapter 3. The membrane-phenotype findings[4], spleen histology[2, 25, 28] and clinical evolution[33] suggest that PLL is a distinct disorder. More recently, the routine use of cell markers for the study of lymphoid malignancies has helped to characterize prolymphocytes of B- and T-lineage and to identify a relatively less common form of the disease: T-cell PLL[7]. In fact, except for some clinical features, namely splenomegaly and high WBC count, and the morphological appearance of the neoplastic lymphocytes, both types of PLL are distinct disorders in their own right. Furthermore, with the study of more cases of T-PLL it has become possible to distinguish subtle morphological differences between B- and T-prolymphocytes[6, 31], findings which will strengthen the concept of B-PLL and T-PLL as separate clinicopathological entities[2a].

The authors' group has now collected data on 150 patients with PLL in the UK. Within the chronic lymphoproliferative disorders the incidence of PLL is about 8%, with B-cell PLL being three times more common than T-PLL. Considering only the B-cell disorders, B-PLL is relatively uncommon (about 5% of cases). However, within the mature T-cell leukaemias, which are, overall, significantly less common than the chronic B-cell ones, T-PLL represents almost one-third of the cases[31]. In this chapter the clinical and laboratory characteristics of both types of PLL are described and the role of cytochemistry in the diagnosis of lymphoid malignancies discussed, with particular reference to the cytochemical differences between B- and T-lineage cells[14, 15].

Clinical and laboratory features

The clinical manifestations described by Galton et al.[21] are characteristic of both forms of the disease, but they refer more particularly to B-PLL. There is a slight predominance of males presenting in the seventh and eighth decades of life[4] with symptoms of short duration: tiredness, weakness, weight loss, sometimes with fever and night sweats. The main physical findings are anaemia and marked splenomegaly, usually with spleens palpated over 10 cm below the left costal margin. Lymphadenopathy is extremely rare in B-PLL but not in T-PLL. The main clinical features of both conditions are compared in Table 5.1. The clinical signs are more florid in T-PLL where, in addition to lymphadenopathy and splenomegaly, skin lesions can be observed, often as discrete nodules and rarely as diffuse erythematous lesions, as well as serous effusions (ascites or pleural effusion).

Table 5.1 Clinical and laboratory differences between two types of PLL

Feature	B-PLL	T-PLL
Relative incidence[a] (%)	75	25
Sex (M:F ratio)	1.6:1	2:1
Age (years)[b]	70 (44–85)	69 (51–90)
Splenomegaly (%)	98	82
Lymphadenopathy (%)	<5	46
Skin lesions (%)	<5	25
Ascites or pleural effusion (%)	<5	20
WBC count (>100 × 10^9/l) (%)	65	82
Hb (<10 g/dl) (%)	70	55
Platelets (<100 × 10^9/l) (%)	72	68
Serum Ig	Low	Normal
Median survival	3 years	<1 year

[a] Earlier analysis suggested a 15% or 20% incidence for T-PLL [4–7]; more recently, the recognition of more cases of T-PLL and the exclusion of a few cases of CLL/PL from the B-PLL group has increased the relative frequency of T-PLL.
[b] The age is given as a mean, with the range in parentheses.

The main laboratory findings are a high WBC count (usually over 100 × 19^9/l) which is more frequent in T-PLL (Table 5.1); two-thirds of T-PLL patients have a WBC count of over 200 × 10^9/l. Anaemia and thrombocytopenia are slightly more common in B-PLL, perhaps reflecting a more slow clinical evolution before diagnosis and/or an earlier involvement of the bone marrow. The proportion of lymphoid cells (prolymphocytes and lymphocytes) in peripheral blood (PB) films is, as a rule, over 90%; the absolute number of neutrophils and monocytes is normal or slightly increased in either form of PLL. Serum uric acid concentrations are frequently above normal and a minority of patients present with abnormal renal and/or liver function tests. Serum immunoglobulins are low in B-PLL, to the same degree as in B-CLL, and normal in T-PLL (Table 5.1). Monoclonal bands of IgM or IgG class are found in the serum of one-third of B-PLL cases. This incidence is higher than in B-CLL where up to 5% of cases may have 'M' bands; these are not seen in T-PLL.

Diagnosis

Light microscopy

The key element for the diagnosis of PLL is the recognition of the prolymphocyte in well-prepared peripheral blood films stained with Romanovsky dyes[4]. The

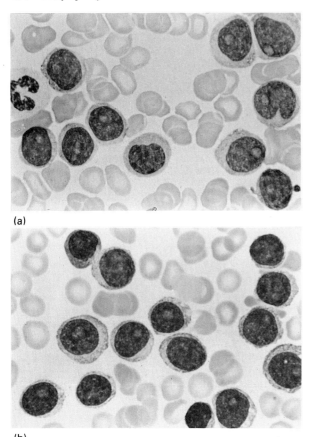

(a)

(b)

Figure 5.1 (a,b) Peripheral blood films from two cases of B-PLL. Note the regular central nucleus with a prominent nucleolus visible in the majority of cells. × 1400, reduced to 56% on reproduction

precise description given by Galton et al.[21] in the original report is still valid today, particularly for the characteristic cell of B-PLL (Figure 5.1). The prolymphocyte is the predominant cell in peripheral blood films and remains so throughout the course of the disease. The distinct features of this cell are: a prominent vesicular nucleolus, relatively well condensed nuclear chromatin (which distinguishes this cell from a blast), and a larger cell size than the CLL lymphocyte, which can be better appreciated by measurement of the cell volume[13, 34]. The B-prolymphocyte also has a more abundant cytoplasm than the small lymphocyte of B-CLL. In addition, some of the smaller cells are also nucleolated and a proportion of larger cells with a finely dispersed nuclear chromatin and a deeply basophilic cytoplasm (immunoblasts) are seen in B-PLL but are rare in T-PLL.

Studies in the authors' laboratory addressing the issue of the distinction between PLL and CLL/PL have shown that more than 55% prolymphocytes in the peripheral blood is the best criterion of definition for the diagnosis of PLL; the mean percentage of these cells found in a series of 22 B-PLL cases was 74%[32]. In PLL, more than in any other lymphoid leukaemia, the appearances of the neoplastic cell (the prolymphocyte) are better recognized in areas of the blood film

Table 5.2 Morphological differences between the two types of PLL[a]

Feature	B-PLL	T-PLL
Light microscopy		
Cell size	Medium–large	Small–medium
Nuclear outline	Regular (65%) or cleft (20%)	Very irregular (50%)
Basophilic cytoplasm	Moderate	Marked
Azurophilic granules	Few (42%)	More numerous (40%)
Acid hydrolases[b]	Negative or moderately positive	Strong in most cells
Electron microscopy		
Golgi apparatus	Inactive	Active (28%)
Endoplasmic reticulum	Short profiles	Long or circular
Ribosomes	Moderate	Prominent
Granules	Small/pale	Large/dense
Vacuoles	Frequent	Rare

[a] Percentages indicate proportion of cases with a particular feature.
[b] Details in Table 5.4.

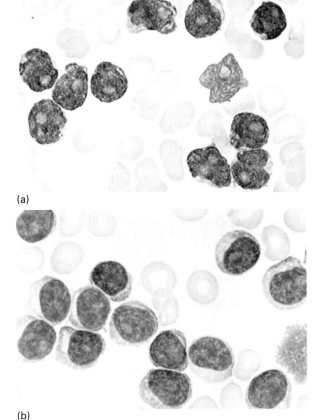

(a)

(b)

Figure 5.2 Peripheral blood films from two cases of T-PLL. In both the prolymphocytes resemble B-PLL cells regarding size and prominence of the nucleolus, although the cells in (a) have a higher N:C ratio and an irregular nuclear outline. × 1500, reduced to 53% on reproduction

in which the cells are well spread. Examination of areas which are either too thick or too thin tend to either obscure the nucleolus, thus resembling a small lymphocyte, or to exaggerate the cell size and the amount of euchromatin, thus giving the impression of a blast cell. In recent years we have also learnt to recognize morphological differences between B- and T-PLL cells and these are summarized in Table 5.2. The cells in half of the cases of T-PLL resemble classic B-PLL, as described above, and have a regular and round nucleus although in general they tend to have less cytoplasm and a higher nucleo-/cytoplasmic ratio than B-prolymphocytes (Figure 5.2). The cells in the remaining T-PLL cases have a very irregular nuclear outline, more irregular than some of the B-PLL cells characterized by a cleft nucleus[11]. In addition, a minority of T-PLL cases have small cells (Figure 5.3a) in which the nucleolus is not easy to see by light microscopic analysis[29, 31]. In general T-prolymphocytes have a deep basophilic

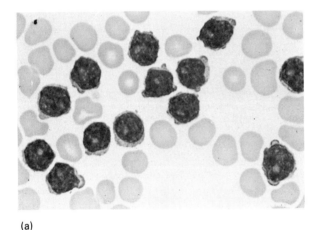

(a)

(b)

Figure 5.3 Peripheral blood films from two other cases of T-PLL. Here the cells are more difficult to recognize as prolymphocytes: they have less cytoplasm (high N:C ratio) which is deeply basophilic. Although a nucleolus is visible in the cells of (a), this is less obvious in the cells of the case illustrated in (b). The cells of (a) are small and represent an example of the small-cell variant (regular) of T-PLL[31]. × 1400, reduced to 53% on reproduction

cytoplasm which sometimes is misleading in suggesting 'plasma-cell' differentiation (Figure 5.3). The morphological heterogeneity of T-PLL accounts for the poor recognition of this form of T-cell leukaemia in many publications where the cases are described as mature T-cell leukaemia, T-CLL with a helper/inducer phenotype or T-CLL of 'knobby' cell type[44].

Electron microscopy

Ultrastructural analysis is necessary for the recognition of the main morphological features of prolymphocytes, in particular the nucleolus, which may not be easily visible at light microscopy in some cases of T-PLL[31]. The differences at electron microscopic level between B- and T-prolymphocytes are summarized in Table 5.2.

B-prolymphocytes (Figure 5.4) are moderately larger than T-PLL cells and significantly larger than CLL lymphocytes[6, 11, 23, 27]. They have a centrally or slightly eccentrically located nucleus; the nuclear outline is often regular and in a minority of cases the prolymphocytes have a nuclear cleft[11]. The heterochromatin is concentrated mainly in the periphery of the nucleus and in the vicinity of the nucleolus. Villi are variable, often more abundant than in CLL cells, but far less than in hairy cells. The moderately villous appearance of B-PLL cells has been recognized by scanning electron microscopy[40]. B-prolymphocytes have few small granules localized in one area of the cytoplasm[6]. The nucleolus is the main morphological feature of prolymphocytes, both B and T (Figures 5.4 and 5.5) and is seen in over 70% of cells. Intracytoplasmic inclusions are well documented in B-PLL cells[10, 25, 27, 42], perhaps with a higher incidence than in other neoplastic B-cells (about 10% of cases). These inclusions can be long and needle-like with periodicity[10], multiple and rectangular, also with periodicity[27], or dense, homogeneous rectangular rods surrounded by a membrane and lacking periodicity[42]. The latter type may correspond to Ig molecules; thus, in this respect, it may be similar to the globular and crystalline inclusions previously described in B-CLL and found to contain IgM molecules (usually IgMλ in the crystalline inclusions)[42].

The cells in half the T-PLL cases have an irregular nucleus (Table 5.2 and Figure 5.5). A proportion of these irregular T-prolymphocytes have a polylobed and almost cerebriform nucleus but without the deep nuclear indentations of Sézary cells[31]. Long and/or circular strands of endoplasmic reticulum associated with clusters of ribosomes and polyribosomes are more prominent in T- than in B-prolymphocytes and account for the marked basophilic cytoplasm seen at light microscopy in T-PLL. Lysosomal granules are large and dense in T-PLL[12, 31] and correlate with the high content of acid hydrolases seen in these cells (see below). Gall bodies are also a feature of these cells and may correlate with the marked dot-like reactivity with α-naphthylacetate esterase (ANAE). The diagnosis of small-cell variant of T-PLL needs always to be confirmed by electron microscopic analysis (Figure 5.5a). These cells are similar in most respects, except for size, to other T-prolymphocytes. The small size, slightly smaller nucleolus and a greater degree of chromatin condensation may be responsible, in some of these cases, for not distinguishing the nucleolus clearly by light microscopic analysis.

Membrane markers

The distinction between B- and T-PLL is now easily achieved by means of membrane phenotype analysis with conventional immunological reagents

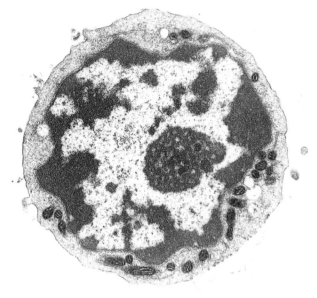

(a)

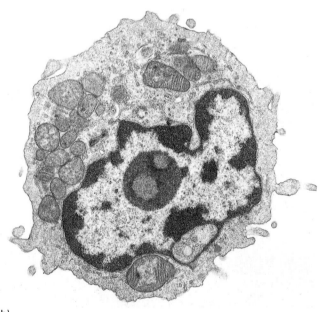

(b)

Figure 5.4 Ultrastructural morphology of prolymphocytes of B-PLL. The cell in (a) has a relatively regular nuclear outline, little cytoplasm, chromatin condensation mainly in the periphery of the nucleus and a distinct 'honeycomb'-type nucleolus. The cell in (b) has more abundant cytoplasm with an active Golgi zone, a more irregular nuclear outline with a 'compact'-type of nucleolus. A nuclear pocket is visible in the inferior part of the cell. × 15 000, reduced to 64% on reproduction

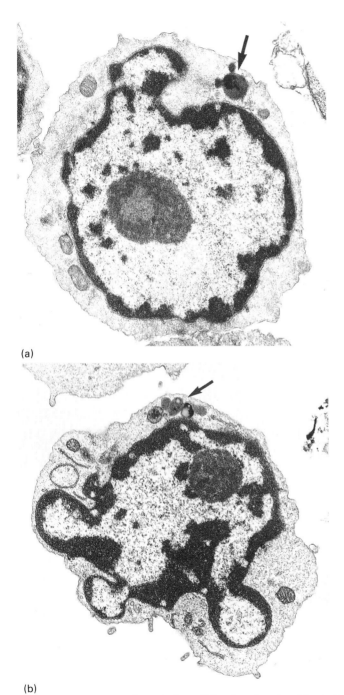

(a)

(b)

Figure 5.5 Ultrastructural morphology of T-prolymphocytes. (a) A typical prolymphocyte with peripheral nuclear chromatin condensation, a large central nucleolus and a large lysosomal granule (arrow). × 22 000, reduced to 69% on reproduction. (b) A T-prolymphocyte with an irregular nucleus, characteristic of some T-PLLs, and a cluster of granules in the cytoplasm (arrow). × 22 000, reduced to 58% on reproduction

**Table 5.3 Membrane phenotype differrences
between two types of PLL**

Marker	B-PLL	T-PLL
SmIg	++	−
CD5	−/+	++
E-rosettes/CD2	−	++
3A1 (CD7)	−	++
CD3, CD4, CD8	−	++[a]
HLA-DR/FMC7	++	−
B-antigens[b]	++	−

[a] Membrane CD3− in 40% (cytoplasmic CD3+ in all cases); CD4
and CD8 co-expressed in 20%; most cases (70%) CD4+, CD8−.
[b] Demonstrated by several monoclonal antibodies (CD19, 20, 22
etc.)

(E-rosettes, SmIg) and a battery of monoclonal antibodies, as summarized in Table 5.3.

The similarities and differences between B-PLL and other chronic B-cell leukaemias were analysed in Chapter 1 (see Table 1.8). The main difference from B-CLL is the strong expression of SmIg, low binding of mouse RBCs[4] and consistent membrane reactivity with FMC7 and mCD22 seen in B-PLL[5, 32]; B-cell antigens are always expressed (Table 5.3) and the CD5 antigen is detected in half of the cases. Staining for CyIg is positive in a proportion of cases. The predominant heavy chains in the membrane of B-PLL are μ and δ, as in B-CLL and CLL/PL. However, the demonstration of γ-chains (IgG) is more frequent in B-PLL (11%) than in CLL/PL (5%) and CLL (2%). All the above features suggest that the B-prolymphocyte is a cell immunologically more mature than the B-lymphocyte of CLL and that it is closer to the plasma cell[5]. The membrane phenotype of B-PLL is also close to that of hairy cell leukaemia and some non-Hodgkin's lymphomas. However, different from hairy cell leukaemia, B-PLL cells do not react with anti-HC2 (see Table 1.4, Chapter 1) and do not express the receptor for interleukin-2 (IL-2), demonstrated by anti-Tac (CD25) (see Table 1.7, Chapter 1). Recent studies in our laboratory with the monoclonal antibody BU11, which reacts with antigens present preferentially in plasma cells, confirm that hairy cells (BU11+) are more mature than B-prolymphocytes (BU11−).

Analysis of high-molecular-weight DNA by Southern blotting techniques and probes for Ig heavy and light chain genes support the findings with membrane markers which suggest that B-CLL, B-PLL and HCL cells derive from lymphocytes at different stages of B-cell maturation. These studies showed that only one allele of the μ heavy chain locus is rearranged in κ-producing CLL whilst both alleles are rearranged in κ-producing B-PLL and HCL[20a]. In addition, a rearrangement of the constant region of the Ig γ-chain gene was detected almost exclusively in HCL, indicating that Ig class switch, a late maturation event, occurs mainly in hairy cells[20a].

The cells in all cases of T-PLL have a mature (post-thymic) phenotype: they are always TdT−, CD1a−, and E-rosette+, CD7+, CD5+ and OKT17+[7, 31]. The expression of other T-cell differentiation antigens is variable: mCD3 was undetectable in 6 of 23 cases[31]; 70% of cases are CD4+ and CD8−; and 20% of cases co-express CD4 and CD8 in the majority of cells. The latter phenotype, in the absence of CD1a and TdT, is rarely seen in other mature T-cell malignancies (see Table 1.10, Chapter 1) and suggests that these T-prolymphocytes originate from a cell of intermediate maturation between thymic and post-thymic cells. Such rare CD4+, CD8+, CD1a−, TdT− cells have been described in minor populations of normal peripheral blood and tonsil lymphocytes[44].

Functional assays

Functional abnormalities of T-lymphocytes in B-PLL are similar to those described in B-CLL and were referred to in Chapter 3. The functional capacity of T-prolymphocytes, in relation to their membrane phenotype, has been reviewed in Chapter 1. Several, but not all of the CD4+, CD8− cases tested have been shown to function in vitro as helper cells[29, 35, 49]. One, presumably T-PLL, with a CD4+, CD8+ was shown to have normal helper activity[44], whilst another lacked such function[29]. The authors are not aware of cases of T-PLL with a CD4−, CD8+ phenotype, which have been studied by functional assays. The relevance of these T-cell functional tests is that they may add important information on the origin of the proliferating cells, in particular as other T4+ proliferations, e.g. adult T-cell leukaemia/lymphoma (ATLL) function in vitro as suppressor cells (see Table 1.13, Chapter 1).

Serology for HTLV-I

Twelve cases of T-PLL were investigated by the authors for the presence of antibodies to HTLV-I, the retrovirus which is closely associated with ATLL (see Chapter 8), and none was found to be positive. Many of them were also tested for the presence of HTLV-I in the neoplastic cells by means of specific monoclonal antibody against the major viral proteins, p19 and p24, in cells cultured for 7–10 days in the presence of phytohaemagglutinin (PHA). Again no positive case was detected despite the fact that the series included two patients of Caribbean origin. Therefore it would appear that there is no evidence for an involvement of HTLV-I in the pathogenesis of T-PLL, confirming the status of the latter as a distinct clinicopathological entity.

Histopathology

There is little information on the histological features of T-PLL, largely because surgical biopsies are almost never required to establish a diagnosis. The pattern of infiltration of the bone marrow in B-PLL is often dense and diffuse[21], and not very different from that of advanced B-CLL. The lymphoid infiltration occupies mainly the intertrabecular space and is different from the paratrabecular concentration seen in follicular lymphoma[28]. A nodular pattern of infiltration has also been described, with some of the nodules having a paratrabecular position[2]. A pure nodular pattern was not observed in bone marrow trephine biopsies from 30 PLLs reviewed in the authors' laboratory[21a]. The most frequent type of infiltration was a mixed interstitial–nodular one encountered in 40% of cases; an interstitial–diffuse pattern, which has not been described in B-CLL, was recorded in five cases of this PLL series[21a]. No major differences in the pattern of infiltration were observed between B- and T-PLL. All cases had increased bone marrow reticulin and this was slightly more marked in the T-PLLs.

The histology of the spleen has been better characterized, particularly in material from splenectomized cases of B-PLL. Both white and red pulp are affected. The predominant site of involvement is the white pulp which shows large proliferative nodules[2, 25, 28], densely packed with prolymphocytes and large cells less heavily clustered in their periphery, with a characteristic bizonal appearance[28]. The red pulp (cords and sinuses) is also heavily infiltrated. This pattern is similar to that of B-CLL, particularly CLL/PL[28], and is different from that seen in hairy cell leukaemia (HCL) and its variant, HCL-V, where the red pulp is exclusively involved with the formation of pseudosinuses, and the white pulp is atrophic. In a case of T-PLL there was diffuse infiltration of the red pulp with obliteration of the white pulp[2] and in another both red pulp and white pulp were involved[28]. Prolymphocytes can be recognized in histological sections by their chromatin pattern and prominent nucleolus, and are best visualized in the red pulp[2, 28]. The apparent nuclear immaturity together with the paucity of mitotic figures was described as characteristic of B-PLL; the few mitoses are seen only in the white pulp.

The lymph nodes of B-PLL are mainly obtained during splenectomy or at post mortem. The histology shows diffuse involvement with a pseudonodular pattern and obliteration of the normal architecture[2, 25] with a pattern different from that of follicular lymphoma[28]. In T-PLL the infiltration is localized predominantly in the paracortical area, leaving areas of residual tissue intact[2]. The liver shows dense infiltration of portal tracts and diffuse involvement of the sinuses[2,25], a pattern not dissimilar to that of hairy cell leukaemia.

Differential diagnosis

This should be considered separately for both types of PLL, because the immunological analysis should determine unequivocally the B- or T-cell nature of the lymphoproliferative process.

B-PLL

The main distinction should be made from CLL presenting with high WBC count, splenomegaly and an increased proportion (20–40%) of prolymphocytes (CLL/PL). Careful examination of peripheral blood films, if well spread, should facilitate the estimation of the percentage of prolymphocytes. The membrane phenotype may indicate whether there is a typical B-PLL profile or some features of B-CLL (high M-rosettes, weak SmIg etc.), although findings in 15% of cases in the CLL/PL group could be very similar to those found in B-PLL[32]. In general, the combination of markers and morphology is sufficient to clarify the diagnosis[34]. In CLL/PL, two morphologically different cell populations are commonly detected[34] and, clinically, lymph node enlargement usually accompanies splenomegaly. A clinical and laboratory score has recently been proposed in which the absolute number of prolymphocytes, the spleen size, the percentage of M-rosettes and the intensity of SmIg were considered as variables[33]. Rare cases with a borderline percentage of prolymphocytes, below the 55% suggested for typical B-PLL, may be considered as compatible with B-PLL if they have a high score and if this includes an absolute number of prolymphocytes above 15×10^9/l. The prognosis of patients with high scores is not different whether the diagnosis is PLL or CLL/PL[33].

Other conditions to consider in the differential diagnosis of B-PLL are: HCL-V, splenic non-Hodgkin's lymphoma (NHL) with villous lymphocytes in the peripheral blood (SLVL) and other forms of NHL with splenomegaly and high WBC count. The HCL-V could present difficulties as the clinical features and marker studies may be similar to B-PLL. In HCL-V, the cells are larger, have a slightly lower nucleo-/cytoplasmic (N:C) ratio and a distinct 'hairy' cytoplasm. The chief difference, if spleen histology is available, is the pattern of infiltration of the leukaemic cells which in HCL-V, as in HCL, affects mainly the red pulp. Cases of SLVL are described in Chapter 7. The villous cells are smaller than prolymphocytes, have a less conspicuous nucleolus by light microscopy, more condensed nuclear chromatin and distinct cytoplasmic villi. The membrane phenotype is also very similar to B-PLL, although the cells are more mature and often show reactivity with BU11, and 60% of patients have an 'M' band (often IgM, sometimes IgG). Other features of these cases are moderate bone marrow infiltration and a WBC count usually below 50×10^9/l. Intermediate NHL is as yet a poorly defined condition from the haematologists' point of view. The main difference from B-PLL is the morphology of the peripheral blood lymphocytes which show a spectrum of cell sizes: the coexistence of large and small cells including some blasts and small cleft cells. Although nucleolated cells are present, they do not constitute the predominant cell type; the homogeneous picture of B-PLL is not seen[2a]. The cells are intermediate in morphology between large lymphocytes and small cleft cells; they are as a rule CD5+ and this may help the distinction from follicular lymphoma (or centroblastic/centrocytic NHL) which is usually CD5−. The latter condition rarely presents with high WBC count, although splenomegalic forms are well documented. Histologically the spleen of follicular lymphoma could be distinguished from the nodular growth of B-PLL, by the absence in the latter of the dual population of centrocytes and centroblasts (or cleft and non-cleft cells)[2, 25].

T-PLL

Difficulties in the diagnosis may arise in cases of T-PLL in which small irregular prolymphocytes predominate[31]. By light microscopic examination the diagnoses of small-cell Sézary syndrome (SS) or of ATLL are often considered. In addition to the detailed morphological analysis, which in some cases ought to include electron microscopic examination, some clinical features are useful. T-PLL has higher counts than SS and lacks the characteristic erythroderma and the epidermotropic pattern of skin infiltration. The authors have seen cases of Sézary cell leukaemia with splenomegaly and without skin involvement. A diagnosis of small cell variant of T-PLL was entertained by light microscopy, but ultrastructural studies were conclusive in showing typical cerebriform cells without nucleoli; of interest was the finding of a CD8+, CD4− membrane phenotype in both cases of Sézary cell leukaemia, which therefore differed from the classic Sézary syndrome by the absence of skin involvement and the phenotype of the neoplastic cells. The convoluted morphology of some T-PLL cases makes it necessary to distinguish the disease from ATLL. The latter generally affects younger individuals and has clinical features different from those of T-PLL, namely hypercalcaemia and more marked lymphadenopathy than splenomegaly. Serology for HTLV-I is positive in most cases of ATLL studied in Japan, in the Caribbean region and in the UK (in Blacks of Caribbean origin) and this test and/or demonstration of the HTLV-I in the leukaemic cells after culture are important for the differential diagnosis of some of these cases. Overall the morphology is more pleomorphic in ATLL, the WBC count rarely exceeds $100 \times 10^9/l$, and nucleolated cells rarely predominate (see also Chapter 8). T-PLL can be distinguished from cases of granular T-CLL by morphology, cytochemistry (see below), marker analyses (see Table 1.10, Chapter 1) and clinical features: T-CLL is characterized by a lower WBC count, a lack of lymphadenopathy and, with few exceptions, a less aggressive clinical course.

Cytochemistry of B- and T-cell leukaemias

The reappraisal of the value of light microscopic cytochemistry for the study of B- and T-cell malignancies began with the observation that lymphoblasts of T-ALL showed a strong localized acid phosphatase reaction. Further advances were made possible by the combination of cytochemical staining and immunological labelling of the cells with monoclonal antibodies, for example with the immunogold method[16], which allowed a better correlation between cytochemical pattern and expression of specific antigens on B- and T-cells.

At least 20 enzymes can be detected by cytochemical reactions in lymphoid cells[14]. Only five of them (Tables 5.4 and 5.5) have been shown to be of value for the differential diagnosis of B- and T- lymphoproliferative disorders. These include the acid hydrolases: acid phosphatase, β-glucuronidase, N-acetyl-β-glucosaminidase, one of the non-specific esterases [α-naphthylacetate esterase (ANAE)] and one of the proteases (dipeptidylaminopeptidase IV or DAP IV). Other proteases which are demonstrated by different substrates, such as DAP I and DAP II, have also been found in variable proportions of lymphocytes[30].

Table 5.4 Cytochemical profile of B-lymphoproliferative disorders

Disease	ANAE	Acid phosphatase	β-Glucuronidase	β-Glucosaminidase	DAP IV
B-CLL	−	−	−/±	−	−
B-PLL	−	−/+ [a]	−/±	−	−
HCL	−/+	++ [a]	−/±	−	−
LPL [b]	+	+	+	+	−
Myeloma	++	++	++	++	−

[a] Tartrate resistant.
[b] Lymphoplasmacytic lymphoma (see Chapter 7), including cases of splenic lymphoma with villous lymphocytes (SLVL).

ANAE: α-naphthylacetate esterase; DAP IV: dipeptidylaminopeptidase IV.

Table 5.5 Cytochemical profile of T-lymphoproliferative disorders

Disease	ANAE [a]	Acid phosphatase	β-Glucuronidase	β-Glucosaminidase	DAP IV
T-ALL/T-LbLy	−/+	++	±	±	−/+
T-PLL	++	+ [b]	++	++	++ [d]
T-CLL	−/±	++ [b]	++	++	−/+ [d]
ATLL	+	+	++	++	−
CTCL [c]	+	+	++	++	−/+

[a] Abbreviation of enzymes as in Table 5.4.
[b] Tartrate resistant in few cases.
[c] Sézary cells.
[d] Negative in CD8+ cases.

From Table 5.4 it is apparent that acid phosphatase is the only enzyme demonstrated consistently in B-cell disorders, in particular the tartrate-resistant isoenzyme 5 characteristic of hairy cell leukaemia. Of interest too is that with increased maturation towards the plasma cell stage most acid hydrolases are strongly expressed in B-cells, except for DAP IV which seems to be found only in a subset of T-cells[1, 8, 16, 18–20]. However, most of these enzymes are strongly expressed in the T-cell disorders[15]. T-PLL is the only disease, in the authors' experience, in which a strong cytochemical reaction can be shown with the five enzymes (Table 5.5, Figure 5.6). The pattern of reactivity in T-cells depends on the enzyme and the stage of maturation of the T-cells[14], acid phosphatase being the first enzyme detected in early T-cells (pre-T-ALL). In late stages of T-cell maturation differences in reactivity have been shown between CD4+ and CD8+ lymphocyte subsets[14], and this is also reflected in the neoplastic T-cells.

α-Naphthylacetate esterase

A characteristic dot-like reaction (NaF resistant) is a feature of T-cells, particularly the CD4+ subset[14, 15]. This pattern of reaction contrasts with that seen in monocytes which is diffuse throughout the cytoplasm and is NaF sensitive[50]. Combined cytochemical and membrane marker studies show that 75–80% of CD4+ cells are ANAE positive, whilst only 40% of CD8+ cells are positive; B-cells are mostly ANAE negative.

As shown in Table 5.4, ANAE activity is only detected, within the B-cell series, in normal and malignant plasma cells. A weak reaction in small granules is seen in B-lineage ALL[1] cells and in other B-cell disorders but, because it is different from the strong dot-like reaction of T-cells, it is usually considered as negative for practical purposes. Within the T-cell malignancies, ANAE expression is variable in T-ALL but it is, as a rule, strongly positive in T-PLL cells. In the latter condition the dot-like reactivity of ANAE does not correlate with the membrane phenotype of the T-PLL cells, i.e. it is seen whether the cells are CD4+ or CD8+ or both CD4+ and CD8+[15]. In T-CLL (granular Tγ, CD8+ lymphocytes, rarely CD4+), ANAE is weak and has a diffuse pattern of reaction. A dot-like pattern is also a feature of other CD4+ disorders, ATLL and Sézary syndrome[1, 15]. The localized pattern in CD4+ cells (Figure 5.6b) relates to the presence in the cytoplasm of gall bodies, a structure which appears to contain the esterase activity. Gall bodies are not seen in large granular lymphocytes which, however, have a high content of lysosomal enzymes, but not ANAE, in the cytoplasmic granules and in the parallel tubular arrays[12].

Acid phosphatase

Early work with acid phosphatase, β-glucuronidase and N-acetyl-β-glucosaminidase identified a high concentration of these enzymes in tissue areas recognized as T-cell associated, i.e. paracortical and interfollicular zones of lymph nodes and periarteriolar sheets in the spleen. Subsequent studies with cell suspensions rosetted with sheep RBCs, have confirmed the T-cell preference of acid phosphatase. However, although this enzyme is more strongly expressed on T-cells, it is not T-cell specific, and degrees of reactivity can be shown also on B-cells. As mentioned above, acid phosphatase increases in content with B-cell maturation being particularly strong in hairy cells and plasma cells. The isoenzyme

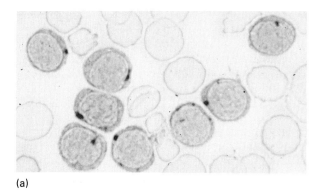

(a)

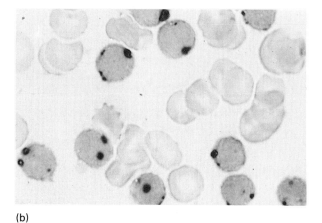

(b)

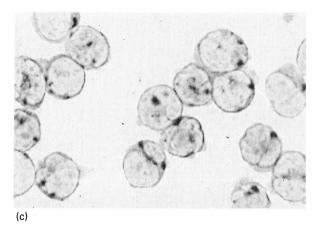

(c)

Figure 5.6 Light microscopy cytochemistry of T-PLL cells showing characteristic positive reactions with three acid hydrolases: (a) acid phosphatase; (b) α-naphthylacetate esterase, with the consistently strong pattern seen in T-PLL; and (c) DAP-IV. × 1400, reduced to 62% on reproduction

5, responsible for the property of resistance to tartaric acid, is also demonstrable in small amounts in some B-PLLs[4, 25] and lymphoplasmacytic lymphomas including a few cases of splenic lymphoma with 'villous' lymphocytes. Acid phosphatase is usually positive (Figure 5.6a) in most T-cell leukaemias and lymphomas, including cases of pre-T-ALL with an immature T-cell phenotype[14].

β-Glucuronidase and N-acetyl-β-glucosaminidase

The pattern of reactivity with these two acid hydrolases is similar to that of acid phosphatase (see Tables 5.4 and 5.5). However, it would appear that N-acetyl-β-glucosaminidase is more T-cell specific (except for plasma cells) than acid phosphatase and β-glucuronidase. Both enzymes are strongly positive in all types of T-cell malignancies (except in T-lymphoblasts), thus they could be considered as 'pan-T' cytochemical markers[15] in situations where immunological marker studies are not available. In this respect they differ from ANAE and DAP IV (see below) which react selectively with some, but not all, types of normal and leukaemic T-cells (see Table 5.5).

Dipeptidylaminopeptidase IV

In contrast to the above enzymes, DAP IV has not been demonstrated in any type of B-cell, including B-lineage lymphoblasts[1, 8, 18, 30]. In normal cells, DAP IV activity is found on 72% of CD4+ lymphocytes and in 41% of CD8+ lymphocytes[16]. Within the T-cell malignancies the reactivity of DAP IV is restricted to some CD4+ proliferations (see Table 5.5)[8, 16, 18, 19, 48]. In the authors' experience CD4+ T-PLL has a consistently strong DAP IV reaction (Figure 5.6c); a similar pattern is seen in T-lymphoblastic lymphoma but not in the less mature blasts of T-ALL[16]. DAP IV is negative in CD8+ leukaemias, including CD8+ T-PLL[1] and, it was seen to be diffusely positive in a case of T-CLL with large granular cells and an unusual membrane phenotype CD4+, CD11b+, Fcγ+. On the other hand, not all cases of CD4+ proliferations are DAP IV positive. Sézary cells[1, 16, 28] are often DAP IV negative, although few positive cases have been described[1, 20]. These findings suggest that DAP IV has a more selective expression in a subset of T-lymphocytes than the other acid hydrolases. Although this enzyme may be more T-cell specific its absence in a number of disorders (see Table 5.5) suggest that the routine use of this cytochemical reaction may be limited. It may be of value to define more precisely the phenotypic and functional properties of the T-subset(s) which is DAP IV positive in order to apply this test with a well-defined indication[1].

Prognosis and treatment

The pattern of clinical evolution of PLL, both in its B- and T-forms, is one of continuous disease progression. In contrast to CLL, the authors are not aware of PLL patients in which the disorder remains static for prolonged periods of time. The clinical and laboratory findings suggest that T-PLL progresses more rapidly, and has an overall more aggressive course with multiorgan involvement, than B-PLL, in which splenomegaly and high WBC count are the main manifestations.

Observations in two patients who were diagnosed by chance at an early stage of their disease illustrate the natural history of untreated PLL well. One of them presented with a non-specific skin rash and laboratory analyses led to the diagnosis of B-PLL. The prolymphocyte count rose steadily from $20 \times 10^9/l$ to $90 \times 10^9/l$ over 2 years, associated with progressive splenomegaly and features of bone marrow failure. The evolution of this patient was illustrated in work by one of the authors (DC[4], Figure 30.4). Treatment was started 2.5 years after diagnosis: the overall survival was 6.5 years. The other patient, diagnosed as T-PLL as a result of a routine blood count, progressed more rapidly. Splenomegaly was noted 2 months later and the WBC count rose from $30 \times 10^9/l$ to $150 \times 10^9/l$ in 1.5 years; he survived 20 months.

By extrapolating Rai's staging system for CLL to PLL, the authors could establish that 30% of B-PLL patients present with stage II (splenomegaly only), 20% with stage III (anaemia and splenomegaly) and 50% with stage IV (thrombocytopenia often also with anaemia and splenomegaly). In T-PLL the majority of patients presents with stage IV.

Analysis of survival in an early series[4] showed that the survival was significantly shorter (7 months) for stage IV patients than for stages II–III (26 months). However, the main reason for this difference is the worse outcome of T-PLL. The survival of PLL in Galton's original series[21] was 17 weeks. A subsequent analysis gave a median survival of 2 years, but more recent results suggest an improved figure of 3 years for B-PLL[33]. This improvement may result from the recognition of early cases but probably also from the success of some therapeutic manoeuvres in B-PLL.

Treatment of B-PLL

A number of modalities have been used for the management of B-PLL patients and all of them have been shown to have a favourable effect, i.e. a good clinical/haematological response, although of variable degree. Randomized comparisons between therapies have not been possible largely because the disease is uncommon and partly because some of the treatments are used in succession on individual patients. For example, we believe that splenectomy is a useful measure in this disease. Nevertheless in patients treated by either splenic irradiation or splenectomy no obvious difference was observed. However, the condition of the patients in both groups was not the same. In general splenectomy was left as a last resource, thus patients who did not respond to other measures, including splenic irradiation, were often subjected to splenectomy.

Splenic irradiation given in weekly (or twice weekly) fractions of 100 cGy for 10 weeks, to a total dose of 1000 cGy, results in a beneficial response in half of the patients[37]. This effect is very similar to that obtained in splenomegalic forms of B-CLL. Because of its simplicity and the fact that it directs the therapy to the main proliferating focus of disease, splenic irradiation should be considered as the first line of therapy, particularly for patients over 60 years of age. In a small proportion of patients (about 25%) a complete remission has been recorded[4, 37]. Successful therapy can be repeated again, if required, after a suitable interval (of at least 6 months). However, it makes sense that if this needs to be repeated more than once due to the enlargement of the spleen, splenectomy should follow a successful irradiation treatment. In fact one of the most prolonged responses the authors observed was in a patient splenectomized following an excellent response to a second course of splenic irradiation[37]. The reason for suggesting further irradiation in such patients before splenectomy is that the treatment has not only a local effect (by reducing the spleen size) but improves directly and/or indirectly the blood counts.

Splenectomy is effective as a debulking procedure in B-PLL, and it is often indicated at some stage in the disease (Figure 5.7). In addition, the hypersplenic component of the cytopenia always benefits to a variable degree from this manoeuvre. Splenectomy should not be considered as an effective measure in itself,

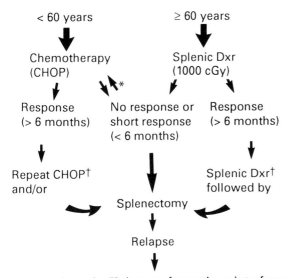

Figure 5.7 Strategy for the management of B-PLL. *CHOP may be considered for non-responders to splenic irradiation. †After relapse

but as part of the overall strategy of treatment of B-PLL. The benefits of splenectomy alone are often short lived and therefore its benefits (blood improvement, reduction in tumour mass) should be followed by other measures. For example, by a further debulking procedure such as leucapheresis, which needs to be carried out intensively, i.e. every week, until significant reduction in the WBC count is obtained[4, 37]. Early splenectomy could, in theory, be more effective than late splenectomy, as there is some evidence that B-PLL behaves like its animal model, the BLC1 leukaemia in mouse. Unfortunately, as mentioned above, early diagnosis is rare.

Response to chemotherapy has been recorded in a number of B-PLL patients[4, 5, 45], largely with the combination CHOP (cyclophosphamide, hydroxydauno-rubicin, oncovin and prednisolone). This therapy is better tolerated by young patients (less than 60 years). One of them, reported in preliminary form in 1979[43], survived 10 years from diagnosis. This patient illustrates well some aspects of the management of B-PLL (Figure 5.7). He achieved a complete remission with eight courses of CHOP which continued for 2 years. A relapse in 1981 was followed by a new complete remission following six further courses of

CHOP. In 1984 a massive spleen was removed followed by normalization of haemoglobin and platelets but with a rising WBC count ($>200 \times 10^9$/l). B-PLL patients are not always responsive to CHOP and only a few patients benefit from chlorambucil and prednisolone as used in B-CLL[4, 22], and very few respond to oncovin and prednisone alone[22]. Other measures such as 2'-deoxycoformycin (DCF) or α-interferon have not been tried extensively in B-PLL. No response was observed to α-interferon in a patient treated following splenectomy but who experienced subsequently a prolonged partial response to DCF (greater than 1 year).

Intrathecal methotrexate may be required for the rare complication of meningeal leukaemia[26].

Treatment of T-PLL

The poor prognosis of T-PLL suggested in the authors' earlier report[4] of eight patients (median survival 7 months), has not improved in a recent analysis of 30 patients (median survival 6 months). The main reasons for this bleak outlook are the aggressive nature of the disease and the poor response to treatment. Good responses to treatment have as a rule been associated with improved survival.

Combination chemotherapy with CHOP has occasionally resulted in complete remission[36]. In our recent experience the complete remission rate with CHOP is less than 30%. Another modality which has been reported to induce remissions in T-PLL is upper mediastinal (thymic?) irradiation with doses around 3000 cGy[41]. The authors are aware of another prolonged complete remission in a case of T-PLL treated in this way by Dr A. Pollock (personal communication).

Exciting recent developments are the responses reported with the adenosine deaminase inhibitor 2'-deoxycoformycin (DCF) used at low doses[17]. Two patients aged 81 and 74 years achieved a good remission, which in one lasted over 1 year with no maintenance. Five other patients have been treated with T-PLL and the results observed were one good response, almost complete remission, two partial remissions (Figure 5.8) and no responses in two. It is early to draw final conclusions about this therapy but the authors' impression is that patients with CD4+ cells respond better to DCF. This is supported by observations of complete remission in a T-CLL with the rare CD4+, CD11b+ membrane phenotype (and the lack of response in one with CD8+, CD11b+ cells), and in a patient with an aggressive form of Sézary syndrome (CD4+). At the low doses of DCF used (4 mg/m^2 every week) the side effects are minimal and the renal toxicity seen with the higher doses of this agent are not observed[16a].

Chromosome abnormalities

The use of specific mitogens for B- and T-cells has facilitated the analysis of chromosome abnormalities in B- and T-cell PLL. With these methods it has been possible, in the last few years, to document changes which may be more common in PLL than in other lymphoid disorders. A feature of both B- and T-PLL (in contrast to B- and T-CLL) is that metaphases are easier to obtain and that clonal chromosome abnormalities are nearly always observed[3, 3a, 38, 39]. In addition, the breakpoints commonly involved in the abnormalities include genes which are specifically rearranged during B- and T-cell differentiation.

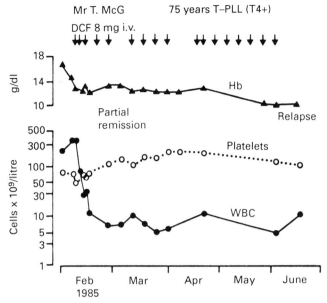

Mr T. McG   75 years T–PLL (T4+)

DCF 8 mg i.v.

Figure 5.8 Haematological chart of the response to 2′-deoxycoformycin (DCF) by a patient with T-PLL. Despite the dramatic fall in the WBC count, there was less effect on the enlarged organs. Drug resistance eventually ensued despite continuation of therapy

Findings in B-PLL

There are few cytogenetic studies in B-PLL. The authors first reported a series of nine cases in which clonal abnormalities involving chromosome 14 at band q32 were seen in seven[39]. A further 14 cases were studied subsequently and this series[3] has confirmed the marker 14q+ as the most frequent abnormality in this disease (16 out of 23 cases). Less frequently, abnormalities involving other chromosomes have been reported (reviewed by Brito-Babapulle et al.[3]): del(3)(q25), t(3;8)(p13;q13), del(6)(q21), del(12)(p12–13), the latter also seen in B-CLL and hairy cell leukaemia[3], and t(6;12)(q15;p13). It is of interest that chromosomes numbers 3q, 11p and 12p have been suggested as sites for the *c-ras* oncogene family[24].

Most of the authors' studies were carried out on peripheral blood prolympho-cytes. Initially pokeweed mitogen (PWM) and lipopolysaccharide B (LPS) were used as mitogens after pre-treatment of the cells with neuraminidase and galactose oxidase[39]. Recently the Epstein–Barr virus has been used as a specific polyclonal B-cell mitogen and the phorbol ester 12-*O*-tetradecanoylphorbol-13-acetate (TPA)[3].

All cases of B-PLL studied have chromosome abnormalities. The common rearrangement involving chromosome 14 has the breakpoint at band q32 where the locus for the Ig heavy chain gene is located. The frequent involvement of 14q32 in B-PLL may relate to the higher frequency of rearrangement of both heavy chain genes in this disease compared with B-CLL[3, 20a].

Of particular interest is the demonstration of the translocation t(11;14)(q13;q32) in 5 of 23 cases. Although this abnormality has also been described in other B-cell disorders, including B-CLL, non-Hodgkin's lymphomas (NHLs) (1.7% of cases)

and plasma cell leukaemia (10% of cases), the incidence in B-PLL (21% of cases) appears to be significantly higher[3]. The breakpoint 11q13 has been cloned and it has been suggested that it is the locus for a putative oncogene, *bcl-1*, which may be involved in the pathogenesis of B-cell malignancies[41a, 47].

Trisomy for chromosome 12, an abnormality characteristic of B-CLL (see Chapter 3), has been observed in two patients with unequivocal B-PLL in the authors' series (10%) and some cases have been reported by others although the possibility that some of them were examples of CLL/PL has not been ruled out. Nevertheless this abnormality emphasizes the relationship between B-lineage CLL and PLL.

In a number of cases of B-PLL the authors have been able to document karyotypic evolution, i.e. the development of new abnormalities which appear to exert a proliferative advantage[3, 39]. By analogy with other disorders in which this process is common, e.g. chronic granulocytic leukaemia, it is likely that the poor prognosis of B-PLL and its poor response to therapy, compared with B-CLL, may relate to the presence of highly resistant clones with multiple chromosome abnormalities.

The use of TPA stimulation and infection in vitro by Epstein–Barr virus (EBV) resulted in the establishment of three B-PLL-derived cell lines (JVM-2, JVM-3 and JVM-13) in the authors' laboratory[33a]. These B-lymphoblastoid cell lines have the same karyotypic abnormalities and identical Ig gene rearrangements as the original leukaemic cells but their immunophenotype shows more mature features. Attempts to establish cell lines from B-CLL by a similar technique have been unsuccessful, except for a cell line derived from a case of CLL/PL (JVM-14)[33a]. Possible reasons for the relatively easy immortalization of B-prolymphocytes in comparison with B-CLL cells include: a more mature membrane phenotype and consistent evidence of structural chromosome abnormalities in prolymphocytes[33a] and/or a specific interaction between the Epstein–Barr virus and the B-PLL cells. Work in Dr Crawford's laboratory[47a] has shown that the high susceptibility for immortalization by EBV of B-PLL lymphocytes correlates with the expression of the latent membrane protein induced by viral genes; this protein is not detected in CLL cells resistant to immortalization. Other changes induced by EBV, such as expression of the EBNA complex, membrane CD23 and HLA-DR, are identical in CLL and PLL B-cells; thus, these do not explain the observed differences in response[47a].

Findings in T-PLL

Analysable metaphases are obtained with T-cell mitogens, chiefly PHA and the phorbol ester TPA. These have allowed, in the first instance, the demonstration of the clonal nature of T-PLL[38, 46]. In an earlier study the authors have documented structural abnormalities in each of six cases studied[38] although without obvious specific features for the disease. Recently a further 19 cases have been studied and showed that rearrangements involving chromosome band 14q11 where the gene for the α-chain of the T-cell receptor has been mapped are very common (68% of cases) in T-PLL[3a, 31a]. Frequently the abnormality consists of an inversion of chromosome 14 with breakpoints at q11 and q32, inv(14)(q11;q32), also reported by Corwin et al. in a case of T-PLL[9], and described in other T-cell leukaemias, some of which may correspond to T-PLL[3a]. A breakpoint at 14q11 is also a feature of T-ALL, but this results in a specific translocation t(11;14)(p13;q11–13).

In another T-cell malignancy (ATLL – see Chapter 8), trisomy or partial trisomy for 7q often involving band 7q35 in which the gene for the β-chain of the T-cell receptor has been located, has been found by the authors in four cases. Other frequent abnormalities seen in T-PLL were del(6), and trisomy 8q[3a]. Again, as in B-PLL, it is likely that the constant presence of complex karyotypic abnormalities in T-PLL is responsible for the more aggressive nature of this disorder. It is too early to be able to ascertain whether certain abnormalities are associated with a worse prognosis.

References

1. Andrews, C., Crockard, A. D., San Miguel, J. F. and Catovsky, D. (1985) Dipeptidylaminopeptidase IV (DAP IV) in B- and T-cell leukaemias. *Clinical and Laboratory Haematology*, **7**, 359–368
2. Bearman, R. M., Pangalis, G. A. and Rappaport, H. (1978) Prolymphocytic leukemia: clinical histopathological and cytochemical observations. *Cancer*, **42**, 2360–2372
2a. Bennett, J. M., Catovsky, D., Daniel, M-T. et al. (1989) Proposals for the classification of chronic (mature) B and T lymphoid leukaemias. *Journal of Clinical Pathology*, **42**, 567–584
3. Brito-Babapulle, V., Pittman, S., Melo, J. V., Pomfret, M. and Catovsky, D. (1987) Cytogenetic studies on prolymphocytic leukemia. I. B cell prolymphocytic leukemia. *Hematologic Pathology*, **1**, 27–33
3a. Brito-Babapulle, V., Pomfret, M., Matutes, E. and Catovsky, D. (1987) Cytogenetic studies on prolymphocytic leukaemia II. T-cell prolymphocytic leukaemia. *Blood*, **70**, 926–931
4. Catovsky, D. (1982) Prolymphocytic and hairy-cell leukemias. In *Leukemia*, 4th edn, edited by F. Gunz and E. Henderson, pp. 759–781. New York: Grune & Stratton
5. Catovsky, D. (1982) Prolymphocytic leukaemia. *Nouvelle Revue Française d'Hematologie*, **24**, 343–347
6. Catovsky, D., Matutes, E., Crockard, A. D., O'Brien, M. and Costello, C. (1984) Prolymphocytic leukemia of B- and T-cell types. Morphological differences by light and electron microscopy. In *Human Leukemias*, edited by A. Polliack, pp. 251–259. Boston: Martinus Nijhoff
7. Catovsky, D., Wechsler, A., Matutes, E. et al. (1982) The membrane phenotype of T-prolymphocytic leukaemia. *Scandinavian Journal of Haematology*, **29**, 398–404
8. Chilosi, M., Pizzolo, G., Semenzato, G., de Rossi, G. and Pandolfi, F. (1984) Heterogeneous expression of dipeptidyl-amino-peptidase (DAP IV) in T-cell chronic lymphocytic leukemia. *Acta Haematologica*, **71**, 277–281
9. Corwin, D. J., Kadin, M. E. and Andres, T. L. (1983) T-cell prolymphocytic leukaemia. *Acta Haematologica*, **70**, 43–49
10. Costello, C., Catovsky, D. and O'Brien, M. (1981) Cytoplasmic inclusions in a case of prolymphocytic leukemia. *American Journal of Clinical Pathology*, **76**, 499–501
11. Costello, C., Catovsky, D., O'Brien, M. and Galton, D. A. G. (1980) Prolymphocytic leukaemia: an ultrastructural study of 22 cases. *British Journal of Haematology*, **44**, 389–394
12. Costello, C., Catovsky, D., O'Brien, M., Morilla, R. and Varadi, S. (1980) Chronic T-cell leukemias. I. Morphology, cytochemistry and ultrastructure. *Leukemia Research*, **4**, 463–476
13. Costello, C., Wardle, J., Catovsky, D. and Lewis, S. M. (1980) Cell volume studies in B-cell leukaemia. *British Journal of Haematology*, **45**, 209–214
14. Crockard, A. D. (1984) Cytochemistry of lymphoid cells: a review of findings in the normal and leukaemic state. *Histochemical Journal*, **16**, 1027–1050
15. Crockard, A. D., Chalmers, D., Matutes, E. and Catovsky, D. (1982) Cytochemistry of acid hydrolases in chronic B and T cell leukaemias. *American Journal of Clinical Pathology*, **78**, 437–444
16. Crockard, A. D., Macfarlane, E., Andrews, C., Bridges, J. M. and Catovsky, D. (1984) Dipeptidylaminopeptidase IV activity in normal and leukemic T cell subpopulations. *American Journal of Clinical Pathology*, **82**, 294–299
16a. Dearden, C., Matutes, E., Brozovic, N. et al. (1987) Response to deoxycoformycin in mature T cell malignancies relates to membrane phenotype. *British Medical Journal*, **295**, 873–875

17. El'Agnaf, M. R., Ennis, K. E., Morris, T. C. M., Robertson, J. H., Markey, G. and Alexander, H. D. (1986) Successful remission induction with deoxycoformycin in elderly patients with T-helper prolymphocytic leukaemia. *British Journal of Haematology*, **63**, 93–104

18. Feller, A. C., Heijnen, C. J., Ballieux, R. E. and Parwaresch, M. R. (1982) Enzymehistochemical staining of Tμ lymphocytes for glycyl-proline-4-methoxy-beta-naphthylamide-peptidase (DAP IV). *British Journal of Haematology*, **51**, 227–234

19. Feller, A. C., Parwaresch, M. R., Bartels, H. and Lennert, K. (1982) Enzyme cytochemical heterogeneity of human chronic T-lymphocytic leukemia as demonstrated by reactivity to dipeptidylaminopeptidase IV (DAP IV; EC 3.4.14.4). *Leukemia Research*, **6**, 801–808

20. Feller, A. C., Ziegler, A., Sterry, W., Goos, M. and Parwaresch, M. R. (1983) Phenotypic heterogeneity of leukemic Sézary cells. *Blut*, **47**, 333–341

20a. Foroni, L., Catovsky, D. and Luzzatto, L. (1987) Immunoglobulin gene rearrangements in hairy cell leukemia and other chronic B cell lymphoproliferative disorders. *Leukemia*, **4**, 389–392

21. Galton, D. A. G., Goldman, J. M., Wiltshaw, E., Catovsky, D., Henry, K. and Goldenberg, J. (1974) Prolymphocytic leukaemia. *British Journal of Haematology*, **27**, 7–23

21a. Hernandez Nieto, L., Lampert, I. A. and Catovsky, D. (1989) Bone marrow histological patterns in B-cell and T-cell prolymphocytic leukemia. *Hematologic Pathology*, **3**, 79–84

22. Hollister, D., Jr and Coleman, M. (1982) Treatment of prolymphocytic leukaemia. *Cancer*, **50**, 1687–1689

23. Huhn, D., Thiel, E., Rodt, H. and Theml, H. (1978) Prolymphocytic leukemia. *Klinische Wochenschrift*, **56**, 709–714

24. Juliusson, G., Robert, K-H., Ost, A. et al. (1985) Del(3)(p13) in B-prolymphocytic leukemia – a new nonrandom chromosomal aberration possibly related to the *c-ras* oncogene. *Cancer Genetics and Cytogenetics*, **14**, 191–195

25. Katayama, I., Aiba, M., Pechet, L., Sullivan, J. L., Roberts, P. and Humphreys, R. E. (1980) B-lineage prolymphocytic leukemia as a distinct clinicopathologic entity. *American Journal of Pathology*, **99**, 399–412

26. Kernoff, L. M. and Coghlan, P. J. (1983) Prolymphocytic leukemia with leukaemic meningitis and extralymphoid tumours. *South African Medical Journal*, **64**, 290–292

27. Kjeldsberg, C. R., Bearman, R. M. and Rappaport, H. (1980) Prolymphocytic leukemia: an ultrastructural study. *American Journal of Clinical Pathology*, **73**, 150–159

28. Lampert, I., Catovsky, D., Marsh, G. W., Child, J. A. and Galton, D. A. G. (1980) The histopathology of prolymphocytic leukaemia with particular reference to the spleen: a comparison with chronic lymphocytic leukaemia. *Histopathology*, **4**, 3–19

29. Lauria, F., Foa, R., Raspadori, D. et al. (1985) T-cell prolymphocytic leukaemia: a clinical and immunological study. *Scandinavian Journal of Haematology*, **35**, 319–324

30. Lojda, A. (1985) The importance of protease histochemistry in pathology. *Histochemical Journal*, **17**, 1063–1089

31. Matutes, E., Garcia Talavera, J., O'Brien, M. and Catovsky, D. (1986) The morphological spectrum of T-prolymphocytic leukaemia. *British Journal of Haematology*, **64**, 111–123

31a. Matutes, E., Brito-Babapulle, V., Worner, I., Sainati, L., Foroni, L. and Catovsky, D. (1988) T-cell chronic lymphocytic leukaemia: the spectrum of mature T-cell disorders. *Nouvelle Revue Française d'Hematologie*, **30**, 347–351

32. Melo, J. V., Catovsky, D. and Galton, D. A. G. (1986) The relationship between chronic lymphocytic leukaemia and prolymphocytic leukaemia. I. Clinical and laboratory features of 300 patients and characterisation of an intermediate group. *British Journal of Haematology*, **63**, 377–387

33. Melo, J. V., Catovsky, D., Gregory, W. M. and Galton, D. A. G. (1987) The relationship between chronic lymphocytic leukaemia and prolymphocytic leukaemia. IV. Analysis of survival and prognostic features. *British Journal of Haematology*, **65**, 23–29

33a. Melo, J. V., Foroni, L., Brito-Babapulle, V., Luzzatto, L. and Catovsky, D. (1988) The establishment of cell lines from chronic B cell leukaemias: evidence of leukaemic origin by karyotypic abnormalities and Ig gene rearrangement. *Clinical and Experimental Immunology*, **73**, 23–28

34. Melo, J. V., Wardle, J., Chetty, M. et al. (1986) The relationship between chronic lymphocytic leukaemia and prolymphocytic leukaemia. III. Evaluation of cell size by morphology and volume measurements. *British Journal of Haematology,* **64**, 469–478

35. Miedema, F., van Oostveen, J. W., Terpstra, F. G. et al. (1985) Analysis of helper activity on PWM- and IL-2-driven immunoglobulin synthesis by neoplastic T4+ cells. *Journal of Clinical Investigation,* **76**, 2139–2143

36. Newland, A. C., Turnbull, A. I., Bainbridge, D. and Jenkins, G. D. (1980) Complete remission in T-cell prolymphocytic leukaemia. *British Journal of Haematology,* **45**, 513–514

37. Oscier, D. G., Catovsky, D., Errington, R. D., Goolden, A. W. G., Roberts, P. D. and Galton, D. A. G. (1981) Splenic irradiation in B-prolymphocytic leukaemia. *British Journal of Haematology,* **48**, 577–584

38. Pittman, S. and Catovsky, D. (1983) Chromosome abnormalities in B-cell prolymphocytic leukemia: A study of nine cases. *Cancer Genetics and Cytogenetics,* **9**, 355–365

39. Pittman, S., Morilla, R. and Catovsky, D. (1982) Chronic T cell leukemias. II. Cytogenetic studies. *Leukemia Research,* **6**, 33–42

40. Polliack, A., Leizerowitz, T., Berrebi, A. et al. (1984) Prolymphocytic leukaemia: surface morphology in 21 cases as seen by scanning electron microscopy and comparison with B-type CLL and CLL in 'prolymphocytoid' transformation. *British Journal of Haematology,* **57**, 577–584

41. Price, P. J. S., Jackson, J. M. and Stokes, J. B. (1982) Thymic irradiation in T-cell prolymphocytic leukaemia. *British Journal of Haematology,* **51**, 498–500

41a. Rabbitts, P. H., Douglas, J., Fischer, P. et al. (1988) Chromosome abnormalities at 11q13 in B cell tumours. *Oncogene,* **3**, 99–103

42. Robinson, D. S. F., Melo, J. V., Andrews, C., Schey, S. A. and Catovsky, D. (1985) Intracytoplasmic inclusions in B prolymphocytic leukaemia: ultrastructural, cytochemical and immunological studies. *Journal of Clinical Pathology,* **38**, 897–903

43. Sibbald, R. and Catovsky, D. (1979) Complete remission in prolymphocytic leukaemia with the combination chemotherapy – CHOP. *British Journal of Haematology,* **42**, 488–490

44. Simpkins, H., Kiprov, D. D., Davis, J. L. III, Morand, P., Puri, S. and Grahn, E. P. (1985) T cell chronic lymphocytic leukemia with lymphocytes of unusual immunologic phenotype and function. *Blood,* **65**, 127–133

45. Taylor, H. G., Butler, W. M., Rhoads, J., Karcher, D. S. and Detrick-Hooks, B. (1982) Prolymphocytic leukemia: treatment with combination chemotherapy to include doxorubicin. *Cancer,* **49**, 1524–1529

46. Thiel, E., Bauchinger, M., Rodt, H., Huhn, D., Theml, H. and Thierfelder, S. (1977) Evidence for monoclonal proliferation in prolymphocytic leukaemia of T-cell origin. *Blut,* **35**, 427–436

47. Tsujimoto, Y., Jaffe, E., Cossman, J., Gorham, J., Nowell, P. C. and Croce, C. M. (1985) Clustering of breakpoints on chromosome 11 in human B-cell neoplasms with the t(11;14) chromosome translocation. *Nature,* **315**, 340–343

47a. Walls, E. V., Doyle, M. G., Patel, K. K., Allday, M. J., Catovsky, D. and Crawford, D. H. (1989) Activation and immortalization of leukaemic B cells by Epstein–Barr virus. *International Journal of Cancer* (in press)

48. Wirthmuller, R., Dennig, D., Oertel, J. and Gerhartz, H. (1983) Dipeptidylaminopeptidase IV (DAP IV) activity in normal and malignant T cell subsets as defined by monoclonal antibodies. *Scandinavian Journal of Haematology,* **31**, 197–205

49. Woods, G. M., Sawyer, P. J., Kirov, S. M., Lowenthal, R. M., Jupe, D. M. and Catovsky, D. (1985) Functional and phenotypic analysis of a T cell prolymphocytic leukemia. *Leukemia Research,* **9**, 587–596

50. Yam, L. T., Li, C. Y. and Crosby, W. H. (1971) Cytochemical identification of monocytes and granulocytes. *American Journal of Clinical Pathology,* **55**, 283–290

Chapter 6

Hairy cell leukaemia

Introduction

Hairy cell leukaemia (HCL) is a chronic lymphoproliferative disorder of the adult age group which accounts for approximately 2% of all forms of leukaemia. First described in 1958 by Bouroucle et al.[2] as leukaemic reticuloendotheliosis, it received several designations until the term 'hairy cell leukaemia', first coined by Shrek and Donnelly [80], was generally adopted. HCL is now a well-defined clinicopathological entity[1, 7, 11, 16] characterized by the proliferation of cells with long cytoplasmic projections, which are best appreciated by phase contrast microscopy and ultrastructural analysis [1, 25, 34, 50, 77, 80].

Numerous studies have been carried out in order to identify the origin of the hairy cell, to define its morphological, cytochemical and immunological features, and to recognize the possible counterpart of the malignant cell in normal tissues. Although great controversy has surrounded the early studies on the nature of the hairy cell, it is now generally accepted that these cells belong to the B-lymphocyte lineage [8, 11, 12, 47, 52, 63, 91]. This disease together will B-CLL and B-PLL represents one of the main clinical types of chronic B-cell leukaemia in humans. Significant strides forward on its treatment have been witnessed in the last 2 years [10, 48, 53, 86, 87].

Clinical and laboratory features (Table 6.1)

HCL affects middle-aged adults (generally over the age of 45), with an approximately four-fold male predominance [1, 35, 81]. Presenting symptoms may be non-specific and most often patients complain only of tiredness and/or dyspnoea on exertion. Haemorrhagic manifestations are only rarely present. In 15% of cases infection may be the initial complaint.

On examination, splenomegaly is the most frequent physical finding. A palpable spleen can be encountered in about 90% of patients. In 50% of them the spleen is palpable several centimetres below the left costal margin. Hepatomegaly is also present in half of the patients and lymphadenopathy is uncommon. Rare cases with massive lymphadenopathy have nevertheless been described both at diagnosis [6] and as a terminal event of the disease [62].

The blood counts always reveal variable degrees of cytopenia; 75% of patients have pancytopenia: anaemia, thrombocytopenia and neutropenia. The anaemia is

Table 6.1 Clinical and laboratory features of HCL[a]

Features		Incidence (%)
Splenomegaly		80–90
Hepatomegaly		50
HB	<12 g/dl	80
Platelets	<100 × 10⁹/l	80
Neutrophils	<1 × 10⁹/l	75
WBC count	<5	60
(× 10⁹/l)	5–10	20
	10–20	20
Hairy cells	<10%	10
(peripheral blood)	10–50%	65
	>50%	25

[a] Based on several reviews [1, 35, 81].

generally normochronic and normocytic. No haemolytic anaemia has been described and the direct antiglobulin test is usually negative. The pathogenesis of the anaemia is multifactorial and relates to bone marrow failure and/or increased splenic sequestration [57] and/or haemodilution due to an increased plasma volume. The white blood count is the most variable haematological parameter, although leucopenia is much more frequent than both a normal or a high count (Table 6.1). Leucocytosis of more than $10 \times 10^9/l$ is seen only in 20% of cases. Monocytopenia is also frequently associated with HCL, and this abnormality has been implicated in the pathogenesis of the atypical infections which characteristically accompany this disease [3, 37, 83].

Hairy cells are present in the peripheral blood of most patients and can be recognized on well-prepared films stained with May–Grünwald–Giemsa. The proportion of circulating hairy cells varies from case to case and only 25% of them have more than 50% hairy cells in the differential count [1, 35, 81]. For this reason a diagnosis of HCL, suspected on the basis of clinical and haematological features, often needs to be confirmed by either cytochemical, ultrastructural, histological or immunological methods. These are often necessary also for the differential diagnosis between HCL and other lymphoproliferative disorders.

Diagnostic features

Morphology

The recognition of the characteristic hairy cell is essential for a correct diagnosis of the disease. Hairy cells (Figure 6.1) are relatively large cells with a diameter of 10–20 µm, abundant cytoplasm and characteristic long villi protruding from the cytoplasm [1, 2, 10, 11, 16]. Occasionally, the cytoplasmic projections may not be obvious. The cytoplasm is weakly basophilic and occasionally shows few azurophilic granules. The nucleus is eccentric and round or indented in shape; nucleoli are only rarely seen. Occasionally, lymphocytes with a 'hairy' cytoplasm but without the other morphological features of hairy cells can be seen in films made from normal blood. Patients with genuine 'hairy' or 'villous' lymphocytes are

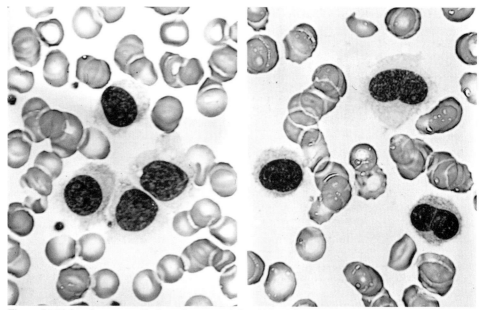

Figure 6.1 Light microscopy of hairy cells on a peripheral blood film from two patients. × 1400, reduced to 67% on reproduction

seen in some non-Hodgkin's lymphomas, chiefly immunocytoma and this is described in Chapter 7.

A rare variant of HCL has been reported [14, 19] (see below). In these cases the morphology of the hairy cells shows intermediate features between those of prolymphocytes (round and centrally placed nucleus and frequently with a nucleolus) and hairy cells (abundant cytoplasm and moderately long villi) (Figures 6.2 and 6.3).

Morphological examination at light microsopy carried out on peripheral blood and/or bone marrow films coupled to clinical features may not be sufficient to diagnose HCL with certainty unless the findings are typical. Additional techniques are often needed to establish the final diagnosis.

Bone marrow aspirate and biopsy

Bone marrow trephine biopsy represents a reliable diagnostic tool and must be performed in all cases in which a diagnosis of HCL is considered, particularly when this is suspected on clinicohaematological grounds but there is a paucity of circulating hairy cells [7, 88]. Bone marrow aspirates are often unsuccessful in HCL (dry tap). This is due to a moderate or marked increase in reticulin fibres as well as to leukaemic infiltration. Sufficient diagnostic material is obtained by aspiration in less than half of the patients. The cells infiltrating the bone marrow are morphologically similar to those seen in the peripheral blood films although the cytoplasmic projections are less prominent in the former.

The bone marrow biopsy shows in most cases a diffuse infiltration by hairy cells, recognized by their blunt nucleus. In a minority of cases patchy infiltration can be

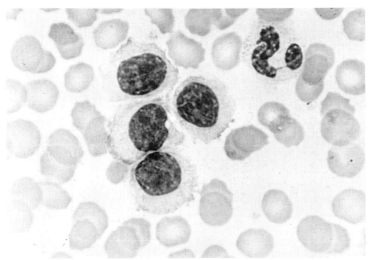

Figure 6.2 Peripheral blood cells from a patient with the HCL-variant, showing a round nucleus and a visible nucleolus in three of them. × 1400, reduced to 61% on reproduction

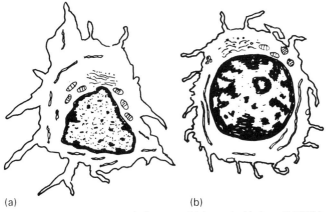

(a)   (b)

Figure 6.3 Diagram of the main features of (a) a typical hairy cell (HCL) and (b) a cell of the HCL-variant

found, more frequently in the early stages of the disease [1]. Hairy cells infiltrate the bone marrow in a characteristic loose fashion with a well-defined rim of cytoplasm which leaves a clear zone around the cells. These appearances facilitate the differential diagnosis from other lymphoproliferative disorders which have either a more heavy and closely packed lymphocyte infiltration, as in B-CLL and B-PLL, or a predominantly paratrabecular arrangement, as in follicular lymphoma. Fibrosis of the bone marrow due to increased reticulin formation is always present, particularly in the areas of neoplastic infiltration [7, 88].

The size and composition of the residual normal haemopoiesis may indicate whether there will be a good recovery of the blood counts following splenectomy, and whether alternative therapies may be required. When the bone marrow is heavily infiltrated (e.g. over 80%) with little residual haemopoiesis, the chances of success with splenectomy alone are minimal.

Spleen histology

Splenectomy is often performed in most patients with HCL at some stage during the course of the disease. In all cases the spleen shows distinct histological features which are clearly different from those observed in other lymphoproliferative disorders [1, 66]. Thus, the spleen histology may be useful to confirm or exclude a diagnosis of HCL in difficult cases.

Microscopically the sections show heavy infiltration of the red pulp and widening of the pulp cords. This accumulation of leukaemic cells often produces an engorgement of the sinuses. The white pulp may also be affected altering the architecture of the malpighian corpuscles and often leading to their atrophy. A characteristic feature of the spleen in HCL is the presence of the so-called 'pseudosinuses' in the red pulp lined by hairy cells [66]. The sinuses are filled with erythrocytes and leucocytes; in some cases these pseudosinuses may resemble haemangiomas. No mitoses are generally seen, nor is any significant degree of extramedullary haemopoiesis observed in the spleen sections.

Liver histology

A liver biopsy is rarely performed for diagnostic purposes. Data on the liver histology in HCL are therefore mainly derived from biopsies carried out at the time of splenectomy or from autopsy specimens. A diffuse infiltration of the hepatic sinuses and of the portal tracts by leukaemic cells has been reported in the majority of cases [1, 16]. The overall architecture of the liver is preserved. In 10–20% of cases no evidence of liver infiltration can be documented.

Lymph node histology

As described above, lymph nodes are enlarged in a minority of patients and therefore a lymph node biopsy is only exceptionally performed in this disease. Data from lymph nodes examined at autopsy or at the time of splenectomy have demonstrated a diffuse infiltration by leukaemic cells in most cases [1].

Cytochemistry

It is now well recognized that a moderately strong acid phosphatase reaction, not inhibited by tartaric acid, is the most typical cytochemical property of hairy cells[93, 94]. This tartrate-resistant acid phosphatase (TRAP) is seen in the form of irregular small granules diffusely distributed throughout the cytoplasm of the cells. The cytochemical reaction has been demonstrated both in buffy coat films and also in tissue sections [40, 66]. Within the different acid phosphatase isoenzymes shown by polyacrylamide gel electrophoresis, it has been shown that the characteristic tartrate-resistance of hairy cells is a property of the isoenzyme 5[93].

The percentage of TRAP+ cells in HCL varies greatly and in some cases it may be extremely low or even completely negative. Although this cytochemical reaction appears to be fairly specific for hairy cells[93], it should be recalled that TRAP activity has been occasionally also documented in other lymphoproliferative disorders of B-cell origin[11] and, rarely, in chronic T-cell leukamia (see Table 5.5, Chapter 5).

Inconsistent results have been reported with the non-specific esterase reactions. Both α-naphthylacetate esterase and butyrate esterase may be weakly to moderately strongly positive in a proportion of cases with a characteristic pattern of fine to coarse granules in the cytoplasm arranged in a crescent configuration [42].

The combined positivity of acid phosphatase and non-specific esterase results in a typical cytochemical profile in hairy cells which is distinct from that seen in other B- and T-chronic lymphoproliferative disorders[23] (see Tables 5.4 and 5.5, Chapter 5).

Electron microscopy

Transmission electron microscopy constitutes a useful tool for the diagnosis of HCL in cases in which the morphology of the cells in films or tissue biopsies is far from typical. The ultrastructural aspect of hairy cells is quite unique and clearly distinguishes this form of leukaemia from other lymphoproliferative disorders (Figures 6.4 and 6.5)[10, 11, 25, 50]. Along with other features, two structures are quite characteristic of hairy cells: first are the cytoplasmic villi which are long, measuring between 0.5 and 4.0 μm, and have a broad base. In some tissues the microvilli may be seen interdigitating with those of neighbouring cells. The other ultrastructural peculiarity of HCL cells is represented by the so-called ribosome–lamella complexes seen in 50% of cases (Figures 6.4 and 6.5). These cylindric structures, formed by numerous parallel membranes containing rows of ribosomes[77], were initially thought to be unique to HCL[50]. However, similar or identical structures have been observed, though less frequently, in B-CLL, monoblastic leukaemia and Waldenström's macroglobulinaemia[5]. In well-stained preparations it is possible to identify ribosome–lamella complexes by light

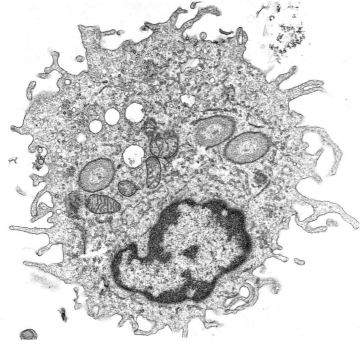

Figure 6.4 Ultrastructure of a typical hairy cell showing three ribosome–lamella complexes and abundant villi. × 16 000, reduced to 74% on reproduction

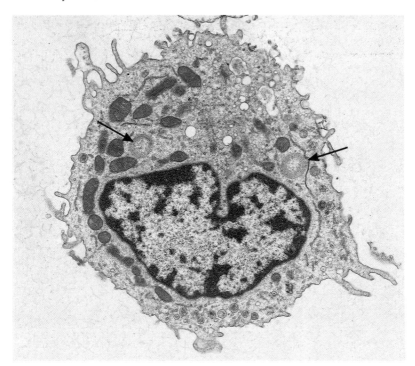

Figure 6.5 Electron microscopic photomicrograph from another HCL also showing two small ribosome–lamella complexes and small numbers of lysosomal granules in the cytoplasm. × 14 000, reduced to 75% on reproduction

microscopy[49]. The nucleus of hairy cells measures 8–12 μm in diameter, is generally oval and often indented. In some cases a small nucleolus may be visible. The cytoplasm is abundant with many free ribosomes and small numbers of electron-dense granules (Figure 6.5). The long cytoplasmic projections explain the large cell volume recorded by flow cytometry which is significantly greater than in cells from B-CLL and B-PLL [4, 22] (see below).

Morphometric analysis of some ultrastructural features could define in a quantitive and objective fashion the morphological characteristics that distinguish hairy cells from other neoplastic B-cells, namely: greater size, lower nucleo-/ cytoplasmic ratio, inconspicuous and/or small nucleolus, greater cytoplasmic contour index and a more irregular nuclear outline[74a].

Scanning electron microscopy demonstrates various types of villous structures, a mixture of the thin villi of B-lymphocytes with the broad-based membrane ruffles of monocytes[34].

Membrane markers

For many years the origin and nature of hairy cells was a matter of controversy. The early data suggesting a monocytic origin and the more recent demonstration of B-cell features will be discussed in more detail at the end of this chapter.

As shown in Chapter 1 (see Table 1.8), cells from HCL have membrane phenotype characteristics similar to other B-cell disorders, especially B-PLL, and other features which are unique and which may be helpful for the purposes of differential diagnosis. The cells in the great majority of cases show monoclonal SmIg with unequivocal light chain restriction. In contradistinction from other conditions, however, hairy cells may express more than one heavy chain isotype on the membrane but with a single light chain[8, 11, 32]. A finding reported by several groups is the presence of IgA in addition to IgG or IgM. The proportion of cases with membrane IgG is higher than in other B-cell leukaemias[11]. In 25% of cases, hairy cells bind mouse erythrocytes[15], although rarely the percentage of M-rosettes is greater than 50%, a feature which is typical of B-CLL (see Chapter 1).

Studies with monoclonal antibodies have shown that hairy cells display a distinctive antigenic make-up. They are always positive with FMC7[12, 47, 63, 91], RFB1[63], anti-Tac (CD25)[52], monoclonal antibodies of the CD22 group (Leu14, To15), and LeuM5 (CD11c), which reacts with an antigen also expressed in monocytes and macrophages. In addition these cells react with monoclonal antibodies against class II HLA determinants (Ia-antigen) and other pan-B reagents such as B4 (CD19) and B1 (CD20) (see Table 1.8, Chapter 1) and with specific anti-HCL monoclonal antibodies: HC1, HC2[69, 70] and B-ly7[87a]. In contrast to B-CLL, hairy cells are usually negative with monoclonal antibodies against the T1 (CD5) antigen (Leu1, T101 etc.)[63] (see also Chapter 1). Because of the presence on the cell membrane of Fc receptors with high affinity for IgG, special care should be taken when performing marker studies on hairy cells, particularly when using monoclonal antibodies. As with monocytes, both the first layer (mouse IgG) or second layer (goat anti-mouse Ig) can bind non-specifically to the Fc receptors. It is recommended that affinity purified $F(ab)_2$ antibodies are always used for the second layer and that the Fc receptors are blocked with 2% human AB serum. Control ascites of the same Ig subclass as that of the primary monoclonal antibodies should always be included as a control. For testing SmIg the use of directly conjugated $F(ab)_2$ antibody and pre-incubation of the sample in serum-free media for 1 or 2 hours at 37°C will help to obtain reproducible results. Part of the early difficulties in characterizing hairy cells was due to unawareness of these technical problems.

Assessment of spleen and bone marrow functions

The degree of splenomegaly in HCL may be extremely variable. Thus, together with patients with massive splenomegaly, some of whom may in fact represent a distinct 'splenic' form of the disease, others show only a modest splenic enlargement.

Because the anaemia in HCL often results from the combined effect of a depressed bone marrow function and an increased splenic pooling, isotope studies to assess the contribution of the spleen and the bone marrow may be useful to evaluate the main mechanism of the anaemia in individual patients. Isotope studies have shown that the splenic red cell pool is greatly increased in HCL compared to patients with other disorders that have a similar degree of splenomegaly[57]. These findings are probably related to the unique histological lesions of the spleen in HCL with its dilated red cords and typical pseudosinuses[57, 66]. Splenic pooling also produces a lengthened exposure of the blood to the phagocytic activity of the reticuloendothelial system. Isotope studies may also be useful to assess the possible beneficial effect of splenectomy.

It is useful to predict whether a particular patient will require further treatment following splenectomy, and for this an assessment of the normal bone marrow haemopoietic reserve is also important. In general a good assessment can be obtained from the trephine biopsies[39] but ferrokinetic studies have also been shown to be useful for this purpose. Patients presenting with very low reticulocyte counts and a low haemoglobin have, as a rule, a compromised bone marrow regardless of the spleen pooling studies.

Differential diagnosis

This should be considered in the context of other conditions that have bone marrow fibrosis, splenomegaly and abnormal lymphocytes in the peripheral blood. The rare splenic form of B-CLL (see Chapter 3) may occasionally present diagnostic difficulties with HCL when the patients have a low white blood cell (WBC) count and a large spleen without lymphadenopathy. The following features should be taken into account for the differential diagnosis between these two disorders:

1. The bone marrow aspirate is often easily obtained in B-CLL and shows increased cellularity with predominant infiltration with small lymphocytes.
2. The bone marrow histology is very different: in B-CLL there is either heavy infiltration with packed small lymphocytes or nodular aggregates and this contrasts with the characteristic loose infiltrate in HCL (see above).
3. The distinct morphology of the circulating cells. Patients with HCL and a high WBC count, in the range of those found in B-CLL, invariably have a high proportion of typical hairy cells in the peripheral blood which can be easily recognized from the small B-CLL lymphocytes.
4. Cytochemistry: acid phosphatase positive cells in HCL and negative in B-CLL.
5. Membrane markers in B-CLL: CD5+, SmIg+ (weak), M-rosettes+ (over 50% of cells) and in HCL: CD5−, SmIg+ (strong), M-rosettes+ (20–40% of cells) as well as expression of other antigens, e.g. CD25, CD11c, HC2 etc. – see Table 1.8, Chapter 1.

The differential diagnosis with B-PLL is generally easy on the basis of the very high WBC count and the prominent nucleoli characteristic of prolymphocytes although occasionally B-PLL cells may show a 'hairy' cytoplasm. The membrane phenotype of hairy cells is very similar to that of B-prolymphocytes (see Table 1.8, Chapter 1) and this may also present diagnostic problems. Some difficulties can also arise with the rare cases of the HCL-variant which have a higher WBC count than typical HCL as well as a large spleen (see Figure 6.2 and see below).

Primary myelofibrosis is sometimes considered in cases with no circulating hairy cells, but the correct diagnosis should not be difficult on the basis of the bone marrow biopsy findings. Waldenström's macroglobulinaemia and immunocytoma are recognized by typical trephine biopsy features as well as by the presence of a distinct monoclonal band in the serum. An IgM or IgG paraprotein, although rare, has been well recognized in HCL[11, 18, 32, 44]. A frequent problem is posed by a lymphoplasmacytic splenic lymphoma (or immunocytoma) with splenomegaly and villous lymphocytes in the peripheral blood (SLVL). This condition, described in detail in Chapter 7, can be distinguished from HCL by the histology of the spleen and bone marrow and the morphology and cytochemistry of the circulating cells. It should be noted that the membrane markers may be very similar in both diseases, although the consistent reactivity with anti-HC2 and anti-Tac (CD25) in hairy cells is not seen in SLVL; CD11c (LeuM5) is also infrequently positive in SLVL.

Prognostic features

Patients with HCL have a variable clinical course and, as a result, their life expectancy may be extremely different, ranging from early deaths, particularly in the first 2 years from diagnosis, to a relatively long clinical course of 10 or more years[1, 10, 35, 36]. In this respect, the search for clinical, haematological or immunological parameters which may bear prognostic implications is of relevance. Such studies have shown that prognosis in HCL is directly correlated with the degree of pancytopenia at diagnosis[35, 45]. Patients with low levels of haemoglobin (<8 g/dl), low neutrophil counts ($<0.5 \times 10^9$/l), and low platelet counts ($<50 \times 10^9$/l) have been shown to require a more prompt therapeutic intervention.

Staging

Jansen and Hermans[46] proposed a clinical staging system on the basis of data from 391 patients included in a multicentre study contributed by 22 institutions. Three aspects were considered. First, several clinico-laboratory features were analysed in order to predict survival time from diagnosis. Secondly, the attention was focused on which patients would benefit from splenectomy and, thirdly, data from splenectomized patients were analysed in order to predict survival postsplenectomy. The latter two aspects will be dealt with in the section on treatment.

The two most important and reliable prognostic parameters for predicting survival in non-splenectomized patients are the level of haemoglobin and the size of the spleen[46]. Based on combinations of these two features a rather complex staging system has evolved[46]. Patients were accordingly grouped in three stages (I, II, III), each including about one-third of the cases. Lack of anaemia with a small spleen was the best group (I); high degree of anaemia with a large spleen was worst (III). A good correlation was observed between staging and the actuarial survival. The weakness of this scheme is that it may not be valid once the patient (i.e. stage III) is splenectomized. Another prognostic feature is represented by the number of circulating hairy cells. Patients with a high proportion of hairy cells appear to fare poorly. Based on this study[46], the neutrophil count does not represent a significant prognostic indicator, despite the fact that infection is the main cause of death in patients with HCL (see below). Persisting neutropenia after splenectomy has, on the other hand, a poor prognosis[35].

The overall median survival in HCL has been of the order of 4–5 years[35, 36]. Improvements in prognosis as a result of new therapies will be discussed in the next section.

Splenic and bone marrow forms

Along with the majority of patients who show bone marrow and spleen involvement, individual cases with atypical features have been reported. Some patients appear to have a pure 'splenic' form of the disease. Five such patients with massive splenomegaly have been described in the literature[1, 11, 65, 66a, 85]. In all these cases the clinicohaematological picture improved dramatically following splenectomy and the patients remained well and in complete remission without evidence of active disease for many years. It is likely therefore that in these cases the disease was mainly confined to the spleen with minimal or no bone marrow involvement.

On the other hand, the presence of pancytopenia in patients with marked marrow involvement and without splenic enlargement suggests that this is mainly due to bone marrow failure. As opposed to the 'splenic' form of HCL, these patients may suffer from a 'bone marrow' form of the disease. To date, however, the authors are not aware of a single case report of HCL with bone marrow involvement and normal spleen histology. Presumably no splenic tissue was examined in such rare cases. It is of interest that the multicentre study reported by Jansen and Hermans[45] concluded that splenectomy did not improve the survival of patients with a small spleen. In such cases it may be important to try to assess carefully the bone marrow and splenic function before any therapeutic measure is decided.

Treatment

Because HCL patient are often symptomatic they will always require some form of treatment. Only a small group of patients may be followed with only close clinical and haematological attention without the need of any form of therapy. The disease in such patients is not aggressive and may remain stable for many years. Golomb et al.[35] identified a small subgroup of patients who are slightly older than average and have only minimal splenomegaly with few hairy cells in the peripheral blood and who may not require any therapeutic intervention.

The four main treatment approaches that have been employed in HCL are splenectomy, chemotherapy, α-interferon and 2'-deoxycoformycin. Other modalities, including a single case treated by syngeneic bone marrow transplantation, have also been attempted.

Splenectomy

Splenectomy remains one of the treatments of choice in the management of HCL, although the effectivity of this procedure is largely dependent on the size of the spleen and the degree of bone marrow infiltration which will determine whether further treatment will be necessary[10, 39]. Splenectomy may not be necessary or effective if anaemia and/or the other cytopenias are only partly due to splenic sequestration and result mainly from bone marrow failure. The main indication for splenectomy is the degree of cytopenia in the presence of splenomegaly. Its main beneficial effect, both in terms of haematological improvement and prognosis, has been documented in several studies[1, 11, 35, 45]. A large multicentre (non-randomized) study[45] has convincingly demonstrated the value of splenectomy in a series of 391 patients. However, correlations between clinical findings and response to surgery indicate that splenectomy is less beneficial in patients with spleens palpable less than 4 cm below the costal margin, with the possible exception of cases showing concomitant anaemia[45]. The benefits of splenectomy are more often evident on the platelet count, followed by the haemoglobin level and, last, by a rise in the neutrophil count.

It is important to be able to predict the long-term benefits of splenectomy. A complete response, judged by an improvement in the three blood parameters (haemoglobin, platelets and neutrophils), reflecting good bone marrow function, is associated with good prognosis[11]. This has been confirmed also in Jansen and Hermans' series[45], in which complete responders were considered to be those who reached values of haemoglobin >11 g/dl, platelets >100 × 10^9/l and neutrophils >1 × 10^9/l after splenectomy. The majority of these patients were alive 5 years after splenectomy. Overall, it can be estimated that 10% of HCL patients may not require any other treatment after a successful splenectomy. Using data from the multicentre study, the same authors[46] suggested a postsplenectomy staging system based on the levels of haemoglobin and neutrophils 2–3 months after surgery. This system allowed them to subdivide splenectomized patients as follows: no cytopenia = best prognosis; moderate anaemia or neutropenia = intermediate prognosis; moderate anaemia and neutropenia or severe anaemia = worst prognosis. A good correlation was observed in that series between the postsplenectomy staging system and the probability of survival[46]. This system should be of value for selecting patients who, following splenectomy, may require alternative therapeutic approaches. On the other hand, using a simple system based on the analysis of trephine biopsies before splenectomy, Golomb and Vardiman[39] found that the core biopsy/hairy cell index correlated well with the platelet recovery after the operation. Furthermore, they suggested that this index could also be used to predict complete or partial responders to splenectomy and thus to foresee patients who will require early chemotherapy.

Chemotherapy

Although the validity of chemotherapy in the management of HCL has been debated in the past, many patients will require at some stage of their illness alternative forms of treatment other than splenectomy. These include those who have a poor response to splenectomy (30–40% of cases), those who relapse some time after splenectomy (another 30%), as well as those considered unsuitable for surgery on the basis of minimal or no splenic enlargement. Early reports of chemotherapy in HCL before splenectomy have been disappointing[1, 27]. Part of the problem has to be ascribed to the lack of adequate supportive care facilities in the 1970s.

Relatively good results have been reported using low-dose continuous chlorambucil (4 mg/day) [33]. Although it has been difficult to obtain a complete remission with this regimen, clinicohaematological improvements have been observed in the majority of patients. A major drawback is that neutropenia rarely improves and this may result in severe infectious complications. An example of the response in a patient treated by the authors is shown in Figure 6.6. Cyclophosphamide has also been used in some patients with similarly good effects[11]. However, the advent of newer, less toxic and more specific forms of therapy (see below) will reduce the indications for alkylating agents to a few special cases in which the new treatments or splenectomy are contraindicated.

A more intensive approach with cytotoxic drugs such as doxorubicin or rubidazone, used either alone or in combination, has resulted in complete or partial remission in most patients treated[26, 60, 61]. This therapy should, however, be considered as third-line treatment and attempted only when other forms of therapy are no longer effective. Furthermore, ablative chemotherapy should be initiated only if adequate and prolonged haematological support of the same quality as those utilized for acute leukaemia patients can be guaranteed.

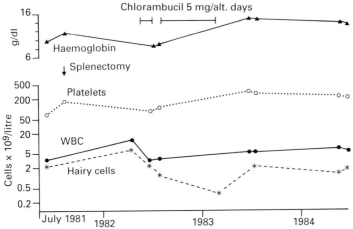

Figure 6.6 Haematological chart illustrating the partial response to chlorambucil therapy in a patient with HCL. Note the significant increase in haemoglobin and platelet count and the reduction in the hairy cell numbers. He relapsed 19 months later and achieved a good partial response to α-interferon (not shown) which lasted 32 months. He achieved later for the first time a complete remission with 2'-deoxycoformycin which is lasting more than 6 months off all therapy at present

α-Interferon

Important results have been reported by using partially purified leucocyte α-interferon in the treatment of HCL. Quesada et al.[73] described three complete and four partial remissions in seven patients aged between 26 and 51 years treated with daily doses of 3 MU of α-interferon intramuscularly. Remissions were maintained for up to 10 months. All patients studied had a clinicohaematological picture of slowly progressive disease; none was profoundly pancytopenic when treatment was commenced. This exciting report on the beneficial effect of α-interferon in HCL has now largely been confirmed in a number of studies (see reviews[10, 87]). Over 200 HCL patients with pancytopenia have been treated in the UK and in Italy with a highly purified (85% pure) preparation of human lymphoblastoid α-interferon [Wellferon (Wellcome)], obtained from the supernatant of a Burkitt's lymphoma-derived cell line which produces α-interferon upon stimulation with the Sendai virus. All patients treated so far showed a significant improvement in the blood counts and a rapid fall in the hairy cell counts[10]. Some of them were resistant to chlorambucil, as in the case illustrated in Figure 6.7. The treatment was given initially with the same schedule as used by Quesada et al.[73], 3 MU daily, and the side effects have been negligible. Other pure preparations of α-interferon obtained by recombinant DNA technology [i.e. Intron (Schering) and Roferon (Roche)] are currently being used[87] with similar success and low toxicity.

After 5 years' experience with α-interferon in the treatment of HCL[10, 87], the status of this biological response modifier can be summarized as follows:

1. Ninety per cent of patients achieve, within 6 months, normalization of blood counts; this includes disappearance of circulating hairy cells, reappearance of monocytes, normal or slightly reduced neutrophil counts (due to an effect of α-interferon on granulopoiesis), normal or higher than normal haemoglobin levels, and normal platelet counts.

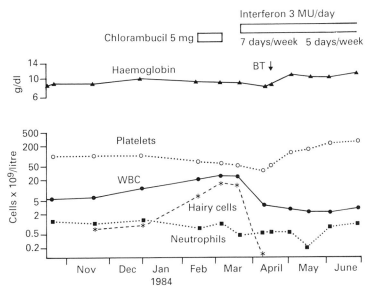

Figure 6.7 Diagram illustrating the response of an HCL patient to α-interferon. This patient had a good response to chlorambucil in 1983 (not shown) but on restarting this therapy in February 1984 showed no response. The administration of Wellferon (Wellcome) resulted in a normalization of the blood counts and a disappearance of the circulating hairy cells

2. Significant reduction of hairy cell infiltration from the bone marrow with complete clinicohaematological remissions in approximately one-third of the cases.

3. Quality and durability of the response seems to depend on the duration of treatment; optimal results require at least 1 year of therapy and these are even better after 2 years.

4. Responses are obtained with daily or 3-weekly injections and also with doses lower than the standard 3-MU injections. Responses are quicker with daily injections; these are often reduced in frequency once blood counts are normalized.

5. Good responses can be obtained without resorting to splenectomy, but these may take longer than in splenectomized patients.

6. The median duration of remission after discontinuation of therapy is 15 months. The majority of patients will relapse slowly off therapy but few seem to relapse on long-term maintenance with 1- or 2-weekly injections.

7. Re-treatment after relapse is usually successful; resistance to α-interferon seems to be rare.

8. Side effects are seen mainly during the first few weeks. There is no evidence yet of any deleterious effect on long-term therapy with this agent.

Despite its remarkable effect on HCL, the exact mechanism of action of α-interferon in this disease is unknown. An indirect action via the stimulation of natural killer cells, whose activity improves with treatment[31a], has been ruled out in favour of a direct effect upon the hairy cells mediated via specific interferon receptors on the cell surface. Hairy cells have higher levels of interferon receptors than cells of other disorders but this difference may not be enough to account for their greater sensitivity. It is of interest that patients with the HCL-variant do not seem to benefit from this treatment and the cells in some of them have low levels of α-interferon receptors (G. Flandrin, personal communication).

Other forms of treatment

Lithium carbonate has been tried in the hope of improving the haemopoietic function, in particular neutropenia, but the overall results have been disappointing. Good results have been reported using intensive leucapheresis in four patients[31, 64] but this procedure is obviously time consuming and may be reserved for the rare cases with high WBC counts. The beneficial effect of leucapheresis lasted for up to 2 years from the procedure.

Splenic irradiation has also been used to treat HCL with some beneficial effects[1, 84]. The response to radiotherapy was observed several weeks after the completion of treatment. Prolonged responses have been reported in a few cases.

An important, but so far unique, approach has been reported by Cheever et al.[21] – the sucessful bone marrow transplant carried out in a 47-year-old patient from his identical twin. At the time of the report the patient, previously splenectomized, had no signs of disease activity and had normal peripheral blood counts 4 years after the transplant. This study demonstrates that high-dose chemotherapy and total body irradiation followed by syngeneic bone marrow transplantation can be effective in eradicating hairy cells successfully for long periods. As hairy cells have a slow proliferative activity, it is still too early to suggest that the patient has been cured. Quesada et al.[71] also described good remissions in seven patients who were given allogeneic mononuclear cells from siblings collected by means of a cell separator. These observations are suggestive of a possible immune-mediated response, although it cannot be excluded that the allogeneic cells may act directly on the bone marrow precursors possibly via the production of growth factors which are reduced or absent in the florid phase of the disease[74]. The main source of these factors is the monocytes which are characteristically impaired in HCL patients[43, 83].

2'-Deoxycoformycin

2'-Deoxycoformycin, also known as Pentostatin, is a potent inhibitor of the enzyme adenosine deaminase (ADA) which has lately been shown to have a remarkable effect in HCL. Three reports[48, 53, 86] have described a high response rate, including a greater proportion of complete remissions, with aspirable bone marrow, than observed with α-interferon. Early work in T-ALL was disappointing because higher doses of DCF were necessary to inhibit the high levels of adenosine deaminase in T-lymphoblasts and this proved too nephrotoxic. The recent reports have shown that lower doses can be effective with less toxicity in HCL where the cellular concentration of adenosine deaminase is very low. Although the drug is only available for controlled trials, these results are highly encouraging. The different doses used by these authors may have a bearing on the toxicity of the agent. Johnston et al.[48] used $4 \, mg/m^2$ per week for 3 consecutive weeks and observed two complete and four partial remissions in eight patients. Kraut et al.[53], with a lower dose ($4 \, mg/m^2$ every 2 weeks), documented nine complete remissions in ten patients. The largest study so far, from the Eastern Cooperative Study Group and reported by Spiers et al.[86], who made the initial observations in

HCL, treated 37 patients of whom 34 were evaluable. Complete remissions were observed in 53% and partial remissions in 38%, with only 9% non-responders. The responses were obtained over a period of 3–4 months and seem to be prolonged, e.g. longer than 1 year in some patients. This study used doses of 5 mg/m^2 given for 3 consecutive days every 4 weeks or for 2 days every 2 weeks and, perhaps predictably, recorded a higher toxicity than the other two. Five patients (15%) died of infections and three suffered life-threatening complications[86].

The authors' experience with DCF has been summarized in two recent reports[28a, 28b]. Forty patients have been treated and followed up for a minimum of 6 months; 33 of them had been previously treated with α-interferon. DCF was administered at the dose of 4 mg/m^2 weekly for the first 4 weeks, but recently the protocol has been modified to one injection every 2 weeks. Upon remission, no further treatment was given. The overall response rate was 97% with 82% complete and 15% partial remissions[28b]. The remissions seem to be long lasting but comparisons with α-interferon are still too early. Severe infections developed in 10% of patients treated with DCF and one died of sepsis before the response could be evaluated. Pre-treatment with α-interferon for 3–6 months immediately prior to the use of DCF, aimed at improving the haematological and clinical status, was associated with fewer infections and the need for less DCF injections than when α-interferon was not given prior to DCF. Although DCF may be more effective than α-interferon it has, at the same time, greater myelotoxicity and immunosuppressive potential. Patients need to have normal renal function, be free of infections and have a relatively good performance status before starting DCF. Infection is, however, not a contraindication for using α-interferon and several patients have been observed whose infections recovered without interrupting this treatment.

It is too early to draw definitive conclusions about the relative merits of these two agents in HCL because comparative trials have not as yet been completed. In fact it is likely that the ideal approach for a cure of this disease should involve first splenectomy (if indicated according to spleen size), then α-interferon to induce a further reduction in the hairy cell mass and to normalize the blood counts and, finally, when bone marrow function has been restored, DCF to eradicate any residual disease[28a].

Monitoring the response to α-interferon and DCF is only possible by means of high quality bone marrow trephine biopsies. Even with good pathological material, the assessment of complete remission may be difficult with standard histology. In the authors' experience, immunocytochemical methods performed on frozen sections with some of the anti-HCL specific monoclonal antibodies, e.g. HC2, CD25 and B-ly 7, significantly improve the results and could indicate the presence of residual disease when the conventional techniques appeared to show none. Some anti-B-cell antibodies can be used in sections from paraffin-embedded biopsies, e.g. L26, and these may also provide useful diagnostic information.

Complications and unusual associations

Infections

These were a frequent accompanying feature of HCL before useful treatments became available and used to represent the primary cause of mortality in this disease[1, 3, 11, 34]. Half of the patients are affected at some stage throughout the course of their illness. A culture-documented infection can be found only in a proportion of cases and this varies from series to series. Pneumonia and septicaemia due to Gram-negative organisms are the most frequent causes of serious infection and often of death. Gram-positive bacteria, fungi, viruses etc. have also been implicated. A surprisingly high frequency of mycobacterial infections has been reported in patients with HCL. The incidence of tuberculosis in the range of 5–10% according to various reports[37, 81, 90] is much higher than in other haematological malignancies. Often the infection is caused by atypical mycobacteria[59, 90] which may show a poor response to conventional treatment. In all patients with a clinical picture of persistent undetermined fever and no positive cultures, also in the absence of documented lung infiltrates, a diagnosis of mycobacterial infection (typical and atypical) should always be considered. In this respect the important diagnostic role of a liver biopsy must be stressed as very often the mycobacterial involvement affects the visceral organs only. Other causes of obscure fever in this disease are *Toxoplasma* and atypical fungal infections.

Both granulocytopenia and monocytopenia play an important role in the pathogenesis of the infective complications frequently seen in HCL. The correlation between neutropenia and infections has been well documented[3, 35, 37]. The incidence of serious infections is significantly higher in patients with a granulocytopenia of less than $0.5 \times 10^9/l$, compared with that of patients with a granulocyte count greater than $0.5 \times 10^9/l$[37]. In addition to granulocytopenia, an impaired leucocyte mobilization may contribute to the frequent occurrence of pyogenic infections[92]. It is likely that monocytopenia[43, 83] plays a major role in the high incidence of non-pyogenic infections, particularly tuberculosis. Together with the quantitative reduction in monocytes, a poor or absent mobilization capacity by mononuclear cells and the presence of inhibitors of normal monocyte chemotactic activity have been reported[92]. However, unlike in other chronic leukaemias, the humoral immunity in patients with HCL is usually normal[54].

Splenectomy does not appear to be a hazardous procedure in HCL as the incidence of infective complications is low in splenectomized patients presumably as a result of the improved blood counts. Other forms of treatment, namely corticosteroids, are known to increase the risk of infections[3]. A common practice in HCL, as well as in other B-cell disorders with impaired immunity, is to institute long-term prophylaxis with oral penicillin after splenectomy because the ability of these patients to mount an antibody response to anti-pneumococcal vaccines may be inadequate.

Infection is a frequent and potentially serious complication which represents the primary cause of death in untreated HCL. Although not all episodes may be severe, it is imperative to consider always HCL patients at risk, and to investigate thoroughly all episodes of fever, bearing in mind the frequent atypical aetiology of the infections.

Association with systemic vasculitis

The first report of a possible association between HCL and systemic vasculitis was that of Elkon et al.[30], who described four cases of HCL with features similar to those of periarteritis nodosa. Thereafter, other cases with a similar or related picture have been described[29, 56] including a patient with HCL, rheumatoid arthritis and high levels of circulating immune complexes[24]. As this association has been observed more frequently in splenectomized patients, it has been suggested that the clinical manifestations may be related to a poor clearance of circulating immune complexes[11].

Osteolytic lesions

In the last few years several investigators have described cases of HCL accompanied by osteolytic lesions[11, 28, 44, 72, 76, 89]. On the basis of the different series the incidence of osteolytic lesions can be estimated to be of the order of 3%. The bone lesions seem to be localized more frequently in the upper femur and may or may not be accompanied by paraproteinaemia[18, 32]. In some cases both osteolytic lesions and paraproteinaemia have been observed[13, 44, 67]. In two of these reports[13, 67] a clearly distinct picture of myelomatosis coexisted with that of typical HCL and the plasma cells were the cells responsible for the osteolysis. In contrast the bone lesions in the two cases reported by Jansen et al.[44] were caused by the hairy cells and in one of them it was possible to demonstrate that the M-protein was also synthesized by these cells.

To date, the occurrence of isolated paraproteinaemia or osteolytic lesions has not been associated with poor prognosis, whilst the cases with both paraproteinaemia and bone lesions had a progressive and rapidly fatal disease[44] . The localized bone lesions in HCL can be treated successfully with local radiotherapy[72, 76].

The evidence of the association of HCL and osteolytic lesions, and/or paraproteinaemia, further points to the B-cell origin of the hairy cells. These manifestations have been also described in other B-lymphoproliferative disorders, such as Waldenström's macroglobulinaemia and B-CLL, in addition to myelomatosis. The possible relationship between hairy cells and plasma cells is also suggested by the rare occurrence of amyloidosis complicating HCL[29, 58].

Atypical forms of HCL

As mentioned previously, lymphadenopathy is a rare finding in HCL. Nevertheless, individual patients with massively or moderately enlarged abdominal lymphadenopathy have been reported[27]. Budman et al.[6] described a patient with generalized lymphadenopathy and an accompanying cutaneous involvement who was unresponsive both to chemotherapy and radiotherapy. Mehta et al.[62] reported a patient with HCL and systemic vasculitis whose clinical course was complicated by massive retroperitoneal lymphadenopathy (histologically showing only HCL) and ascites.

Hairy cell variant

Cawley et al.[19] first described two patients with a distinct chronic lymphoproliferative disorder as a variant of HCL. A further case with similar characteristics has been reported by the authors[14]. These patients have a chronic course and marked splenomegaly and in contrast to typical HCL cases, have a high WBC count (range $47-110 \times 10^9$/l) without monocytopenia or neutropenia and a bone marrow that is easy to aspirate. It is of interest that the three reported cases had IgG on the cell membrane. The neoplastic cells show a 'hairy' morphology with a nucleo-/cytoplasmic ratio higher than in typical HCL and have a centrally placed round nucleus with prominent nucleolus (see Figure 6.3). The TRAP activity is positive but weaker than in typical HCL. The ultrastructural features of these 'intermediate' hairy cells can be appreciated in Figure 6.8. A detailed comparison between B-PLL, HCL and HCL-variant has been reported elsewhere [14]. Based on clinical, morphological and immunological studies the authors have postulated that this variant may represent an intermediate disease between HCL and B-PLL [14]. Cell volume studies with a Coulter ZBI linked to a Coulter Channelizer [22] demonstrate that the volume of the variant cells is larger than the volume of B-CLL and B-PLL cells (Figure 6.9) and is similar to that of typical hairy cells (Figure 6.10). The membrane phenotype of the HCL-variant cells is more similar to that of B-prolymphocytes than to hairy cells. For example, HC2 (see Chapter 1) and CD25 (Tac) are as a rule negative. It is of interest that IgG is the main heavy chain demonstrable in these cells. Patients with the HCL-variant may respond to chlorambucil and have a good prognosis despite the high WBC count. However, they do not respond to α-interferon or DCF, as do typical HCL cases.

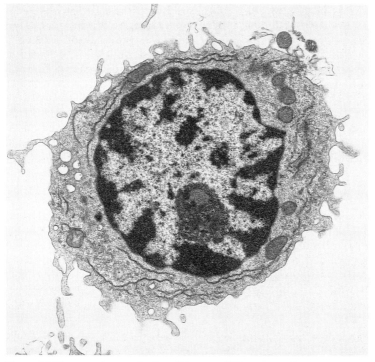

Figure 6.8 Electron micrograph of a cell from an HCL-variant. The nucleus is more uniformly round than the cell of Figures 6.4 and 6.5 and shows a prominent nucleolus. Note that the cytoplasmic villi are less broad. × 14 000, reduced to 78% on reproduction

The origin of hairy cells

In view of its unique morphological and cytochemical characteristics, the nature of the hairy cell, as well as its site of origin and its possible 'normal' counterpart, have been a subject of great interest. The main debate has centred initially on the

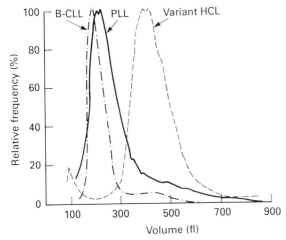

Figure 6.9 Diagram illustrating the cell volumes from a case of B-CLL, one of B-PLL and one of HCL-variant recorded by a Coulter Model ZBI linked to a Coulter Channelizer[22]

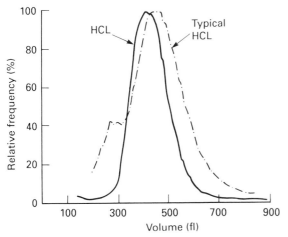

Figure 6.10 Similar cell volumes in a case of typical HCL (·–·–) and one of HCL-variant (—)

lymphocytic or monocytic nature of hairy cells. The belief that the hairy cell could be closely related to the monocytic compartment was based mainly on its phagocytic ability[25] and on equivocal immunological findings. However, it appears that both mouse and human lymphocytes may also express, under certain conditions, a phagocytic potential[17].

Following the advances in the phenotypic characterization of normal and leukaemic cells resulting from the use of more specific immunological reagents, it has become increasingly clear that hairy cells are related to the B-cell lineage. First of all they have easily recognizable SmIg on the cell membrane and their monoclonality is demonstrated consistently by the presence of a single light chain, as described above. The presence of multiple heavy chain determinants, including IgG and IgA, on the membrane of the hairy cells can be interpreted as reflecting

B-cells at a late stage of maturation. Although the capacity to form M-rosettes is not a constant feature of hairy cells, it also suggests that these cells are of B-cell origin because no other haemopoietic cells are known to bind specifically mouse RBCs. Thus SmIg expression and M-rosette formation are strongly suggestive that hairy cells are B-lineage cells. In addition in a minority of cases, Ig can also be demonstrated in the cytoplasm of hairy cells.

The advent of monoclonal antibodies has improved the possibilities for a better characterization of these cells. The cells in all cases have class II HLA determinants and are positive with several B-lineage-specific monoclonal antibodies which are demonstrated either on fresh cells or following in vitro culture[47, 63, 91]. However, using specific monocyte/macrophage monoclonal antibodies, hairy cells are unreactive. The monoclonal antibody FMC7, which reacts only with a subset of B-cells, is positive in HCL and B-PLL. This suggests a close relationship between the cells in these two disorders suggesting that they probably arise from a similar stage of B-cell differentiation, different from that of B-CLL lymphocytes which are, as a rule, FMC7−.

Recently, Posnett et al.[69] have described two new monoclonal antibodies showing specificity for hairy cells. One of them in particular, HC2, seems in the authors' experience to be consistently positive in HCL and not in other disorders (see Chapter 1, Table 1.4). This monoclonal antibody does not appear to cross-react with the cells of other B-cell malignancies, i.e. B-CLL, B-PLL and non-Hodgkin's lymphoma. Studies with this monoclonal antibody appear to provide both a reliable diagnostic tool and also some clues about the origin of hairy cells. Further studies by Posnett and Marboe[70] have shown that HC2 reacts with 2% of SmIg+ normal blood lymphocytes and that the proportion of HC2+ cells is higher in B-cell-enriched populations. B-cell differentiation induced by pokeweed mitogen (PWM) and helper T-cells increases the percentage of HC2+ cells after 4–5 days in culture. These authors[70] concluded that HCL represents a malignancy of activated B-cells and that this stage of differentiation is demonstrated by the monoclonal antibody HC2.

Further evidence of the B-cell origin of hairy cells derives from the demonstration that these cells show rearrangement of the heavy and light Ig chain genes[52]. As DNA rearrangement of both heavy and light Ig chains is a prerequisite event during B-cell development only exceptionally seen within other haemopoietic lineages, this, together with the previously documented B-cell marker positivity, establishes the B-lineage nature of the hairy cells.

It is of interest that Korsmeyer et al.[52] found that cells from all HCL cases were recognized by the monoclonal antibody anti-Tac (CD25) which reacts with the receptor for interleukin-2 (or T-cell growth factor)[55]. The authors have confirmed this finding in all but one of the cases of HCL tested with this monoclonal antibody (see Chapter 1, Table 1.7). In most cases of B-CLL the cells become reactive with anti-Tac following mitogenic or IL-2 stimulation. This further supports the concept that hairy cells may represent activated B-cells.

The above observations may be of value in the attempts to identify counterparts of hairy cells in normal blood and/or in other lymphoid tissues. Studies carried out in the authors' laboratory[75] have shown that 10% of the peripheral blood B-lymphocytes have morphological similarities to hairy cells. Furthermore, by means of the immunogold method and monoclonal antibodies, it was possible to establish a membrane phenotype similarity between these normal 'hairy' cells and those from HCL by their reactivity with anti-HLA-DR, FMC7, HC1 and HC2[75].

Although in the great majority of patients the pathological cells have B-lineage features, rare cases of T-HCL have also been reported[20, 41, 79, 82]. All these cases have been studied prior to the advent of monoclonal antibodies, thus preventing a more precise characterization of the T-cell subset involved. On the basis of receptors IgG (Tγ) and IgM (Tμ), Semenzato et al.[82] found that their case showed a marked increase in Tγ-cells with an almost absent proportion of Tμ-cells. Cases with the apparent combined expression of T- and B-cell markers have also been described[9]. Of interest is that a cell line derived from the case described by Saxon et al.[79] seems to harbour a rare member of the family of human T-cell leukaemia retroviruses (HTLV-II) (see Chapter 8).

Special studies

Chromosome abnormalities

There have been few reports of clonal chromosome abnormalities in HCL[38, 51, 78]. Spontaneous mitoses are rare and metaphases of the neoplastic cells can best be obtained by means of polyclonal B-cell mitogens[68]. Early studies using T-cell mitogens (phytohaemagglutinin, PHA) yielded mainly normal karyotypes. Nevertheless abnormalities of chromosome 12 were observed in two cases[38]. A marker 14q+ was reported in two other cases[51, 78]. The authors' experience using PWM, following the treatment of the cells with neuraminidase and galactose oxidase (see Chapter 3), suggests that a marker 14q+, with breakpoint at 14q32, can be demonstrated in one-third of patients[68]. In more recent experience using other polyclonal B-cell mitogens the authors demonstrated clonal chromosome abnormalities in 12 of 15 patients with HCL in whom adequate metaphases were obtained from peripheral blood samples[4a]. Of these, five had a marker 14q+ with breakpoint at 14q32, a finding common to other B-cell malignancies. No consistent translocation was, however, identified[4a]

Studies of T-lymphocytes in HCL

There have been several reports on the membrane phenotype and the functional properties of the T-cells in this disease. These cells show essentially a normal response to phytohaemagglutinin and a preserved helper function although abnormalities in the cytotoxic function have been observed. All these features are described in detail with the findings on B-CLL and B-PLL in Chapter 3.

References

1. Bouroncle, B. A. (1979) Leukemic reticuloentheliosis (hairy cell leukemia). *Blood,* **53**, 412–436
2. Bouroncle, B. A., Wiseman, B. K. and Doan, C. A. (1958) Leukemic reticuloendotheliosis. *Blood,* **13**, 609–630
3. Bouza, E., Burgaleta, C. and Golde, D. W. (1978) Infections in hairy-cell leukemia. *Blood,* **51**, 851–859
4. Braylan, R. C., Jaffe, E. S., Triche, T. J. et al. (1978) Structural and functional properties of the 'hairy' cells of leukemic reticuloendotheliosis. *Cancer,* **41**, 210–227
4a. Brito-Babapulle, V., Pittman, S., Melo, J. V., Parreira, L. and Catovsky, D. (1986) The 14q+ marker in hairy cell leukaemia. A cytogenetic study of 15 cases. *Leukemia Research,* **10**, 131–138

5. Brunning, R. D. and Parkin, J. (1975) Ribosome–lamella complexes in neoplastic hematopoietic cells. *American Journal of Pathology*, **79**, 565–578

6. Budman, D. R., Koziner, B., Arlin, Z., Lampen, N. and Gee, T. (1979) Massive lymphadenopathy mimicking lymphoma in leukemic reticuloendotheliosis. *American Journal of Medicine*, **66**, 160–162

7. Burke, J. S. (1978) The value of the bone marrow biopsy in the diagnosis of hairy cell leukemia. *American Journal of Clinical Pathology*, **70**, 876–884

8. Burns, G. F., Cawley, J. C., Worman, C. P. et al. (1978) Multiple heavy chain isotypes on the surface of the cells of hairy cell leukemia. *Blood*, **52**, 1132–1147

9. Burns, G. F., Worman, C. P. and Cawley, J. C. (1980) Fluctuations in the T and B characteristics of two cases of T-cell hairy-cell leukaemia. *Clinical and Experimental Immunology*, **39**, 76–82

10. Catovsky, D. (1986) Leukemia and myeloma. In *Cancer Chemotherapy 8*, edited by H. M. Pinedo and B. A. Chabner, pp. 224–261. Amsterdam: Elsevier Science Publishers BV

11. Catovsky, D. (1982) Prolymphocytic and hairy cell leukemias. In *Leukemia*, 4th edn, edited by F. Gunz and E. S. Henderson, pp. 759–781. New York: Grune & Stratton

12. Catovsky, D., Cherchi, M., Brooks, C., Bradley, J. and Zola, H. (1981) Heterogeneity of B-cell leukemias demonstrated by the monoclonal antibody FMC7. *Blood*, **58**, 406–408

13. Catovsky, D., Costello, C., Loukopoulos, D. et al. (1981) Hairy cell leukemia and myelomatosis: chance association or clinical manifestations of the same B-cell disease spectrum. *Blood*, **57**, 758–763

14. Catovsky, D., O'Brien, M., Melo, J. V., Wardle, J. and Brozovic, M. (1984) Hairy cell leukemia (HCL) variant: An intermediate disease between HCL and B prolymphocytic leukemia. *Seminars in Oncology*, **11**, 362–369

15. Catovsky, D., Papamichail, M., Okos, A., Miliani, E. and Holborow, E. J. (1975) Formation of mouse red cell rosettes by 'hairy' cells. *Biomedicine*, **23**, 81–84

16. Catovsky, D., Pettit, J. E., Galton, D. A. G., Spiers, A. S. D. and Harrison, C. V. (1974) Leukaemic reticuloendotheliosis ('hairy' cell leukaemia): a distinct clinico-pathological entity. *British Journal of Haematology*, **26**, 9–27

17. Catovsky, D., Sperandio, P., O'Brien, M., Cherchi, M. and Galton, D. A. G. (1977) Phagocytic potential of leukaemic B-lymphocytes. *Scandinavian Journal of Haematology*, **19**, 211–216

18. Cawley, J. C., Burns, G. F., Bevan, A. et al. (1979) Typical hairy-cell leukaemia with IgGk paraproteinaemia. *British Journal of Haematology*, **43**, 215–221

19. Cawley, J. C., Burns, G. F. and Hayhoe, F. G. J. (1980) A chronic lymphoproliferative disorder with distinctive features: a distinct variant of hairy-cell leukaemia. *Leukemia Research*, **4**, 547–559

20. Cawley, J. C., Burns, G. F., Nash, T. A., Higgy, K. E., Child, J. A. and Roberts, B. E. (1978) Hairy-cell leukemia with T-cell features. *Blood*, **51**, 61–69

21. Cheever, M. A., Fefer, A., Greenberg, P. D. et al. (1982) Treatment of hairy-cell leukemia with chemoradiotherapy and identical-twin bone marrow transplantation. *New England Journal of Medicine*, **307**, 479–481

22. Costello, C., Wardle, J., Catovsky, D. and Lewis, S. M. (1980) Cell volume studies in B-cell leukaemia. *British Journal of Haematology*, **45**, 209–214

23. Crockard, A. D., Chalmers, D., Matutes, E. and Catovsky, D. (1982) Cytochemistry of acid hydrolases in chronic B- and T-cell leukaemias. *American Journal of Clinical Pathology*, **78**, 437–444

24. Crofts, M. A. J., Sharp, J. C. and Joyner, M. V. (1979) Rheumatoid arthritis and hairy-cell leukaemia. *Lancet*, **ii**, 203–204

25. Daniel, M. T. and Flandrin, G. (1974) Fine structure of abnormal cells in hairy cell (tricholeukocytic) leukemia, with special reference to their in vitro phagocytic capacity. *Laboratory Investigation*, **30**, 1–8

26. Davis, T. E., Waterbury, L., Abeloff, M. and Burke, P. J. (1976) Leukemic reticuloendotheliosis. Report of a case with prolonged remission following intensive chemotherapy. *Archives of Internal Medicine*, **136**, 620–622

27. Davies, G. E. and Wiernik, P. H. (1977) Hairy cell leukemia with chylous ascites. *Journal of the American Medical Association*, **238**, 1541–1542

28. Demanes, D. J., Lane, N. and Beckstead, J. H. (1982) Bone involvement in hairy cell leukemia. *Cancer*, **49**, 1697–1701

28a. Dearden, C. and Catovsky, D. (1988) Current treatment of hairy cell leukaemia. *European Journal of Haematology*, **41**, 193–196

28b. Dearden, C. and Catovsky, D. (1990) Treatment of hairy cell leukaemia with 2'-deoxycoformycin. *Leukemia and Lymphoma* (in press)

29. Dorsey, J. K. and Penick, G. D. (1982) The association of hairy cell leukemia with unusual immunologic disorders. *Archives of Internal Medicine*, **142**, 902–903

30. Elkon, K. B., Hughes, G. R. V., Catovsky, D. et al. (1979) Hairy cell leukaemia with polyarteritis nodosa. *Lancet*, **ii**, 280–282

31. Fay, J. W., Moore, J. O., Logue, G. L. and Huang, A. T. (1979) Leukopheresis therapy of leukemic reticuloendotheliosis (hairy cell leukemia). *Blood*, **54**, 747–749

31a. Foa, R., Fierro, M. T., Lusso, P. et al. (1987) Effect of alpha-interferon on the immune system of patients with hairy cell leukemia. *Leukemia*, **1**, 377–379

32. Golde, D. W., Stevens, R. H., Quan, S. G. and Saxon, A. (1977) Immunoglobulin synthesis in hairy cell leukaemia. *British Journal of Haematology*, **35**, 359–365

33. Golomb, H. M. (1981) Progress report on chlorambucil therapy in post splenectomy patients with hairy cell leukemia. *Blood*, **57**, 464–467

34. Golomb, H. M., Braylan, R. and Polliak, A. (1975) 'Hairy' cell leukaemia (leukaemic reticuloendotheliosis): a scanning electron microscopic study of eight cases. *British Journal of Haematology*, **29**, 455–460

35. Golomb, H. M., Catovsky, D. and Golde, D. W. (1978) Hairy cell leukemia. A clinical review based on 71 cases. *Annals of Internal Medicine*, **89**, 677–683

36. Golomb, H. M., Catovsky, D. and Golde, D. W. (1983) Hairy cell leukemia: a five-year update on seventy-one patients. *Annals of Internal Medicine*, **99**, 485–486

37. Golomb, H. M. and Hadad, L. J. (1984) Infectious complications in 127 patients with hairy cell leukemia. *American Journal of Hematology*, **16**, 393–401

38. Golomb, H. M., Lindgren, V. and Rowley, J. D. (1978) Chromosome abnormalities in patients with hairy cell leukemia. *Cancer*, **41**, 1374–1380

39. Golomb, H. M. and Vardiman, J. W. (1982) Response to splenectomy in 65 patients with hairy cell leukemia: an evaluation of spleen weight and bone marrow involvement. *Blood*, **61**, 349–352

40. Grouls, V. (1980) Diagnosis of hairy-cell leukaemia by tartrate-resistant acid phosphatase activity in paraffin-embedded tissue sections. *Journal of Clinical Pathology*, **33**, 552–554

41. Hernandez, D., Cruz, C., Carnot, J., Dorticos, E. and Espinosa, E. (1978) Hairy cell leukaemia of T-cell origin. *British Journal of Haematology*, **40**, 504–506

42. Higgy, K. E., Burns, G. F. and Hayhoe, F. G. J. (1978) Identification of the hairy cells of leukaemic reticuloendotheliosis by an esterase method. *British Journal of Haematology*, **38**, 99–106

43. Janckila, A. J., Wallace, J. H. and Yam, L. T. (1982) Generalized monocyte deficiency in leukaemic reticuloendotheliosis. *Scandinavian Journal of Haematology*, **29**, 153–160

44. Jansen, J., Bolhuis, R. L. J., van Nieuwkoop, J. A., Schuit, H. R. E. and Stenfer Kroese, W. F. (1983) Paraproteinaemia plus osteolytic lesions in typical hairy-cell leukaemia. *British Journal of Haematology*, **54**, 531–541

45. Jansen, J. and Hermans, J. (1981) Splenectomy in hairy cell leukemia. A retrospective multicenter analysis. *Cancer*, **47**, 2066–2076

46. Jansen, J. and Hermans, J. (1982) Clinical staging system for hairy-cell leukemia. *Blood*, **60**, 571–577

47. Jansen, J., LeBien, T. W. and Kersey, J. H. (1982) The phenotype of the neoplastic cells of hairy cell leukemia studied with monoclonal antibodies. *Blood*, **59**, 609–614

48. Johnston, J. B., Glazer, R. I., Pugh, L. and Israels, L. G. (1986) The treatment of hairy-cell leukaemia with 2'-deoxycoformycin. *British Journal of Haematology*, **63**, 525–534

49. Katayama, I., Nagy, G. K. and Balogh, K. Jr (1973) Light microscopic identification of the ribosome-lamella complex in 'hairy cells' of leukemic reticuloendotheliosis. *Cancer*, **32**, 843–846

50. Katayama, I. and Schneider, G. B. (1977) Further ultrastructural characterization of hairy cells of leukemic reticuloendotheliosis. *American Journal of Pathology*, **86**, 163–182

51. Khalid, G., Li, Y-S., Flemans, R. J. and Hayhoe, F. G. J. (1981) Chromosomal abnormalities in a case of hairy cell leukaemia. *Leukemia Research,* **5**, 431–435
52. Korsmeyer, S. J., Greene, W. C., Cossman, J. et al. (1983) Rearrangement and expression of immunoglobulin genes and expression of Tac antigen in hairy cell leukemia. *Proceedings of the National Academy Sciences of the USA,* **80**, 4522–4526
53. Kraut, E. H., Bouroncle, B. A. and Grever, M. R. (1986) Low-dose deoxycoformycin in the treatment of hairy cell leukemia. *Blood,* **68**, 1119–1122
54. Lang, J. M., Giron, C., Oberling, F., Goetz, M. L. and North, M. L. (1976) Normal humoral immunity in hairy cell leukaemia. *Biomedicine,* **25**, 41–43
55. Leonard, W. J., Depper, J. M., Uchiyama, T., Smith, K. A., Waldmann, T. A. and Green, W. C. (1982) A monoclonal antibody that appears to recognize the receptor for human T-cell growth factor; partial characterization of the receptor. *Nature,* **300**, 267–269
56. Le Pogamp, P., Ghandour, C. and Le Prise, P. Y. (1982) Hairy cell leukaemia and polyarteritis nodosa. *Journal of Rheumatology,* **9**, 441–442
57. Lewis, S. M., Catovsky, D., Hows, J. M. and Ardalan, B. (1977) Splenic red cell pooling in hairy cell leukaemia. *British Journal of Haematology,* **35**, 351–357
58. Linder, J., Silberman, H. R. and Croker, B. P. (1982) Amyloidosis complicating hairy cell leukemia. *American Journal of Clinical Pathology,* **78**, 864–867
59. Manes, J. L. and Blair, O. M. (1976) Disseminated *Mycobacterium kansasii* infection complicating hairy cell leukaemia. *Journal of the American Medical Association,* **236**, 1878–1879
60. Marty, M., Calvo, F., Castaigne, S. and Flandrin, G. (1981) Leucemie à tricholeucocytes à la phase d'insuffisance medullaire severe. Remission complete apres polychimiotherapie chez deux malades. *La Nouvelle Presse Médicale,* **10**, 2977–2979
61. McCarthy, D. and Catovsky, D. (1978) Response to doxorubicin in hairy cell leukaemia. *Scandinavian Journal of Haematology,* **21**, 445–447
62. Mehta, A. B., Catovsky, D., O'Brien, C. J., Lott, M., Bowley, N. and Hemmingway, A. (1983) Massive retroperitoneal lymphadenopathy as a terminal event in hairy cell leukaemia. *Clinical and Laboratory Haematology,* **51**, 259–263
63. Melo, J. V., San Miguel, J. F., Moss, V. E. and Catovsky, D. (1984) The membrane phenotype of hairy cell leukemia: A study with monoclonal antibodies. *Seminars in Oncology,* **11**, 381–385
64. Mielke, C. H., Dobbs, C. E., Winkler, C. F. and Yam, L. T. (1982) Therapeutic leukapheresis in hairy cell leukaemia. *Archives of Internal Medicine,* **142**, 700–702
65. Myers, T. J., Ikeda, Y., Schwartz, S., Pharmakidis, A. B. and Baldini, M. G. (1981) Primary splenic hairy cell leukemia. Remission for 21 years following splenectomy. *American Journal of Hematology,* **11**, 229–303
66. Nanba, K., Jaffe, E. S., Soban, E. J., Braylan, R. C. and Berard, C. W. (1977) Hairy cell leukemia. Enzyme histochemical characterization, with special reference to splenic stromal changes. *Cancer,* **39**, 2323–2336
66a. Ng, J-P., Hogg, R. B., Cumming, R. L. C., McCallion, J. and Catovsky, D. (1987) Primary splenic hairy cell leukaemia: A case report and review of the literature. *European Journal of Haematology,* **39**, 349–352
67. Noseda, G., Reiner, M. and Scali, G. (1980) Haarzell-leukamie und myelom. *Schweizerische Medizinische Wochenschrift,* **110**, 1494–1498
68. Pittman, A. (1984) Cytogenetic studies in human B-cell malignancies. *PhD Thesis,* London University
69. Posnett, D. N., Chiorazzi, N. and Kunkel, H. G. (1982) Monoclonal antibodies with specificity for hairy cell leukemia cells. *Journal of Clinical Investigation,* **70**, 254–261
70. Posnett, D. N. and Marboe, C. C. (1984) Differentiation antigens associated with hairy cell leukemia. *Seminars in Oncology,* **11**, 413–415
71. Quesada, J. R., Hersh, E. M., Keating, M., Zander, A. and Hester, J. (1981) Hairy cell leukemia: clinical effects of the methanol extraction residue (MER) of BCG, lithium carbonate and mononuclear cell-enriched leukocyte transfusions. *Leukemia Research,* **5**, 463–476
72. Quesada, J. R., Keating, M. J., Libshitz, H. I. and Llamas, L. (1983) Bone involvement in hairy cell leukemia. *American Journal of Medicine,* **74**, 228–231
73. Quesada, J. R., Reuben, J., Manning, J. T., Hersh, E. M. and Gutterman, J. U. (1984) Alpha

interferon for induction of remission in hairy-cell leukemia. *New England Journal of Medicine*, **310**, 15–18

74. Resnitzky, P., Barak, Y., Karov, Y., Berrebi, A. and Sharon, R. (1982) Hairy cell leukemia: defective production of granulocyte-macrophage colony-stimulating factor by peripheral blood cells. *Israel Journal of Medical Sciences*, **18**, 845–848

74a. Robinson, D., Lackie, P., Aber, V. and Catovsky, D. (1989) Morphometric analysis of chronic B-cell leukaemias – an aid to the classification of lymphoid cell types. *Leukemia Research*, **13**, 357–365

75. Robinson, D. S. F., Posnett, D. N., Zola, H. and Catovsky, D. (1985) Normal counterparts of hairy cells and B-prolymphocytes in the peripheral blood. An ultrastructural study with monoclonal antibodies and the immunogold method. *Leukemia Research*, **9**, 335–348

76. Rosenthal, R. L., Steiner, G. C. and Golub, B. S. (1979) Hairy cell leukemia: historical aspects of bone involvement. *Mount Sinai Journal of Medicine*, **46**, 237–242

77. Rosner, M. C. and Golomb, H. M. (1980) Ribosome–lamella complex in hairy cell leukemia. Ultrastructure and distribution. *Laboratory Investigation*, **42**, 236–247

78. Sadamori, N., Han, T., Kakati, S. and Sandberg, A. A. (1983) Chromosomes and causation of human cancer and leukemia. LI. A hairy cell leukemia case with 14q+ and ring chromosomes: significance of ring chromosomes in blood disorders. *Cancer Genetics and Cytogenetic*, **10**, 67–77

79. Saxon, A., Stevens, R. H. and Golde, D. W. (1978) T-lymphocyte variant of hairy-cell leukemia. *Annals of Internal Medicine*, **88**, 323–326

80. Schrek, R. and Donnelly, W. J. (1966) 'Hairy' cells in blood in lymphoreticular neoplastic disease and 'flagellated' cells of normal lymph nodes. *Blood*, **27**, 199–211

81. Sebahoun, G., Boufette, P. and Flandrin, G. (1978) Hairy cell leukemia. *Leukemia Research*, **2**, 187–195

82. Semenzato, G., Basso, G., Cartei, G., Pezzatto, A. and Cocito, M. G. (1980) Hairy cell leukaemia with T cell features. *British Journal of Haematology*, **46**, 491–492

83. Seshadri, R. S., Brown, E. J. and Zipursky, A. (1976) Leukemic reticuloendotheliosis. A failure of monocyte production. *New England Journal of Medicine*, **295**, 181–184

84. Sharp, R. A. and MacWalter, R. S. (1983) A role for splenic irradiation in the treatment of hairy-cell leukaemia. Case report and review of the literature. *Acta Haematologica*, **70**, 59–62

85. Slater, N. G. P., Barkhan, P. and Williams, H. J. H. (1979) Hairy cell leukemia – apparent cure with reversal of marrow fibrosis. *Clinical and Laboratory Haematology*, **1**, 65–68

86. Spiers, A. S. D., Moore, D., Cassileth, P. A. et al. (1987) Remissions in hairy-cell leukemia with pentostatin (2′-deoxycoformycin). *New England Journal of Medicine*, **316**, 825–830

87. Thompson, J. A. and Fefer, A. (1987) Interferon in the treatment of hairy cell leukemia. *Cancer*, **59**, 605–609

87a. Visser, L., Shaw, A., Slupsky, J., Vos, H. and Poppema, S. (1989) Monoclonal antibodies reactive with hairy cell leukemia. *Blood*, **74**, 320–325

88. Vykoupil, K. F., Thiele, J. and Georgii, A. (1976) Hairy cell leukemia. Bone marrow findings in 24 patients. *Virchows Archiv A, Pathological and Anatomy and Histology*, **370**, 273–289

89. Weh, H. J., Katz, M., Bray, B., Rodat, O., Degos, L. and Flandrin, G. (1979) Lesions osseuses au cours des leucemies à tricholeucocytes. *Nouvelle Presse Médicale*, **8**, 2253–2254

90. Weinstein, R. A., Golomb, H. M., Grumet, G., Gelmann, E. and Schechter, G. P. (1981) Hairy cell leukemia: association with disseminated atypical mycobacterial infection. *Cancer*, **48**, 380–383

91. Worman, C. P., Brooks, D. A., Hogg, N., Zola, H., Beverley, P. C. L. and Cawley, J. C. (1983) The nature of hairy cells. A study with a panel of monoclonal antibodies. *Scandinavian Journal of Haematology*, **30**, 223–226

92. Yam, L. T., Chaudhry, A. A. and Janckila, A. J. (1977) Impaired marrow granulocyte reserve and leucocyte mobilization in leukemic reticuloendotheliosis. *Annals of Internal Medicine*, **87**, 444–446

93. Yam, L. T., Janckila, A. J., Li, C-Y. and Lam, W. K. W. (1987) Cytochemistry of tartrate-resistant acid phosphatase: 15 years' experience. *Leukemia*, **1**, 285–288

94. Yam, L. T., Li, C. Y. and Lam, K. W. (1971) Tartrate-resistant acid phosphatase isoenzyme in the reticulum cells of leukemic reticuloendotheliosis. *New England Journal of Medicine*, **284**, 357–360

Chapter 7

The leukaemic phase of non-Hodgkin's lymphoma

Introduction

In the study of lymphoid malignancies it is apparent that a number of cases are not primarily leukaemias but represent spill-over to the blood and bone marrow of non-Hodgkin's lymphomas (NHLs), these being tissue-based tumours arising commonly from lymph nodes and, rarely, from the spleen. Such cases often present problems of differential diagnosis with the de novo lymphoid leukaemias described in other chapters. Most NHLs may evolve with a leukaemic phase [2, 5, 30, 35a, 48] and some of them, e.g. follicular lymphoma, may present with a high WBC count and a blood picture which resembles CLL [29, 42]. NHLs or lymphoid leukaemias may originate from B- and T-cells at similar or closely related stages of maturation. Despite this superficial resemblance, it is likely that subtle changes in membrane receptors, and/or the tissue of origin, may result in a lymphoid malignancy behaving like a leukaemia or as a lymphoma. It is for this reason that differences in immunophenotype can be detected by monoclonal antibodies in NHLs and the primary leukaemias, e.g. between T-lymphoblastic lymphoma and T-cell ALL. Similarly the very rare occurrence of an NHL with a phenotype indentical to that of common-ALL suggests that either the proliferating cells arise only from the bone marrow or that their biological properties make them evolve almost exclusively as a leukaemia.

Both B- and T-derived NHLs may develop a leukaemic blood picture. Some of the T-cell tumours with a frequent leukaemic phase or 'lymphoma/leukaemia syndromes' are being dealt with in other chapters as they constitute distinct entities (T- lymphoblastic lymphoma in Chapter 2, adult T-cell leukaemia/lymphoma or ATLL in Chapter 8, and Sézary syndrome in Chapter 9). The features of the other NHLs, mainly B-derived, presenting with blood and bone marrow involvement will be discussed in this chapter.

The classification of non-Hodgkin's lymphomas

A brief look at the current classification of NHLs is necessary as a background against which some of the leukaemic manifestations will be discussed. Rappaport's classification [36] was used for many years and was based on the presence or absence of a nodular (or follicular) pattern and the predominant cell type (well or poorly differentiated and histiocytic). This classification was found to be clinically useful and reproducible. However, it did not reflect accurately the heterogeneity of the lymphoid system which was being unveiled by the development of immunological markers. New classifications evolved in which function and cell types (B and T) were taken into account[23, 25], but still their recognition was based on morphological criteria. This renders them poorly reproducible and too complex for practising pathologists. To bring uniformity to the chaos created by widely different classifications, each with its own positive aspects, the National Cancer Institute set up a study group which published new proposals or working formulation in 1982[39] based on a clinical and histopathological review of over 1000 cases of NHLs from three centres in the USA and one in Italy. The working formulation consists of three main categories based on prognosis[38] – low grade (median survival 6 years), high grade (1.3 years) and intermediate grade (3.5 years) – and on the morphology of the predominant cell. This classification does not employ immunological markers, although it is possible to expand it or improve upon it by introducing immunological criteria now that marker techniques are widely used and some reagents can also be used on paraffin-embedded tissues. The Kiel classification[23] is widely used in Europe and recently it has been the object of a major modification, which has divided the NHLs into B- and T-types[44], recognizing and/or suggesting that immunological marker studies should be part of the diagnostic procedure in NHLs. In addition a number of distinct types of peripheral T-cell NHLs, not recognized specifically in the working formulation or in the previous Kiel proposals, are now part of the classification[45b].

Here a simplified approach which aims at describing the features of the NHLs which more frequently evolve with blood and bone marrow involvement will be followed. These are usually low or intermediate grade NHLs of B-cell type which could be confused with B-CLL or the other chronic B-cell leukaemias (Table 7.1, groups 1–4). The high grade B-cell NHLs have less frequent leukaemic manifestations (Table 7.1, groups 5 and 6). One type not included in Table 7.1 is B-lymphoblastic (SmIg+, non-Burkitt's) which is not so well characterized as a

Table 7.1 Leukaemic phase of B-cell non-Hodgkin's lymphomas[a]

Group	Cell type
1	Follicular lymphoma (centrocytes/small cleaved)
2	Intermediate/mantle zone NHLs (medium and large lymphocytes)
3	Splenic lymphoma (villous lymphocytes)
4	Lymphoplasmacytic lymphoma (lymphoplasma cells)
5	Burkitt's lymphoma (L3 or Burkitt cells)
6	Large cell NHLs (centroblasts/large non-cleaved cells; immunoblasts)

[a] Cell type in peripheral blood films is given in parentheses.

leukaemia and will therefore not be discussed here. There is little difference histologically between the splenic lymphoma with circulating villous lymphocytes (SLVL) (Table 7.1, group 3) and lymphoplasmacytic NHL or immunocytoma, which includes Waldenström's macroglobulinaemia (described in Chapter 10). However, the different clinical presentation and paraprotein levels, which reflect the primary involvement of the spleen in SLVL and the greater degree of plasma cell differentation in immunocytoma, together with the different haematological features (high WBC count in SLVL and more bone marrow infiltration in immunocytoma), justifies the separate description of these disorders. The B-cell disorders which are considered as leukaemias rather than primary nodal malignancies, such as B-CLL, B-PLL and hairy cell leukaemia, are dealt with in separate chapters.

The T-cell NHLs which constitute 'leukaemia/lymphoma syndromes' are described in other chapters. In this chapter only T-immunoblastic NHLs (HTLV-I negative) which may sometimes have a leukaemic phase are referred to. ATLL, a disease caused by HTLV-I (see Chapter 8), is not specifically described in the working formulation, perhaps because such pathology was not included in the review of cases from Europe and the USA, and it is included in three different categories in the updated Kiel classification of T-cell NHLs (pleomorphic, small cell; pleomorphic medium and large cell; and immunoblastic). The latter reflect the heterogeneity of the lymph node histology in ATLL which has been confirmed in the authors' experience in patients of Caribbean origin, but do not justify the inclusion of ATLL as separate disease entities.

The separation between T-lymphoblastic NHLs and T-cell ALLs is not always possible. The age of incidence and the histological appearances are very similar with convoluted or non-convoluted blasts[23]. In practice T-lymphoblastic lymphoma refers to tumours with no bone marrow or peripheral blood (PB) involvement or with less than 25% blasts in the bone marrow; a higher percentage of blast and a leukaemic phase usually corresponds to T-ALL (discussed in Chapter 2). There are some subtle differences in membrane phenotype which may determine whether or not thymic-derived malignancies will evolve as a leukaemia. In T-lymphoblastic lymphoma, in contrast to T-ALL, the blasts are often CD1a+(OKT6+) and they frequently co-express CD4 and CD8, corresponding to the phenotype of common (cortical) thymocytes. In T-ALL the cells correspond to an earlier stage of thymic differentiation in two-thirds of cases and to common or late thymocytes in the remaining one-third. It is not clear whether in the latter cases the clinical features are more akin to those of a lymphoma (anterior mediastinal mass, lymphadenopathy) or a leukaemia (diffuse bone marrow infiltration and high WBC count).

Laboratory investigations for the study of NHLs in leukaemic phase

The diagnosis of the leukaemic phase of NHLs in cases without a preceding lymphomatous stage (e.g. presenting as leukaemia) may not be straightforward and requires a number of diagnostic steps for the full and accurate characterization of the neoplastic process (Table 7.2). These involve methods discussed in more detail in other parts of this book, which are used for the characterization of leukaemic cells and some steps which are specific for NHLs.

Morphology

Careful examination of peripheral blood and bone marrow films could help identify or suspect any of the disorders listed in Table 7.1 and distinguish them from one of the leukaemias. Details will be discussed with each particular NHL. A common feature to these disorders, in contrast to the lymphoid leukaemias, is the relative pleomorphism of the blood picture with the cells of varying size and nuclear shape which, according to the WBC count, may be seen coexisting with normal leucocytes. The most frequent problems of differential diagnosis are seen between follicular lymphoma and B-CLL, intermediate lymphoma with CLL/PL or, rarely, PLL, splenic lymphoma (SLVL) with hairy cell leukaemia (HCL), lymphoblastic lymphoma with ALL, and some of the large cell NHLs with some acute myeloid leukaemias, in particular the monoblastic (M5a) type.

Table 7.2 Laboratory investigations for the diagnosis of NHLs in leukaemic phase

Morphology of the lymphoma cells
Cell volume studies
Histology
   Lymph node
   Bone marrow
   Spleen
Membrane markers
Immunocytochemistry
Karyotype of the malignant cells
DNA analysis
   T-cell receptor and immunoglobulin gene rearrangement
   Polymerase chain reaction for chromosome breakpoints, e.g. t(14;18)
Protein electrophoresis
   Paraprotein (serum)
   Free light chain (urine)

   There are very distinct morphological features in each of the NHLs which facilitate the diagnosis. The additional techniques of Table 7.2, in particular membrane markers, may establish the diagnosis with more certainty. In a minority of follicular lymphomas (about 10%), the circulating cells do not show the characteristic morphology of small cleaved cells or centrocytes. In such cases the diagnosis of follicular lymphoma on the membrane phenotype can be suspected because it is quite different from that of B-CLL (see below). Confirmation of the diagnosis should always be attempted by histological examination of lymph nodes or splenic tissue.

Cell volume

Differences in cell size may be accurately estimated by cell volume estimations. Large cell components can be easily identified in this way in NHLs presenting or evolving with a leukaemic blood picture (Figure 7.1). From these studies it is apparent too that mixtures of cells are frequent. In follicular lymphoma the circulating cells have a smaller volume (median <200 femtolitres, fl) than CLL lymphocytes (211 fl) on account of their almost complete absence of cytoplasm.

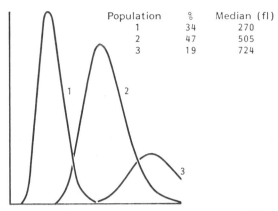

Population	%	Median (fl)
1	34	270
2	47	505
3	19	724

Figure 7.1 Cell volume estimation in a case of large cell NHLs in leukaemic phase. The measurements were done by a Coulter Model ZBI counter linked to a Coulter Channelizer. The fitted curves correspond to the three populations observed in the peripheral blood: (1) normal lymphocytes, (2) large blast-like cells and (3) very large cells (illustrated in Figure 7.8)

The volume of the villous lymphocytes of SLVL (median = 356 fl) is smaller than in typical hairy cells (526 fl). There is no information on the cell size of the circulating cells in the intermediate or mantle zone lymphoma, because the leukaemic phase has not been studied in many cases. It is likely that these cells will come out on these measurements as larger than CLL lymphocytes and closer to the size of prolymphocytes (between 300 and 350 fl). Immunoblasts and other large cells measure well above 500 fl.

Histology

The histological analysis of pathological lymph nodes and, in some cases, of the spleen is essential for the precise diagnosis and classification of the type of NHL. Often such material is not available and splenectomy may not be a good proposition simply for diagnostic purposes. The pattern of lymphocytic infiltration in the spleen provides useful information in order to distinguish hairy cell leukaemia (HCL) from SLVL and the other chronic B-cell leukaemias. In HCL and its variant (see Chapter 6) the spleen involvement affects exclusively the red pulp whilst in SLVL, B-PLL and B-CLL the infiltration always affects the white pulp, although in some cases it may also involve significantly the red pulp.

The histological pattern of lymphocytic infiltration in the bone marrow may also provide important diagnostic information. For example, a paratrabecular pattern is a feature of follicular lymphoma which is not seen in B-CLL. In cases of follicular lymphoma presenting with a high WBC count[29], the infiltration may be diffuse as seen in advanced CLL. In such instances the bone marrow biopsy pattern does not discriminate between these two B-cell disorders. A paratrabecular pattern of infiltration may also be seen in intermediate (or diffuse centrocytic) NHL, but more information about the bone marrow status of this NHL in relation to its leukaemic phase is required. T-cell lymphomas often show a diffuse as well as a paratrabecular pattern whilst in B-cell lymphomas the pattern is more often nodular[21]. Osteoclast activation is also a feature of T-cell NHLs, particularly in ATLL when associated with hypercalcaemia. The relationship of B-CLL with the well-differentiated lymphocytic lymphoma (WDLL) condition which, by definition, has no leukaemic blood picture, has been debated[34]. In 10–20% of CLL cases the bone marrow shows a nodular pattern of lymphocytic infiltration whilst this is the rule in most cases of WDLL[34]. In SLVL the bone marrow aspirate may be normal in half of the cases, with less than 30% lymphocytes, but the trephine biopsy shows patchy nodular infiltrate in two-thirds of cases. In the remaining one-third the bone marrow biopsy may look normal, confirming that this NHL is of splenic origin[28].

Immunocytochemistry of histological material should complement the information of the morphological study[22, 26a, 45, 47]. It will confirm the B- or T-cell nature of the NHL and whether the lymphocyte infiltrates, particularly in the bone marrow if only partially involved, correspond to a monoclonal B-cell proliferation. Such studies are now also possible in paraffin sections with lineage-associated monoclonal antibodies[26a].

Membrane markers

These are essential to establish the B- or T-cell nature of the process and to define its distinct phenotype. Studies with flow cytometry, in particular of the κ/λ ratio, have been able to define discrete monoclonal populations in the peripheral blood, in cases with otherwise normal WBC count or without apparent lymphocytosis. Table 7.3 summarizes the results in B-cell lymphoproliferative disorders, contrasting the findings in two B-cell leukaemias, CLL and HCL, with the NHLs which commonly present with a leukaemic phase: follicular lymphoma, intermediate NHLs and SLVL. The phenotype of B-CLL was discussed in detail in Chapter 3. It is apparent from Table 7.3 that the intermediate NHL is the only B-cell disorder, other than B-CLL and WDLL[1], which consistently expresses CD5[16, 18, 35a, 45, 49].

The pan-B-markers CD19, CD20 and CD24, as well as class II major histocompatibility complex (MHC) antigens (HLA-DR, Ia), can be used to

Table 7.3 Markers in B-cell leukaemias and NHLs

Marker	Leukaemia		NHL in leukaemic phase		
	CLL	HCL	FL	Intermediate[b]	SLVL
SmIg	±	++	++	+/++	++
M-rosettes	++	−/+	−/+	−/+	−
CD5(T1)	++	−	−	++	−
CD19/20/24	++	++	++	++	++
FMC7/CD22[a]	−/+	++	++	++	++
CD10(cALLa)	−	−	++	−/+	−
CD25(Tac)	−	++	−	−	−/+
CD11c(LeuM5)	−	++	−	−	−/+

[a] Membrane staining (on cell suspensions); when tested on fixed cells (cytoplasmic plus membrane staining) CD22 is positive in all B-cell malignancies.
[b] Intermediate or mantle zone NHL or diffuse centrocytic.

establish the B-cell nature of the NHL, but do not allow the differential diagnosis between the various types. CD10 (anti-cALLa) is characteristic of follicular lymphoma (centroblastic/centrocytic in the Kiel classification) as well as of normal germinal centre cells which are the counterparts of follicular lymphoma lymphocytes[16, 37, 45]. Thus CD5 and CD10 have a different pattern of reactivity in intermediate NHL[22, 45] and in follicular lymphoma; both these conditions, if presenting as a leukaemia, could be distinguished from B-CLL by the strong membrane expression of Ig, FMC7 and CD22 (Table 7.3). In intermediate NHL the expression of SmIg is stronger than in CLL but weaker than in follicular lymphoma cells[6]. CD5 and CD10 appear to be mutually exclusive in B-cell lymphomas[3, 22]. However, the expression of CD10 in intermediate NHL has been conflicting with the differences reflecting the use of different techniques[35a, 46]. For example Jaffe's group[6, 18] found some CD10+ cases by the study in cell suspensions with the monoclonal antibody J5 (perhaps detecting weak expression of the cALL antigen), whilst Stein et al.[45], referring to centrocyte lymphoma, and Weisenburger et al.[49] failed to demonstrate CD10 reactivity by immunocytochemistry on frozen sections.

Follicular lymphoma is the only B-cell lymphoma whose cells express membrane IgG as often as IgM[45]; rare cases, up to 15% in some studies[17], may be SmIg−[15]. The Tac antigen (CD25, IL-2 receptor) which is characteristic of hairy cell leukaemia (Table 7.3) and ATLL cells, can be demonstrated in cells of 50% of B-cell lymphomas of low or intermediate grade, using a sensitive immunoperoxidase technique[22]. Large cell lymphomas which may also be SmIg−, express the transferrin receptor (OKT9) and CD38 (OKT10) more consistently than other NHL types[1]. Terminal transferase is useful to distinguish T-lymphoblastic lymphoma (TdT+) from other lymphomas[19] and, in particular, from the peripheral types of T-cell NHLs which are always TdT−.

DNA analysis

Ig gene rearrangements were investigated in peripheral blood samples of low grade B-cell NHLs as an alternative to the morphological identification of neoplastic cells in the circulation and clonal rearrangements were demonstrated in 76% of cases (22 out of 29) investigated[17]. It is of interest that in more than half of these cases there were no indentifiable NHL cells in peripheral blood films and some of them had no other evidence of disease activity. Unfortunately this study from Standford[17] did not compare the sensitivity of DNA analysis against that of staining with anti-light chain reagents and did not provide enough information on WBC counts and differential counts. Nevertheless, it is an important observation, particularly as they suggest that the sensitivity of the technique may be greater than that of flow cytometry.

DNA analysis is also important for the demonstration of clonality and B-cell lineage in cases of NHL with negative SmIg. Similarly, in T-cell NHL clonality could be best demonstrated by the rearrangement of T-cell receptor (TCR) genes than by membrane markers. In rare instances evidence for more than one neoplastic clone can be shown by these molecular techniques[41]. In addition, they can demonstrate identity between the circulating NHL cells with those of the affected lymph nodes. The drawbacks of the DNA hybridization techniques for clinical practice, e.g. time consuming, use of radioactivity, lack of quantitation, background due to partially degraded DNA etc., have been recognized[17].

Incidence of a leukaemic phase

The frequency by which NHLs present and/or evolve with a leukaemic blood picture is of the order of 15% [5, 27, 30, 48] but this has varied in the published series according to the criteria used to define leukaemia, e.g. the level of circulating lymphoma cells and/or the method used to evaluate the presence of such cells in blood samples.

It is agreed that involvement of the bone marrow without the peripheral blood should not be considered as leukaemic in a strict sense. On the other hand, peripheral blood involvement nearly always presupposes bone marrow infiltration, the only exception being cases of the splenic lymphoma, SLVL, where the bone marrow may be normal even by examination of a trephine biopsy. One-third of cases of NHL with bone marrow involvement are expected to have peripheral blood 'spill-over' [30]. The use of a strict definition is difficult in practice as this may also depend on the type of NHL. For example, the criterion used to separate T-lymphoblastic lymphoma from T-ALL is based mainly on the degree of bone marrow involvement and not necessarily on the presence of blasts in the peripheral blood. This criterion is used by paediatric haemato-oncologists to decide on a particular treatment strategy and to evalute prognosis. However, in follicular lymphoma and some other 'chronic' or low grade NHLs, bone marrow infiltration is relatively common and, therefore, the trend is to consider a leukaemic phase only when there is significant peripheral blood lymphocytosis.

The level of spill-over to the blood to consider in the B-cell NHL will vary according to whether a clonal excess of $\kappa+$ or $\lambda+$ cells is demonstrable only by flow cytometry or if the circulating lymphoma cells are so abnormal morphologically as to become apparent by examination of peripheral blood films. Here too the appearance of the cells may influence the defining criteria. For instance, in a large cell NHL, the presence of 10% or more of abnormal cells in the peripheral blood will be recognized easily and should probably be considered pathological regarding the level. However, in cases of low grade NHL where the circulating cells resemble small lymphocytes, the criterion used will consider only an excess over the normal levels, e.g. above $5 \times 10^9/l$, as leukaemia. In borderline cases, with 'normal-looking' cells the additional information provided by marker studies will be invaluable. In follicular lymphoma, Morra et al. [30] quote an incidence of 1.6% blood involvement whilst in Come's [5] and Spiro's [42] series the incidence is significantly higher, of the order of 25–30%. Furthermore, some histological subtypes of follicular lymphoma, according to the Kiel classification, may correlate with the chances of a leukaemic manifestation. A large Italian study of 645 cases of NHL, reported by Mazza et al. [27], found that only 3% of the 'follicular types' of centroblastic/centrocytic NHLs had blood involvement at presentation, contrasting with 24% in the 'follicular and diffuse type', including in the latter 5% of cases with a late leukaemic phase. However, such a correlation was not observed by Lennert himself [23]. In follicular lymphoma it is also important to distinguish the early blood involvement, which consists of typical small-cleaved cells, from that seen in the late stages of the disease in which a blastic population predominates [5, 42].

Prognostic significance

There are a number of factors which contribute to the prognosis of NHLs. The clinical significance of a leukaemic phase depends on the histological types of lymphoma and on whether it is an early or a late feature of the disease[30]. Follicular lymphoma presenting with a moderately raised WBC count and a peripheral blood lymphocytosis up to $30 \times 10^9/l$ does not necessarily have a worse prognosis[5, 30, 43, 48]. Similar conclusions can be drawn in other types of low-grade NHLs, specially those with lymphoplasmacytic differentiation. On the other hand, cases of follicular lymphoma which present with a WBC count greater than $40 \times 10^9/l$ usually have bulky disease and appear to fare worse[29]. The less frequent late blastic phase is also associated with poor prognosis[42]. In high-grade NHLs, particularly lymphoblastic lymphoma, blood involvement is a poor prognostic feature[30, 48]. In large cell NHLs the development of a late leukaemic phase has a poor prognosis[5], but this may not be so when seen early in the disease. It is clear nevertheless that the probability of a cure will be negligible in large cell NHLs with blood involvement at any stage of the disease.

When combination chemotherapy, e.g. COP, CHOP (C = cyclophosphamide, H = hydroxydaunorubicin, O = oncovin, P = prednisolone) or M-BACOD (with methotrexate, folinic acid [Leucovorin] rescue, bleomycin, doxorubicin [Adriamycin], cyclophosphamide, oncovin and dexamethasone) is given to NHL in leukaemic phase the remission rate and the duration of that remission are likely to be shorter than in lymphomas of similar histology but without blood involvement[48]. In general, achievement of a complete remission correlates with a better prognosis in all types of NHL[27], rather than partial or minimal responses.

The leukaemic phase of follicular lymphoma

In a seminal study, Spiro et al.[42], singled out the following features as characteristic of follicular lymphoma:

1. A higher incidence in females confirmed in the series of Lennert[23]; this contrasts with B-CLL which has a male predominance.
2. A history of symptomless lymphadenopathy.
3. Extensive disease at presentation, specially in patients below 40 years of age, the latter being a rare feature in B-CLL.
4. Lymphocytosis $>5 \times 10^9/l$, which could be confused with B-CLL, and recognized as part of follicular lymphoma by the presence of notched nucleus cells. This was seen in that study in 17 out of 75 of cases at presentation and in 10 others during the evolution of the disease, giving an overall incidence of 36%.
5. Good response to radiotherapy and low dose alkylating agents.
6. A long survival.
7. The existence of a rapidly fatal malignant transformation during which the disease behaves like an invasive tumour or an acute leukaemia.

Before the era of surface markers, cases of follicular lymphoma in leukaemic phase were described as 'lymphosarcoma cell leukaemia'. This designation is now considered imprecise because it does not indicate the precise type of NHL or the cell lineage (B or T) of the tumour. Follicular lymphoma is now recognized as a distinct histological entity both in the working formulation[39] and the Kiel classification[23]. The latter subclassifies follicular lymphoma (centroblastic/ centrocytic) according to:

1. The pattern of growth in: follicular (73%); the most common form, follicular and diffuse (23%); and the rare, diffuse pattern (4%).
2. The predominant cell type is small or large.

Follicular lymphoma is included in the working formulation as: follicular small cleaved cell, follicular mixed small cleaved and large cell and, in the group of intermediate prognosis, as diffuse with predominantly small-cleaved cells[38, 39].

Follicular lymphoma is the most common type of NHL (20–25%) in Western countries but is relatively rare in Japan, Africa and India. Although some authors found a correlation between the incidence of a leukaemic phase with a particular pattern of tumour growth[30], this has not been the experience of Lennert[23], who observed the follicular pattern in 19 out of 22 cases studied. The series of Spiro et al.[42] described cases with counts up to $30 \times 10^9/l$. The awareness of this syndrome and the routine use of membrane markers, not available in 1975, allowed the authors to recognize cases of follicular lymphoma presenting with WBC counts greater than $40 \times 10^9/l$[29]. In these, the lymph node histology was follicular with predominantly small cells in four out of seven cases, mixed in one and diffuse in two[29].

Morphology of circulating follicular lymphoma cells

The follicular lymphoma cells described as notched nuclei cells[42], small cleaved cells[25] or centrocytes[23], have distinct features in blood and bone marrow films (Figure 7.2) which are summarized in Table 7.4. These allow the recognition from B-CLL – disease which is often confused with follicular lymphoma although sometimes this distinction could be difficult. All the features listed in Table 7.4 are

Table 7.4 Morphology of circulating cells in follicular lymphoma (see Figure 7.2)

1. Small size, often the diameter of an erythrocyte, rarely less
2. Narrow rim of cytoplasm hardly visible in peripheral blood films; very high N/C ratio
3. Homogeneously condensed nuclear chromatin
4. Irregular nuclear outline with one or two narrow clefts originating in sharp angles from the nuclear surface and sometimes dividing the nucleus in two
5. Absent or inconspicuous nucleolus

From the literature [5, 23, 25, 29, 42].

equally important; the nuclear cleft is only one of them and may, in fact, not be easily visible in some cases. In Spiro's series[42], the peripheral blood cells were not characteristically notched in half of the cases. In a recent series of the authors with higher WBC counts[29], the proportion of such cells varied from 10% to 88%, being greater than 30% in 7 of 10 cases and from 5% to 20% in 3. 'Smudge cells', a feature of CLL, are not seen in follicular lymphoma; the nuclear clefting could be seen occasionally in B-CLL cases with high WBC count, but they rarely constitute more than 10% of the circulating cells.

Ultrastructural analysis is important to recognize the distinct features of follicular lymphoma cells. The proportion of typical cleft cells is always higher in such preparations. This is easy to understand because the narrow nuclear clefts may be below the threshold of visibility of the light microscope in such small cells. Follicular lymphoma cells have a high nucleo-/cytoplasmic (N/C) ratio and, invariably, show one or more deep nuclear clefts (Figures 7.3 and 7.4); nuclear pockets are also common (Figure 7.3). These cellular features are quite different

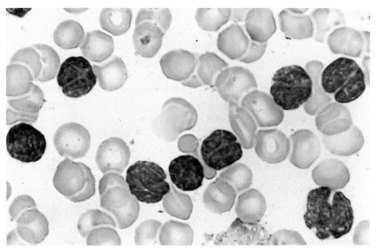

Figure 7.2 Peripheral blood film from a case of follicular lymphoma presenting with a high WBC count. The lymphocytes are of small size with no visible rim of cytoplasm and have distinct nuclear clefts, small cleaved cells of Lukes and Collins[25] and centrocytes of Lennert[23], which seem to divide the nucleus in half. × 1200, reduced to 80% on reproduction

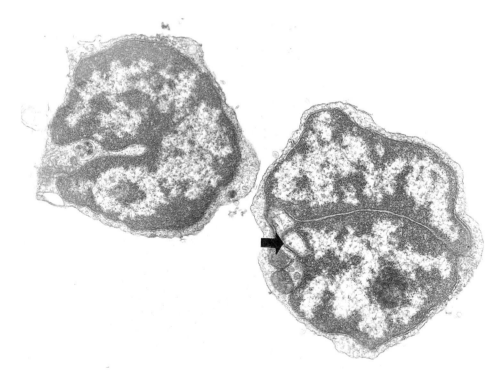

Figure 7.3 Electron micrograph of two circulating small cleft cells from a case of follicular lymphoma in leukaemic phase. The very narrow and deep indentation of one of the cells is not visible by light microscopy. Ultrastructural analysis is a very sensitive technique to identify these cells. Note the scanty cytoplasm in both cells and a nuclear pocket (arrow). × 16 000, reduced to 74% on reproduction

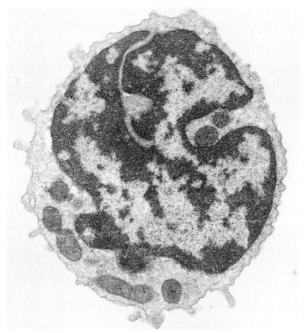

Figure 7.4 Circulating small follicular centre cell from another case of follicular lymphoma with high WBC count. Features are similar to the cells in Figure 7.3, except for a slightly more abundant cytoplasm; the nucleolus is not visible and there is abundant heterochromatin. × 18 400, reduced to 74% on reproduction

from those of the blastic phase of follicular lymphoma, which is a terminal event in 10% of cases [42] and may be seen in patients without previous blood involvement. The blast cells may be pleomorphic or large and undifferentiated, often with one or two prominent nucleoli and a deeply basophilic cytoplasm.

Bone marrow histology

The bone marrow is frequently involved in follicular lymphoma. Cases with a leukaemic phase always show involvement, usually with a paratrabecular and diffuse pattern. The paratrabecular infiltrate of small-to-medium size cells is sometimes clearly separated from the rest of the haemopoietic tissue; a nodular pattern of infiltration may be seen in some cases. In parallel with the upward trend of the WBC count the bone marrow pattern becomes more diffuse. The reticulin is usually increased in direct relationship to the degree of cellular infiltrate. Semithin sections of paraffin- and plastic-embedded material allow good appreciation of the morphology of the follicular centre cells.

Clinical features

As in uncomplicated follicular lymphoma these are: extensive lymphadenopathy, involving areas like the preauricular, mastoid and epitrochlear regions which are rarely involved in diffuse NHL or in B-CLL. CT scan and/or lymphography may show pelvic and para-aortic nodes; mesenteric nodes are also frequently involved.

The physical findings in the ten cases with high WBC count that the authors studied were as follows: splenomegaly in all of them (palpable 3–16 cm below the left costal margin), hepatomegaly in eight (4–12 cm below the right costal margin) and generalized lymphadenopathy in eight. Of interest, and contrasting with the findings of Spiro et al.[42], is the high incidence of splenomegaly in this series. It is possible that splenomegaly is a feature always seen in cases with high counts. However, cases of the rare splenic form of follicular lymphoma may not have a raised WBC count. The age range of the patients, 38–69 years, is consistent with that of other series of follicular lymphoma.

Haematological findings

Out of the authors' ten patients five had anaemia (Hb <10 g/dl), four thrombocytopenia (platelets <100 × 10^9/l), and the range of the WBC count was between 45 and 220 × 10^9/l, with a median of 102 × 10^9/l. The report of Spiro et al.[42] included cases with a WBC count between 5 and 30 × 10^9/l; only one case developed later a WBC count of 64 × 10^9/l, but this was during the terminal blastic phase.

Marker studies

These were discussed in detail above and summarized in Table 7.3. Of the authors' cases with WBC count greater than 40 × 10^9/l[29], one had more than 50% M-rosettes (as in B-CLL), two had 50% or more CD5+ cells, seven had 45% or more FMC7+ cells (a rare feature in B-CLL), and seven had 50% or more CD10+ cells. In addition, SmIg was strong (++ to +++) in all cases. None of the ten cases had the combination of membrane markers seen in B-CLL (see Table 7.3). The role of the membrane phenotype in the diagnosis of this condition was demonstrated by one of the patients from our series, who presented with a WBC count of 113 × 10^9/l, and a low proportion of identifiable small cleaved cells. Only the phenotype: SmIg++, M-rosettes 0%, CD5 28%, FMC7 50%, and CD10 30%, suggested an NHL, which was subsequently confirmed as follicular lymphoma by lymph node biopsy.

Course of the disease

Several reports[5, 42] suggested that a leukaemic phase, with a predominance of small lymphocytes, does not convey a poor prognosis in follicular lymphoma. Spiro et al.[42] discussed several patterns of evolution:

1. In some patients the count could decrease spontaneously and even become normal.
2. In others, it could decline following therapy and remain normal thereafter.
3. In others, it falls with the treatment and raises again during relapse.

This was in fact the authors' experience with several patients.

Patients with follicular lyphoma presenting with high WBC count and splenomegaly may represent a more aggressive form of the disease. Half of the patients in the authors' series[29] were dead within 3 years of diagnosis. This contrasts with the overall median survival of 8 years in CLL and greater than 5 years in follicular lymphoma, with or without a moderate lymphocytosis. Several patients received intensive courses of combination chemotherapy, e.g. CHOP, and although some complete remissions were documented[29], these were short-lived. Except for this group, the overall prognosis of follicular lymphoma is relatively good[39], although cures are rare, and the disease follows a chronic course with a pattern of remissions and relapses. There is as yet no good published evidence that combination chemotherapy with four or more agents is better than the combination of chlorambucil and prednisone, or than chlorambucil alone. An ongoing National Cancer Institute study is comparing the use of intense combination chemotherapy plus total nodal irradiation with a policy of no treatment but of 'watch and wait' until there is evidence of disease progression[52a]. No differences in survival have yet emerged in the published data but this has shown that the initial aggressive therapy is associated with a high complete remission rate (78%) and a prolonged remission duration (median greater than 45 months). Patients in the 'watchful' arm of the study had a lower complete remission rate (43%) when they were crossed over to the intensive therapy arm[52a], thus suggesting that primary resistance to treatment in follicular lymphoma relates more to disease progression than to previous chemotherapy. It is apparent, too, that delaying treatment does not prevent the evolution to transformation of some follicular lymphomas.

Intermediate or mantle zone (or centrocytic) NHL

There are few detailed reports of the leukaemic manifestation of this NHL[35a]. Lennert[23] refers to the leukaemic variant of centrocytic lymphoma as one of the conditions earlier included under the term 'lymphosarcoma cell leukaemia' and also comments that the involvement of the bone marrow (presumably also the peripheral blood) is more frequent in this condition than in follicular lymphoma. The paucity of descriptions of the leukaemic phase of this NHL relates partly to the fact that this condition has only recently been recognized and that there is still some confusion about its relationship with CLL and follicular lymphoma. Part of the confusion is the use of the term 'centrocyte'[23] or 'small cleaved cell'[39] for a cell which appears to be immunologically distinct from the small cleft cell of follicular lymphoma and may originate from the follicular mantle zone[18, 45]. In the working formulation[39] this condition is given as of intermediate prognosis and as equivalent to malignant lymphoma centrocytic of the Kiel classification[23].

The term 'intermediate NHL' is also a source of confusion. For example Evans et al.[10] identified a subgroup of small lymphocytic lymphomas with a relatively high mitotic rate (>30 mitoses per 20 high power fields) in lymph node biopsies, which had a worse prognosis than those with lower mitotic rates. Weisenburger et al.[49] recognize intermediate NHL as a distinct type between the small lymphocytic and small cleaved (follicular lymphoma) type with diffuse pattern of infiltration, and with a course similar to the diffuse small cleaved (or centrocytic) NHL. Although they recognize that some cases have a mantle zone pattern, these authors distinguish the disease they call intermediate lymphocytic lymphoma from mantle zone lymphoma. On the other hand the National Cancer Institute (NCI) group coined the term 'NHL of intermediate grade of differentiation and morphology' and recently defined very precisely the features of this distinct type of NHL, which they describe as identical to centrocytic lymphoma, and suggest the designation in future studies of mantle zone lymphoma[18], in agreement with other reports[35].

Leukaemic phase of mantle zone NHL

Blood involvement has been observed in between 20% and 50% of cases but a WBC count greater than $5 \times 10^9/l$ has been reported as infrequent[18]. However, the authors have recently identified 11 cases in which the WBC count was greater than $50 \times 10^9/l$, with some presenting with counts above $100 \times 10^9/l$[35a]. In other studies, mainly originating from pathological material, the WBC count was usually only moderately raised. Of the 15 cases described by Swerdlow et al.[46], 8 had lymphocytosis, 4 between 4.1 and $15 \times 10^9/l$ and 4 greater than $15 \times 10^9/l$. These cases represented 2.5% of all NHLs studied at St Bartholomew's Hospital, London. Five of the 12 (42%) described by Weisenburger et al.[49] had more than $5 \times 10^9/l$. These authors describe the cells as atypical prolymphocytes rather than small lymphocytes. Four of the 19 cases described by Narang et al.[32] presenting with splenomegaly and histology of intermediate NHL, had lymphocytosis from 5.2 to $6.2 \times 10^9/l$.

Morphology

The predominant cell in peripheral blood is of medium size with condensed nuclear chromatin and nuclear irregularities with indentations which are not so deep as those of follicular lymphoma. There is often an admixture of small round and small cleaved lymphocytes with others of medium size (which predominate) and larger cells with little cytoplasm. A nucleolus is visible in some of these cells but it is rarely large or very prominent as in prolymphocytes. The peripheral blood film is usually pleomorphic without the uniformity seen in CLL or PLL. Some cases resemble follicular lymphoma, if the cleft cells are conspicuous; more often they resemble cases of B-CLL in transformation, with more than one cell size. However, in contrast to CLL/PL, in mantle zone lymphoma the predominant cells are not small lymphocytes.

Histology

There is very little information on the bone marrow appearances in this tumour. This is surprising since involvement of the bone marrow is quite frequent[23, 46]. Bone marrow trephine biopsies usually show diffuse lymphocytic infiltration with cells larger than CLL lymphocytes and show an irregular nuclear outline. A paratrabecular pattern of infiltration may be seen in some cases. More information is clearly necessary on this point, because the bone marrow histology may be an important feature to consider in cases presenting in leukaemic phase. The lymph node histology shows a diffuse or vaguely nodular pattern with lymphocytes that efface the normal architecture[18, 46]. The nodular aspect is the result of the expansion of the mantle zone around 'naked' germinal centres which, in contrast to those seen in CLL, are seen abundantly in the lymph node sections. Also in contrast to the intact germinal centres seen in T-cell malignancies, in mantle zone NHL they lack the normal lymphoid cuffs[18, 35a]. The infiltrating cells are small, show nuclear irregularity and indentation[49], but may rarely be slightly larger with a fine chromatin pattern which can also be seen during progression of the disease[18]. In any case, as those seen in peripheral blood films, nucleoli are inconspicuous. The number of mitotic figures is rarely greater than 30 per 20 high power fields[18, 46]. The spleen is frequently involved (see below) and involvement is seen predominantly in the white pulp which is uniformly expanded with variable red pulp involvement. The white pulp comprises widened mantle zones of small lymphocytes with an irregular nuclear outline surrounded by larger cells in the marginal zone[32]. This phenomenon of margination is seen also in the closely related splenic lymphoma with circulating villous cells or SLVL[28].

Clinical features

Like most low-grade lymphomas, intermediate NHL affects mainly adults. Two-thirds of cases are older than 50 years and about 10% are younger than 40 years. The male:female ratio is 2:1 or greater. Main disease features are: generalized lymphadenopathy in 95%, which includes superficial, hilar, mediastinal and para-aortic nodes, and splenomegaly. Most patients have stage IV disease according to the Ann Arbor classification as shown by pathological involvement of the liver and the bone marrow[18]. In the authors' series of 11 patients presenting with high WBC count (range 26–269 × 10^9/l; median 45 × 10^9/l) splenomegaly (2–10 cm below the costal margin) was noted in 8, hepatomegaly in 5 and lymphadenopathy in 9. Splenomegaly was also recorded in 9 out of 12 cases described by Weisenburger et al.[49], 5 of which had lymphocyte counts above 5 × 10^9/l, and in 11 out of 15 cases reported by Swerdlow et al.[46], 8 of which had lymphocytosis greater than 4 × 10^9/l. In a study of NHL presenting with splenomegaly, Narang et al.[32] described intermediate lymphocytic lymphoma as the largest group – 19 out of 31 cases. In this group only 2 had peripheral lymphadenopathy and 4 had lymphocyte counts above 5 × 10^9/l.

Constitutional symptoms such as sweating, weight loss and fever are present in 30–40% of patients[46]. The gastrointestinal tract, the skin and the central nervous system may be affected in some cases. Anaemia and thrombocytopenia are seen in a variable number of patients. In the authors' series of 11 cases with high WBC count, 6 had haemoglobin less than 10 g/dl and 3 had platelets less than 100 × 10^9/l.

Marker studies

Mantle zone or intermediate NHL is a B-cell malignancy and monoclonal SmIg of moderate to strong density is demonstrated in all cases. In the majority IgM only is expressed on the malignant cells[18, 45], but rarely IgM and IgD are co-expressed sharing a single light chain. In contrast to follicular lymphoma, the residual germinal centres in intermediate lymphoma are not part of the malignancy as shown by the lack of a monoclonal staining pattern with anti-Ig reagents. A distinct feature of this tumour, in common with B-CLL and different from follicular lymphoma, is the consistent expression of CD5 in the majority of cells (see Table 7.3). In 9 of the 11 cases in leukaemic phase, more than 50% of circulating lymphocytes were CD5+ and, in common with other B-cell NHLs, were also FMC7+. The question of the variable expression of CD10 in this lymphoma has been discussed above. The cells may be positive when tested in suspension and this was also the authors' experience in blood samples: three cases had 44–90% positive lymphocytes, three 16–39% positive cells and three were negative. Results in frozen sections by immunocytochemical methods are, as a rule, negative. Stein et al.[45] have argued against the mantle zone origin of centrocytic lymphoma because of the lack of expression of the antigen detected by the monoclonal antibody TU1, whilst normal mantle zone lymphocytes and CLL cells are TU1+. This reagent has not been tested extensively by other workers, so this point will need confirmation in cases classified as mantle zone NHL.

Clinical course

The disease has a variable course which depends on how extensive the organ involvement is at presentation. The median survival is between 2.5 and 4 years which is significantly shorter than in follicular lymphoma; in the series from the NCI[18] the median survival was somewhat longer. In the analysis leading to the working formulation[39] diffuse small cleaved cell NHL, which corresponds to or includes mantle zone lymphoma, was considered of intermediate prognostic grade with a median survival of 3.4 years, contrasting with follicular lymphoma which, in that study, had median survivals of 5 years (for the small cleaved and large cell type) and 7 years (for the small cleaved cell type). The complete remission (CR) rates were also higher in follicular lymphoma (65–73%) than in the diffuse small cleaved type (56%). Relapse after remission is, on the other hand, common for this lymphoma and for follicular lymphoma. The prognosis of the authors' patients with high WBC count appears to be significantly worse than that of patients presenting without leukaemia. A report from St Bartholomew's Hospital, London[46] also showed a significantly shorter survival in patients with lymphocytosis (median 17 months) than those without lymphocytosis (median 52 months). There is not a well-established treatment modality for this NHL. The trend has been to treat with combination chemotherapy but there is not enough information about which regimen is better or whether more intensive protocols are beneficial and result in improved patients' survival.

Lymphoplasmacytic lymphoma

Lymphomas of low grade malignancy in which the cells show morphological and/or functional features of Ig secretion are classified as lymphoplasmacytic lymphoma (LPL). In a high proportion of cases (about 65%) the NHL is associated with moderate lymphocytosis above 4×10^9/l; cases with high WBC count are rare. This disorder according to Lennert represents 16% of all NHLs[23]. Although the histopathological diagnosis is often relatively easy when there are clear features of plasma cell differentation, when no histology is available and a monoclonal band is not detectable in the serum and/or urine as free light chain (which may occur in 60–70% of cases), the differential diagnosis with CLL and other B-cell leukaemias may present problems. In some studies the criteria are not very strict and over-classification of cases in the category of LPL rather than CLL may distort the statistics. Lennert himself[23] has a low threshold for a diagnosis of LPL even by the sole evidence of globular PAS (periodic acid–Schiff) inclusions in the nucleus or cytoplasm of lymphoid cells in lymph node sections. In addition to the morphological and serological criteria, evidence of plasmacytic differentiation provided by cell marker studies may be useful, particularly in relation to the distinction from B-CLL, disease in which up to 5% of cases may have a small 'M' band.

LPL may manifest itself with several clinicopathological syndromes, namely:

1. Waldenström's macroglobulinaemia, characterized by a major IgM band (usually over 20 g/l), lymphoplasmacytic cells in the peripheral blood and bone marrow, increased bone marrow fibrosis and prominent mast cells (this condition is described in more detail in Chapter 10).

2. LPL other than Waldenström's macroglobulinaemia in which the clinical pathological features may be similar but the paraprotein is IgG or rarely IgA; such cases have an agressive clinical course and may be confused with plasma cell leukaemia.
3. Splenic lymphoma with circulating villous lymphocytes (SLVL), a condition which will be described in more detail below.

From the point of view of LPL a purely splenomegalic form represents 10% of all cases; however, SLVL may be more common in cases presenting with a leukaemic blood picture. Two-thirds of cases of SLVL have a monoclonal band which is often IgM, but it could also be IgG or only free light chains[28]. As distinct from Waldenström's macroglobulinaemia the concentration of the 'M' band is always, in the authors' experience, below 20 g/l, in SLVL.

Some of the reasons why differences still exist between different groups in the classification of leukaemia/lymphoma syndromes relate to the source of diagnostic material and whether the analysis is reported by pathological or haematological/ clinical groups. For the latter, peripheral blood and bone marrow morphology, surface markers and clinical information may suffice. Lymph node histology is not always available, sometimes because a biopsy is not possible and sometimes because it is deemed to be non-essential. Clinical details and peripheral blood and bone marrow morphology are not, however, always included in pathology studies. There is clearly a need to define more precisely the conditions included in the large group of LPLs and to spell out clearly the morphological, histological and other biological features of the disease in order to draw better conclusions which could be relevant to patient management.

Splenic lymphoma with villous lymphocytes

Neiman et al. [33] first described in 1979 a group of 10 patients with massive spleen, minimal lymphadenopathy, circulating cells with 'hairy' cytoplasm and an 'M' band in the serum of half of them. Despite the clinical features suggestive of hairy cell leukaemia with low WBC count ($3–18 \times 10^9$/l in this series) and spleen weights of 1.1–3.6 kg, the spleen histology showed white nodules up to 1 cm in diameter and neoplastic cells always involving the white pulp with variable involvement of the red pulp. This clearly was different from the exclusive red pulp involvement of hairy cell leukaemia in which the white pulp is completely unaffected. A number of other groups (see reviews[28, 43]) have now characterized this disorder further, emphasizing as Neiman did, that the main difference from HCL was the nodular involvement of the spleen and also often of the bone marrow.

Morphology

Circulating SLVL cells are larger than CLL lymphocytes and smaller than hairy cells. The nucleus is regular (round or ovoid) and has clumped chromatin; the nucleo-/cytoplasmic (N/C) ratio is relatively high. This intermediate size was confirmed in cell volume studies[28]. A distinct feature of SLVL cells is the presence of numerous short villi or long and thin cytoplasmic projections which are concentrated in one or both poles of the cell (Figure 7.5). When the cytoplasmic villi are not prominent SLVL can be confused with the splenomegalic form of CLL.

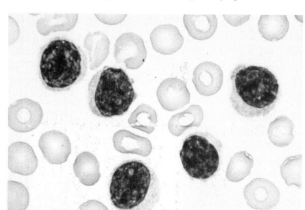

(a)

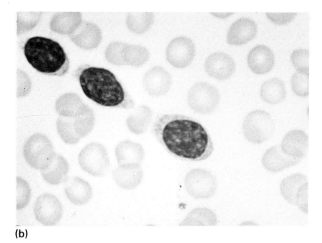

(b)

Figure 7.5 Peripheral blood from patients with splenic lymphoma with circulating villous lymphocytes (SLVL). The lymphocytes have condensed nuclear chromatin with moderate amount of cytoplasm. Some of the cells in (a) show short villi and an irregular membrane outline. Cells in (b) are elongated and tend to have villi in one pole of the cytoplasm. × 1400, reduced to 68% on reproduction

The cytoplasm is less abundant than in hairy cells and is always moderately basophilic; plasmacytic features are apparent in 5–10% of these cells. The nucleolus is prominent in a proportion of cases giving rise to problems of differential diagnosis with B-PLL and the variant form of HCL[28].

A positive tartrate-resistant acid phosphatase (TRAP) was reported by Neiman et al.[33] and Spriano et al.[43] but has not been the authors' experience[28]. Under carefully controlled conditions and using samples of HCL as positive controls, the authors showed acid phosphatase activity in up to 30% of cells but the reaction weakened in the presence of tartaric acid in most cases[28].

Ultrastructural studies carried out by Dr Daniele Robinson from the authors' group confirmed the two types of villous projections seen in these cells: abundant and short, and scanty and long, the high N/C ratio, and the absence of

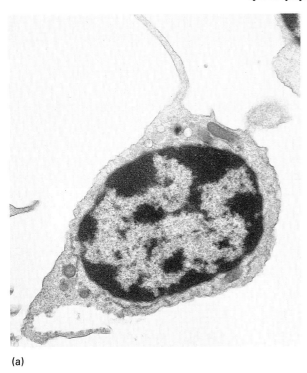

(a)

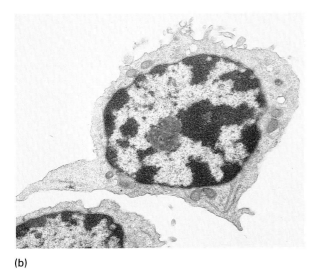

(b)

Figure 7.6 Electron micrographs of two villous lymphocytes from a case of SLVL. These cells have few long cytoplasmic projections. The nuclear chromatin is dense (mature cells) and only one (b) has a visible small nucleolus. No other distinct cytoplasmic features are apparent. (a) ×12 600, reduced to 77% on reproduction; (b) × 15 000, reduced to 63% on reproduction

ribosome–lamella complex (a feature of HCL) and of parallel arrangements of endoplasmic reticulum (as seen in plasma cells), as well as the presence of a small nucleolus in the majority of cells from half of the cases (Figure 7.6)[29a, 38a].

Histopathology

As mentioned above, a characteristic feature of SLVL and other B-cell leukaemias is the involvement of the splenic white pulp[33, 43]. In the authors' experience the infiltration always affects the white and red pulp but predominates in one of them. However, and in contrast to HCL, there is never exclusive involvement of the red pulp with preservation or atrophy of the white pulp; the infiltrating cells are also not arranged in a regular spaced manner as in HCL. The spleen shows nodular infiltration with a mixture of small and medium-sized cells with clumped nuclear chromatin. The white pulp nodules show the phenomenon of margination, i.e. the concentration of larger cells in the periphery and smaller cells in the centre[28]. Features of lymphoplasmacytoid differentiation are always apparent[43] and this, plus the frequent demonstration of an 'M' band, supports the relationship of SLVL with LPL (or immunocytoma). PAS+ material is often found in the central areas of the lymphoid nodules. Peripheral lymph nodes are rarely enlarged but abdominal nodes are often removed during splenectomy[33]. These show infiltration and effacement of the normal architecture with involvement of the cortical, paracortical and medullary nodal areas[33, 43]. The histology of the lymph nodes resembles that of other low grade NHLs with a predominance of well-differentiated lymphocytes plus lymphoplasmacytic differentiation and PAS intranuclear inclusions.

The bone marrow shows a nodular or a patchy diffuse pattern on infiltration. In some cases the infiltration is minimal with a diffuse interstitial or slightly paratrabecular pattern. The bone marrow aspirate did not show an excess of lymphocytes (less than 30%) in half of the authors' cases[28]. In some of the latter, however, the bone marrow trephine biopsy confirmed infiltration by NHL but in others the biopsies failed to show unequivocal evidence of lymphocytic infiltration, confirming that SLVL is primarily a splenic lymphoma. The bone marrow is abnormal in 75% of cases and may be uninvolved in 25% of cases. In contrast to HCL bone marrow aspirates in SLVL are usually successful and do not show the pattern of infiltration characteristic of HCL (see Chapter 6).

Clinical and laboratory features

A summary from the cases reported by the authors[28] is given in Table 7.5. There is a slight predominance of males and the mean age at diagnosis is 72 years. The presenting symptoms are non-specific and in some patients the diagnosis is made by chance. The main physical sign is splenomegaly; rarely a diagnosis of SLVL is made in the absence of a palpable spleen. In contrast to HCL, thrombocytopenia, neutropenia and monocytopenia are uncommon in SLVL, reflecting preservation of the bone marrow function. Moderate anaemia (Hb <12 g/dl) can be seen in half of the patients. Main laboratory features are a moderate lymphocytosis (rarely above $40 \times 10^9/l$) with the morphological features described above and the presence of a monoclonal band in the serum and/or the urine. This constellation of features is unique to SLVL and, if anything, it more often resembles CLL than

Table 7.5 Clinical and laboratory features of SLVL

Feature		Incidence (%)
Splenomegaly		90
Hepatomegaly		45
Lymphadenopathy		22
Hb	<11 g/dl	28
Platelets	<100 × 10⁹/l	20
Lymphocytes	>10 × 10⁹/l	60
	>15 × 10⁹/l	36
Paraprotein[a]		60
Bone marrow	none	28
involvement	mild	22

[a] In serum and/or urine.

HCL. Autoimmune haemolytic anaemia or immune thrombocytopenia may be seen in a minority (about 5%) of cases.

Marker studies

The membrane phenotype of SLVL cells is similar to that of mature late B-cells and, in this respect, is not very different from that of B-PLL or follicular lymphoma. SLVL cells express strongly SmIg, FMC7 and membrane CD22 and are usually CD5− and CD10−. On the other hand, they do not express the hairy cell marker HC2, but may react as HCL with LeuM5 (30% of cases) and CD25 (10% of cases). The evidence of plasmacytic differentiation is confirmed by the reactivity with CD38 (OKT10), a plasma cell marker, in 25% of cases and with BU11 in the majority of cases. In contrast to plasma cells, SLVL cells always express in their membrane the pan-B-cell antigens (CD19, CD20) as well as class II major histocompatibility antigens (HLA-DR).

Differential diagnosis

The distinctive features of a group of B-lymphoproliferative disorders with a large spleen, with particular relevance to SLVL, are analysed in Table 7.6. These details are important because in the authors' patients, as in those from other series[33, 43], a diagnosis of SLVL was not made or suspected at presentation[28], but instead one or other of the B-cell disorders shown in Table 7.6 was diagnosed. SLVL has clinical features in common with all the other disorders, but the combination of clinical and laboratory findings, including membrane markers and spleen and bone marrow histology, suggest that it constitutes a distinct clinicopathological entity. The presence of a paraprotein in the serum and/or of light chains in the urine constitutes a strong element for suspecting SLVL or another form of immunocytoma. Table 7.6 confirms that the membrane phenotype of HCL is unique and different from that of the other B-cell disorders, in particular from B-CLL – disease which, at the other extreme, also has a distinct immunophenotype (see also Table 7.3). The authors have occasionally experienced difficulties in the differential diagnosis between SLVL and HCL-variant when the circulating cells have a slightly abundant villous cytoplasm and a prominent nucleolus.

Table 7.6 Differential diagnosis of B-cell disorders with a large spleen

Feature	CLL	PLL	SLVL	HCL-V	HCL
M:F ratio	2:1	1.6:1	1.9:1	4:1	4:1
Age (years)[a]	64	70	72	61	55
WBC count ($\times 10^9$/l)[a]	97	175	17	85	10
Cell volume (fl)[b]	211	307	356	433	526
Paraprotein (%)	5	30	60	0	10
Spleen size	+	++	++	++	+/++
Lymph nodes	++	−	±	−	−
TRAP	−	−	−/+	−	++
Tac (CD25)	−	−	−	−	++
anti-HC2	−	−	−	−	++
LeuM5 (CD11c)	−	−	−/+	+	++
BU11	−	−/±	++	++	++
SmIg					
Class[c]	MD	MD	MD(AG)	G	MDAG
Intensity	±	++	++	++	++
White pulp[d]	++	++	++	−	−
Red pulp[d]	±	+	+	++	++

[a] Mean values; [b] median values; [c] heavy chains sharing single light chain; [d] spleen involvement; HCL-V: variant form of HCL; TRAP: tartrate-resistant acid phosphatase.

Prognosis and treatment

The disease has a chronic course and, unless the spleen is very large and/or the cytopenia severe, the clinical features may remain stable. Ten per cent of patients may not require any treatment at all for long periods of time. Usually the spleen tends to enlarge and this often leads to a splenectomy or other measures to reduce the spleen size, e.g. splenic irradiation. These two measures have resulted, in the authors' experience, in prolonged haematological and clinical remissions. As Spriano et al.[43] observed, a consistent reduction in the WBC count following splenectomy in some patients has been observed by the authors. When the WBC count is still high and/or the bone marrow shows infiltration after splenectomy, treatment with chemotherapy to reduce further the tumour mass (e.g. chlorambucil as in B-CLL) may be necessary. This type of chemotherapy when given prior to splenectomy has not, however, been very successful. In only one patient treated with a low continuous daily dose of chlorambucil for 2 years were a significant reduction in spleen size and the disappearance of the paraprotein observed. The authors' policy is to observe first the pattern of the disease (in order to decide whether it is stable or progressive) and consider splenectomy as the first line of treatment. If this is contraindicated on clinical grounds or refused by the patient, splenic irradiation is the authors' second choice, followed later on, if indicated, by chlorambucil given intermittently in high doses ($60\,\text{mg/m}^2$ given over 3 or 4 days every month). The effect of treatment with any of these modalities can be monitored by the spleen size, the lymphocyte count, the size of the 'M' band and the correction of the anaemia. There has been no opportunity yet to treat SLVL patients with α-interferon or 2′-deoxycoformycin and therefore the authors are not aware whether these agents are effective in this disease; there are also no published data on their use in this relatively new B-cell disorder.

Burkitt's lymphoma

A leukaemic manifestation is not common in Burkitt's lymphoma. A minority of non-endemic cases present as an acute leukaemia (ALL-L3) and others have bone marrow involvement with some frequency. Burkitt's lymphoma is a high grade NHL in the working formulation (malignant lymphoma, small non-cleaved cell, Burkitt's)[38, 39] and the Kiel classification (lymphoblastic, Burkitt type)[23, 44]. The term 'small non-cleaved cells' is a relative one by comparison with large non-cleaved cells. The cells in Burkitt's lymphoma have a uniform round nucleus; the nuclear membrane is prominent and the chromatin is irregularly distributed; two to five nucleoli are usually present[51]. The cytoplasm is intensely basophilic (pyroninophilic) and a 'starry-sky' pattern given by the macrophages around the tumour cells is characteristic[39, 45]; mitoses are abundant. When seen in bone marrow aspirates and/or lymph node imprints or rarely in peripheral blood films, the cells are moderately large blasts with a deep basophilic cytoplasm which contains numerous vacuoles. Most features of Burkitt's lymphoma have attracted great scientific interest: the histopathology[50], epidemiology[8], chromosome translocations[9, 20, 40, 54], molecular biology[7], the relationship to malaria[8] and the resulting cellular immunodeficiency[52], and, foremost, the possible aetiological role of the Epstein–Barr virus (EBV) in this remarkable disease[8, 26].

Two types of Burkitt's lymphoma

A number of clinical and laboratory findings (summarized in Table 7.7) suggest strongly that there are two distinct types of Burkitt's lymphoma, which can be distinguished by their epidemiology (endemic or sporadic), some of the clinical features and prognosis, and the role that EBV and holoendemic malaria play in their pathogenesis. Features in common are B-cell markers, L3 morphology and chromosome translocations (Table 7.7), although observations on Burkitt's

Table 7.7 Clinical and laboratory features of two types of Burkitt's lymphoma[a]

	Feature	Endemic (African)	Sporadic (non-African)
Similarities	L3 morphology	+	+
	B-cell markers	+	+
	t(8;14) (8q24;14q32)[b]	+	+
Differences	C3b and EBV receptors	+	−
	EBNA	+	−
	Localization (%)		
	Abdomen	58	91
	Jaw	58	7
	Bone marrow	7	20[c]
	Long-term survivors (%)	50[d]	Variable[d]

[a] Based on published data [26, 45].
[b] Typical translocation in 85% of cases; variant translocations t(2;8) (p11;q24) and t(8;22) (q24;q11) seen in 15% of cases [7, 9, 20, 24, 54].
[c] Presenting as ALL-L3 (B-ALL) [20] (see also Chapter 2).
[d] According to disease stage. The median survival of ALL-L3 is 5 months [26].

lymphoma-derived cell lines suggest phenotypic differences between African and non-African cases[11]. Studies by Croce[7] suggest a different molecular lesion resulting from the disease evolving from B-cells at different stages of differentiation. The leukaemic manifestations are seen more often in Caucasians with the sporadic (non-endemic) form of Burkitt's lymphoma. These cases present as ALL-L3 type, or B-cell ALL, which is the leukaemic phase of Burkitt's lymphoma (see also Chapter 2). ALL-L3 shares most biological features with the non-endemic cases, except perhaps the extensive abdominal nodal involvement which is frequent only in the non-leukaemic forms of Burkitt's lymphoma[20]. CNS leukaemia is slightly more frequent in non-endemic (14%) than in African cases (10%)[26].

Relation to Epstein–Barr virus

EBV is associated with African Burkitt's lymphoma in 97% of cases as demonstrated by high antibody titres against viral antigens (eight- to ten-fold greater geometric mean titres than in control groups without Burkitt's lymphoma)[26] and by the presence of EBV DNA, EBV nuclear antigen (EBNA) and the EBV membrane antigenic complex in fresh tumour cells as well as in Burkitt's lymphoma-derived cell lines. EBV has also been isolated from cultured Burkitt's lymphoma cells which release infectious viral particles. Infection with EBV occurs months or years before the development of Burkitt's lymphoma; children with the highest antibody titres appear to be at a greater risk of developing it. The oncogenic potential of EBV is demonstrated by the easy immortalization in vitro of normal B-lymphocytes and the establishment of lymphoblastoid cell lines which lack the chromosome translocations characteristic of Burkitt's lymphoma. Only in a minority of cases of non-African Burkitt's lymphoma (about 15–20%) has an association with EBV been demonstrated. It is now generally accepted that the infection with EBV is only one of the multiple steps which results in Burkitt's lymphoma. Holoendemic malaria is the most important cofactor in the pathogenesis supported by the identical geographical distribution of both conditions in equatorial Africa. A mechanism by which malaria facilitates the action of EBV has recently been suggested. Whittle et al.[52] have shown that following an acute attack of malaria caused by *Plasmodium falciparum*, the balance of T-cell subsets is altered dramatically resulting in a low CD4/CD8 ratio, a loss of virus-specific cytotoxic T-lymphocytes, and in the abnormal proliferation of EBV-infected B-cells which secrete large amounts of Ig and antibodies. Thus the immune response which operates against EBV infections in normal individuals is profoundly affected after acute attacks of malaria.

Membrane phenotype of Burkitt's lymphoma cells and cell lines

Burkitt-type lymphoblasts have a moderately immature B-cell phenotype: they express SmIg, nearly always IgM, and most pan-B antigens (CD19, CD20, CD24), they are often CD10+ but only exceptionally TdT+, and are negative with monoclonal antibodies against CD5 and CD23 (TU1, BL13)[26, 45]. Some differences in maturation stage or of cell origin between African and non-African (sporadic) cases have been suggested as a result of studies with Burkitt's lymphoma (BL)-derived cell lines. Magrath[26] indicated that cells from non-African Burkitt's lymphoma are slightly more immature than cells from African cases. Favrot et al. [11] examined the phenotype of 28 BL cell lines and concluded that some African Burkitt's lymphoma-derived lines have characteristics of follicular centre cells, like centroblasts (CD23+, CD10−, CD24−/+, SmIg−/+, Cyt IgM+) or like centroblastic/centrocytic NHL cells (CD23+, CD10+, CD24+, SmIg+), whilst cell lines from Caucasian Burkitt's lymphoma are CD23−, CD10+, CD24++ which suggests a bone marrow origin. Almost all the cell lines are CD5− and CD20+.

The antigen profile of BL cell lines was correlated, in another study [9], with the types of chromosome translocation. The cell lines carrying variant translocations, t(2;8) or t(8;22), are CD10− and BLA− (a Burkitt's lymphoma antigen), tend to express cytoplasmic rather than membrane Ig, and were thought to consist of more mature B-cells [9]. In contrast, cell lines with the typical t(8;14) are either CD10+ and/or BLA+ or BLA−. As these translocations probably occur as a result of errors during the rearrangement of Ig genes and the rearrangement of heavy chain genes (in chromosome 14) precedes the rearrangement of light chain genes (in chromosome 2 for κ or 22 for λ), the cytogenetic and immunological findings of that study [9] are compatible with the concept that the variant translocation affects more differentiated B-cells than those with the typical t(8;14) translocation.

Clinical course

The prognosis of Burkitt's lymphoma depends on the stage of the disease which in turn reflects the tumour burden. Intra-abdominal disease (stage C), particularly with multiple extra-abdominal sites (stage D) has the worst prognosis [26]. Bone marrow involvement, especially if the percentage of blasts is greater than 25%, is also a bad prognostic feature. The non-endemic form of Burkitt's lymphoma is the one associated with the worst prognostic features. Some biochemical measurements in the serum such as lactic dehydrogenase and uric acid levels tend to correlate with tumour burden. A leukaemic phase, heavy bone marrow involvement, with or without peripheral blood blasts, has the highest risk for early death. Treatment strategies have evolved from single agent chemotherapy, of which cyclophosphamide appears to be the best drug, to intensive combination protocols which include 42-hour infusions of methotrexate in the NCI studies [26]. Patients presenting as ALL-L3 have the worst prognosis by comparison with other lymphoblastic leukaemias. The only chance of cure in such patients, at the present time, is to achieve complete remission and then be treated by total body irradiation, high dose cyclophosphamide and an allogeneic bone marrow transplant.

Large cell NHL in leukaemic phase

The incidence of a frank leukaemic phase in cases of large cell NHL is probably low although precise statistics are lacking. The incidence of bone marrow involvement is of the order of 10% but circulating lymphoma cells are seen in a much lower proportion of cases. The authors have been able to study several patients who presented with large blast cells in the peripheral blood suggesting initially a diagnosis of acute leukaemia. The cells often resemble monoblasts because of their large size, abundant cytoplasm, prominent nucleolus and lack of cytoplasmic granules. Cells of such a large size can be detected by cell volume estimations (see Figure 7.1) and can probably also be identified by the systems used currently for

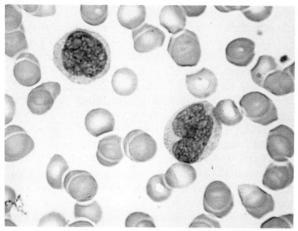

Figure 7.7 Circulating blast-like cells from a case diagnosed as large cell lymphoma in leukaemic phase. Morphologically these cells may correspond to centroblasts[23] or large non-cleaved cells[25]. × 1400, reduced to 65% on reproduction

differential counting based on cell volumes. Cases of large cell NHL have either a B-cell phenotype and correspond to centroblasts or B-immunoblasts (Figures 7.7 and 7.8) or are T-immunoblastic lymphomas which often present with bone marrow involvement as the primary site (Figure 7.9).

Cell markers

The cells in 80% of cases have a mature B-cell phenotype. The majority of cases are SmIg+, CD19+, CD20+, but 10% do not express SmIg[12]. In a case studied by the authors which presented with a WBC count of 90 × 10⁹/l and morphology resembling monoblastic leukaemia, the cells expressed monoclonal SmIg and this was confirmed by the demonstration of rearranged Ig genes by DNA analysis. In the seven cases with a T-cell phenotype tested, the circulating large lymphoma cells formed rosettes with sheep erythrocytes (Figure 7.10) in five, and were either CD4+ or CD8+ and had features of transformed T-lymphocytes: reactivity with CD38 (OKT10) and expression of class II major histocompatibility antigens (HLA-DR), absence of immature (thymic) markers (CD1a−, TdT−), and frequent lack of expression of membrane CD3. Natural killer markers, CD16 and/or CD11b, were positive in two of seven cases (Dr E. Matutes, unpublished data).

Prognosis of large cell NHL

Tumour bulk, presence or absence of B-symptoms, splenic enlargement, involvement of extranodal sites, chiefly bone marrow, liver and pleura are all features of a poor prognosis. Information about prognostic factors facilitates the interpretation of clinical trials. The achievement of complete remission in cases with good prognostic features is associated with prolonged disease-free survival which in many patients represents clinical cures. In the authors' experience a complete remission is difficult to achieve in cases with blood and bone marrow involvement. The evolution in T-cell immunoblastic lymphomas is more aggressive

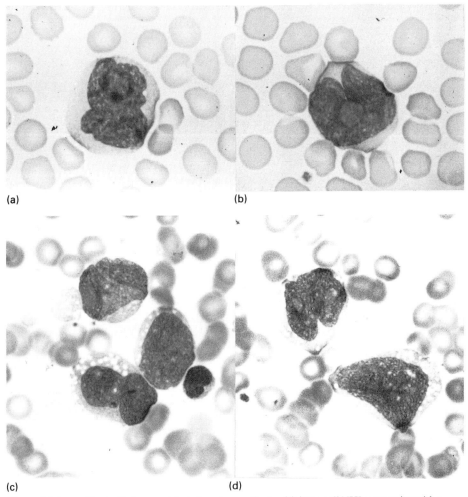

(a)   (b)

(c)   (d)

Figure 7.8 Large blast cells/immunoblasts from two patients with large cell NHL presenting with a leukaemic blood picture. Cells on a and b correspond to the cells with a very large volume of curve 3, Figure 7.1. The blasts in both cases had a mature B-cell phenotype. × 1400, reduced to 78% on reproduction

and is associated with systemic symptoms. Cases with a B-cell phenotype have a better survival despite also not achieving complete remission.

Treatment of NHLs

It is beyond the remit of this chapter to review the treatment of NHLs. The advances and the guidelines will only be outlined when relevant to the management of cases in leukaemic phase. The distinction made above between the different clinical significance of blood and bone marrow involvement when seen in low grade NHLs (where it is frequent) and in high grade NHLs (where it has bad prognostic implications) should be borne in mind. (For a comprehensive review of the treatment strategies for NHLs see Gobbi and Cavalli[14].)

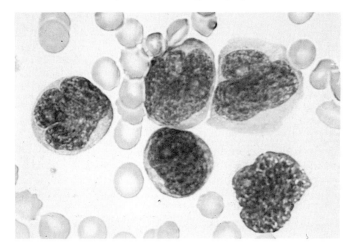

Figure 7.9 Blasts from a case of large cell NHL (T-immunoblastic) who developed a rapidly progressive leukaemic phase shortly after diagnosis. These cells had deep basophilic cytoplasm and membrane phenotype of activated cells (TdT−, E+, CD4+, CD38+, Ia+). × 1500, reduced to 64% on reproduction

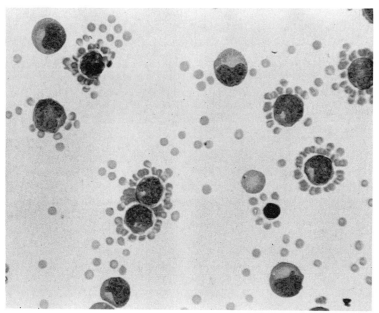

Figure 7.10 Cytospin slides from peripheral blood showing E-rosettes from the case of T-immunoblastic NHL illustrated in Figure 7.9. × 450, reduced to 74% on reproduction

Low grade NHLs

The alternative of delaying therapy in cases presenting with high WBC count rarely arises because the disease always has a progressive course. However, it has been possible to observe the clinical course without active treatment in a few patients with SLVL with stable disease. In high count follicular lymphoma, which usually correlates with bulky disease, the question is whether single agent chemotherapy, e.g. chlorambucil, as used in less advanced cases without leukaemia, may be sufficient, or whether these patients require more intensive treatment. There is no evidence that the addition of vincristine and prednisone to cyclophosphamide (as in COP) has any advantage over chlorambucil alone in follicular lymphoma (or in B-CLL). In follicular lymphoma presenting with a WBC count greater than 40 × 10^9/l, it may be necessary to employ combinations of four or more agents, e.g. the addition of hydroxydaunorubicin (doxorubicin) to COP (as in CHOP), as employed for the treatment of high grade NHLs, because the prognosis is otherwise poor. There are no good data to support this view and more controlled clinical studies are necessary.

In low-grade NHLs, it is important to consider also the potential benefit of other treatment modalities which may be suitable to particular subsets of cases. For example, splenic irradiation or splenectomy, in SLVL and the splenomegalic forms of follicular lymphoma or of mantle zone NHL, are often associated with prolonged remissions; these measures are, however, not curative but they could also facilitate the subsequent use of more radical therapy. One new treatment modality which still needs to find its role in the management of low grade NHLs is α-interferon which could, for example, be given to patients in complete remission or be used in combination with other drugs.

Intermediate grade NHLs

There is little information about the clinical course of patients with mantle zone lymphoma in leukaemic phase. In general they seem to respond poorly to single agent chemotherapy or COP-like combinations. CHOP or the more intensive five or six drug combinations may be indicated[14].

High grade NHLs

Here it is important to distinguish two types of tumours: lymphoblastic lymphoma and large cell NHLs. Lymphoblastic NHL includes T-lymphoblastic and Burkitt's lymphoma and both diseases are nowadays better treated with protocols of the type used in ALL, with little or no gaps during therapy, and should include measures for central nervous system (CNS) prophylaxis. The prognosis of lymphoblastic lymphoma without blood or bone marrow involvement is better than in cases in leukaemic phase. The treatment of Burkitt's lymphoma presenting as ALL-L3, referred to also in Chapter 2, is quite unsatisfactory even with ALL-like modalities. Such cases can achieve prolonged remissions or even cures only by means of allegeneic or syngeneic bone marrow transplantation.

Large cell NHLs are biologically and morphologically heterogeneous tumours with the worst prognosis seen in immunoblastic lymphoma, especially those with T-cell markers. The last decade has witnessed major advances in the treatment of large cell NHLs with the advent of more intensive chemotherapy protocols[14]. These have resulted in a higher proportion of cures and more prolonged periods of disease-free survival. The initial progress was obtained with CHOP, a combination which raised the plateau level of the survival curves to 40–50% from 20% with COP or CVP. New agents were later added to the basic four drug components of

CHOP to improve these results further, for example bleomycin, at doses lower than 15 mg/m^2 to avoid lung toxicity, in CHOP-bleomycin and BACOD, and methotrexate at high (3 g/m^2) or moderate (200 mg/m^2) doses with folinic acid (Leucovorin) rescue, in M- and m-BACOD, respectively. With these combinations, complete remission rates over 50% and long periods of disease-free survival were documented. Recently, even more intensive and sophisticated regimens have evolved which use either the same six drugs as in m-BACOD, but given in alternate weekly rotations to overcome the development of resistance, e.g. MACOP-B, or use eight drugs in rotation, e.g. adding etoposide, nitrogen-mustard and procarbazine (PROMACE-MOPP) or other agents such as cytosine arabinoside (PROMACE-CYTA BOM) plus 5-fluorouracil (F-MACHOP) etc. Although the latter combinations have also increased toxicity, they appear to have moved the plateau level in large cell NHLs to 70%, with complete remission rates of 80%. There are no details about the result of treatment with these modalities in cases of large cell NHL in leukaemic phase. The authors' experience suggests that remissions are difficult to obtain in such cases, with the survival of T-cell lymphomas (large cell) being depressingly short.

The need of CNS prophylaxis in the treatment strategy for NHLs has long been debated. The overall incidence of this complication is low (about 5%) although it is higher in cases with bone marrow involvement. The more frequent use of high dose methotrexate (which crosses the blood–CNS barrier) in current regimens for large cell NHLs in fact constitutes a form of CNS prophylaxis.

Further advances in the treatment of NHLs are likely to evolve from modalities which incorporate autologous bone marrow transplantations for cases without initial bone marrow involvement or for those in which a bone marrow harvest has been possible after a complete remission has been obtained. Encouraging results were reported in a series of relapsed B-cell NHLs which were first treated to a state close to complete remission, with less than 5% lymphoma cells in the bone marrow, followed by high dose chemoradiotherapy and reinfusion of the bone marrow which has been purged by means of the pan-B monoclonal antibody B1 (CD20) and complement[31]. There are a number of other trials using the same principle which are in progress at the present time.

Chromosome abnormalities in NHLs

A number of specific cytogenetic abnormalities are found in NHLs (Table 7.8). There is little information about lymphomas in leukaemic phase, except for ALL-L3 where the same translocation, t(8;14), found in Burkitt's lymphoma is always demonstrated. Recently, the authors have studied a case of large cell lymphoma (B-cell type) presenting with high WBC count and all the metaphases obtained from a peripheral blood sample have been shown to have the same abnormality: t(11;18)(q13;q23). The breakpoint 11q13 is frequently affected in B-cell malignancies[7], commonly in t(11;14) (Table 7.8 and see below), and the breakpoint 18q23 has also been found involved in non-random translocations in large cell NHLs.

Most B-cell malignancies carry reciprocal chromosome translocations which involve a breakage in chromosome 14 at band 14q23, which is the locus of the Ig heavy chain gene. Alterations of chromosome 14 are usually manifested as a marker 14q+[4, 13, 54] and this often results from reciprocal translocations with other chromosomes, chiefly, 8q24, 11q23 and 18q21 (Table 7.8).

Table 7.8 Consistent chromosome translocations in non-Hodgkin's lymphomas of B-cell type

Lymphoma	Abnormality	Incidence (%)	References
Follicular	t(14;18)(q32;q21)	85	[53, 54]
Intermediate and	t(11;14)(q13;q32)	30	[49]
lymphocytic[b]	Trisomy 12	30	[49, 54]
Burkitt	t(8;14)(q24;q32)	85	[7, 9, 40, 54]
	t(2;8)(p11;q24)	} 15	[7, 9, 24]
	t(8;22)(q24;q11)		
Large cell	t(14;18)(q32;q21)	28[a]	[50]
	t(1;14)(q21–23;q32)		[13]
	t(8;14)(q24;q32)		[40, 54]

[a] Demonstrated by molecular analysis with *bcl-2* probes; a minority of cases had a history of follicular lymphoma.
[b] Includes cases with lymphoplasmacytic differentiation. Trisomy 12 is the most common abnormality found in B-CLL (see Chapter 3) and t(11;14) in B-PLL (see Chapter 5).

A common feature of the translocation found in Burkitt's lymphoma is the breakpoint in chromosome 8 at band q24, where the proto-oncogene *c-myc* has been mapped. Somatic cell hybridization experiments have shown that *c-myc* remains intact in chromosome 8 in the variant translocations t(2;8) and t(8;22) where it becomes adjacent to the Ig light chain loci transposed from chromosome 2p11 (κ) and chromosome 22q11 (λ), respectively. In the typical t(8;14), *c-myc* is translocated to 14q32 and involves directly the Ig heavy chain gene[7]. As a result *c-myc* becomes deregulated, does not respond to its transcriptional control and is constitutively expressed at high levels. This is turn allows the neoplastic B-cells to proliferate indefinitely without maturation. It has been suggested that *c-myc* may be driven by enhancer sequences from the Ig genes[7]. The translocation t(8;14) is rare in other NHLs, but it has also been demonstrated in cases classified as B-immunoblastic lymphoma[40, 54] and small non-cleaved (non-Burkitt's)[54]; the latter probably corresponds to atypical forms of non-endemic Burkitt's lymphoma.

In follicular lymphoma, the characteristic translocation t(14;18) involves the juxtaposition of the Ig heavy chain locus at 14q32 and a gene localized on chromosome 18 at the breakpoint in band q21, designated *bcl-2*[7]. DNA probes of this breakpoint region 18q21 have been used to detect rearrangements in the majority of follicular lymphomas and in a proportion of large cell NHLs, which probably result from the transformation of low grade follicular lymphoma[50, 53]. Southern blotting analysis with these and other probes may be particularly valuable in cases where no metaphases can be obtained or when a marker, 14q+, is detected without an obvious origin for the translocation. This situation is analogous to the demonstration of rearrangements of the *bcr* gene in Philadelphia-negative chronic granulocytic leukaemia. The technique of polymerase chain reaction (PCR) now provides a rapid, sensitive and specific assay to amplify the breakpoint of the translocation t(14;18), i.e. the unique DNA sequence which results from the juxtaposition of *bcl-2* and the joining region of the Ig heavy chain[33a]. Two breakpoint regions have been recognized in t(14;18): a major region, or *mbr*, is involved in 60% of cases and a minor cluster region, or *mcr*, is involved in 35% of cases. Studies with the PCR technique are simple and economical and are becoming the standard method to detect t(14;18) in human tissues. In particular, this technique has wide applications for detecting minimal or occult disease[45a] after remission has been induced by chemotherapy.

Chromosome abnormalities, in addition to t(14;18), can be documented in follicular lymphomas and these result from clonal evolution of the tumour and are usually reflected in clinical progression, e.g. deletion 6q, trisomy 12 or partial trisomy 7[53]. Also of interest is the apparent association of deletion 13q32 in cases of follicular lymphoma with small cleaved cells and a leukaemic evolution. Other changes, such as trisomy 3, 18 or 21, are associated with follicular lymphomas of the large cell type[53]. Of particular interest is the association of t(14;18) and the Burkitt's translocation t(8;14) reported in a few cases. Some of them presented as acute lymphoblastic leukaemia (ALL) with L2 or L3 morphology. The authors have recently documented a case presenting as ALL-L3 with a mature B-cell phenotype, SmIg+, TdT−, in which all but one of the bone marrow metaphases analysed had a t(14;18)(q32;q21) and t(8;14)(q24;q32); a single metaphase had t(14;18)(Dr V. Brito-Babapulle, unpublished data). This and previous cases in which the malignant cells had an immature (TdT+) B-cell phenotype, suggest that t(14;18) is an early event, developing during the rearrangement of the Ig heavy chain gene and results in the disease follicular lymphoma upon further maturation of the B-cells (which become TdT−). The t(8;14) occurs at a later stage as a second chromosomal change involving the second chromosome 14, and affects the immature (TdT+) blast rather than the maturing B cell. The activation of the proto-oncogene c-myc, as a consequence of t(8;14), results in a high grade malignancy[18a]. This sequence of events has been documented over a period of time in at least one patient with a diagnosis of follicular lymphoma who subsequently developed a pre-B-ALL[13a]. The association of these two translocations in the same neoplastic cells and, in particular, the evidence for t(8;14) in follicular lymphoma, supports the concept of a follicular centre origin for Burkitt's lymphoma, suggested also by immunological findings.

Further studies are necessary to confirm the incidence of trisomy 12 and t(11;14) reported in some cases of intermediate NHLs[49]. These abnormalities are also a feature of B-CLL (see Chapter 3) and B-PLL (see Chapter 5), respectively, and have been found in other related types of lymphocytic lymphoma[54] (see Table 7.8). Molecular analysis of the translocation t(11;14) has shown that it results also from juxtaposition of the Ig heavy chain gene with another candidate proto-oncogene located at 11q13, and designated bcl-1[7]. DNA probes of this breakpoint region are currently being employed to demonstrate the frequency of this rearrangement in B-cell leukaemias and lymphomas.

The demonstration of specific chromosome abnormalities in NHLs has given a great impetus to studies aimed at clarifying the molecular mechanisms involved in pathogenesis and disease causation and have, in turn, introduced new techniques with profound implications in diagnosis and with potential for introducing more objective criteria in the classification of NHLs. For example the typical finding in follicular lymphoma – t(14;18) and/or the rearrangement of the bcl-2 gene – is not found in other B-lymphocytic tumours, such as CLL or intermediate NHLs, which can often be confused with the leukaemic phase of follicular lymphoma. However, in those disorders, but not in follicular lymphoma, it is possible to find other abnormalities, such as trisomy 12 or t(11;14)[49, 54]. Such findings would result not only in a better characterization of the respective disease but would also suggest a different pathogenetic mechanism.

References

1. Aisenberg, A. C., Wilkes, B. M. and Harris, N. L. (1983) Monoclonal antibody studies in non-Hodgkin's lymphoma. *Blood*, **61**, 469–475
2. Almici, C., Scaluggia, R., de Giuli, M. and Almici, C. A. (1984) Leukemic lymphomas. *Haematologica*, **69**, 188–193
3. Al Saati, T., Laurent, G., Caveriviere, P., Rigal, F. and Delsol, G. (1984) Reactivity of Leu1 and T101 monoclonal antibodies with B cell lymphomas (correlations with other immunological markers). *Clinical and Experimental Immunology*, **58**, 631–638
4. Catovsky, D., Pittman, S., Lewis, D. and Pearse, E. (1977) Marker chromosome 14q+ in follicular lymphoma in transformation. *Lancet*, **ii**, 934
5. Come, S. E., Jaffe, E. S., Andersen, J. C. et al. (1980) Non-Hodgkin's lymphomas in leukemic phase: clinico-pathologic correlations. *American Journal of Medicine*, **69**, 557–674
6. Cossman, J., Neckers, L. M., Hsu, S-M., Longo, D. and Jaffe, E. S. (1984) Low-grade lymphomas. Expression of developmentally regulated B-cell antigens. *American Journal of Pathology*, **115**, 117–124
7. Croce, C. M. and Nowell, P. C. (1985) Molecular basis of human B cell neoplasia. *Blood*, **65**, 1–7
8. de The, G. (1979) The epidemiology of Burkitt's lymphoma: evidence for a causal association with Epstein–Barr virus. *Epidemiologic Reviews*, **1**, 32–54
9. Ehlin-Henriksson, B. and Klein, G. (1984) Distinction between Burkitt lymphoma subgroups by monoclonal antibodies: relationships between antigen expression and type of chromosomal translocation. *International Journal of Cancer*, **33**, 459–463
10. Evans, H. L., Butler, J. J. and Youness, E. L. (1978) Malignant lymphoma, small lymphocytic type. A clinicopathologic study of 84 cases with suggested criteria for intermediate lymphocytic lymphoma. *Cancer*, **41**, 1440–1455
11. Favrot, M. C., Philip, I., Philip, T. and Dore, J. F. (1984) Possible duality in Burkitt lymphoma origin. *Lancet*, **i**, 745–746
12. Freedman, A. S., Boyd, A. W., Anderson, K. C. et al. (1985) Immunologic heterogeneity of diffuse large cell lymphoma. *Blood*, **65**, 630–637
13. Fukuhara, S., Ueshima, Y., Kita, K. and Uchino, H. (1984) 14q+ marker-positive lymphoid cancer and its subclasses. *Acta Haematologica (Japan)*, **47**, 1579–1590
13a. Gauwerky, C. E., Hoxie, J., Nowell, P. C. and Croce, C. M. (1988) Pre-B-cell leukemia with a t(8;14) translocation is preceded by follicular lymphoma. *Oncogene*, **2**, 431–435
14. Gobbi, P. G. and Cavalli, C. (1986) Treatment of adult non-Hodgkin's lymphomas. *Haematologica*, **71**, 321–344
15. Gregg, E. O., Al-Saffar, N., Jones, D. B., Wright, D. H., Sevenson, F. K. and Smith, J. L. (1984) Immunoglobulin negative follicle centre cell lymphoma. *British Journal of Cancer*, **50**, 735–744
16. Harris, N. L., Nadler, L. M. and Bhan, A. K. (1984) Immunohistologic characterization of two malignant lymphomas of germinal center type (centroblastic/centrocytic and centrocytic) with monoclonal antibodies. Follicular and diffuse lymphomas of small-cleaved-cell type are related but distinct entities. *American Journal of Pathology*, **117**, 262–272
17. Hu, E., Trela, M., Thompson, J., Lowder, J., Horning, S., Levy, R. and Sklar, J. (1985) Detection of B-cell lymphoma in peripheral blood by DNA hybridisation. *Lancet*, **ii**, 1092–1095
18. Jaffe, E. S., Bookman, M. A. and Longo, D. L. (1987) Lymphocytic lymphoma of intermediate differentiation. Mantle zone lymphoma: A distinct subtype of B-cell lymphoma. *Human Pathology*, **18**, 877–880
18a. de Jong, D., Voetdijk, B. M. H., Beverstock, G. C., van Ommen, G. J. B., Willimze, R. and Kluin, P. M. (1988) Activation of the *c-myc* oncogene in a precursor-B-cell blast crisis of follicular lymphoma, presenting as composite lymphoma. *New England Journal of Medicine*, **318**, 1373–1378
19. Koziner, B., Filippa, D. A., Mertelsmann, R. et al. (1977) Characterization of malignant lymphomas in leukemic phase by multiple differentiation markers of mononuclear cells. Correlation with clinical features and conventional morphology. *American Journal of Medicine*, **63**, 556–567
20. Knuutila, S., Elonen, E., Heinonen, K. et al. (1984) Chromosome abnormalities in 16 Finnish patients with Burkitt's lymphoma or L3 acute lymphocytic leukemia. *Cancer Genetics and Cytogenetics*, **13**, 139–151

21. Kurihara, K., Yoshida, S. and Hashimoto, N. (1985) Bone and bone marrow histology in non-Hodgkin's lymphomas. Autopsy cases. *Journal of Kyushu Hematological Society*, **33**, 23–37
22. Laurent, G., Al-Saati, T., Olive, D., Laurent, J. C., Poncelet, P. and Delsol, G. (1986) Expression of Tac antigen in B cell lymphomas. *Clinical and Experimental Immunology*, **65**, 354–362
23. Lennert, K. (1978) *Malignant Lymphomas Other than Hodgkin's Disease*. Berlin: Springer-Verlag
24. Lenoir, G. M., Preud-homme, J. L., Bernheim, A. and Berger, R. (1982) Correlation between immunoglobulin light chain expression and variant translocation in Burkitt's lymphoma. *Nature*, **298**, 474–476
25. Lukes, R. J. and Collins, R. D. (1974) Immunologic characterization of human malignant lymphomas. *Cancer*, **34**, 1488–1503
26. Magrath, I. (1984) Burkitt's lymphoma: clinical aspects and treatment. In *Diseases of the Lymphatic System. Diagnosis and Therapy*, edited by D. W. Molander, pp. 103–139. New York: Springer-Verlag
26a. Mason, D. Y. and Gatter, K. C. (1987) The role of immunocytochemistry in diagnostic pathology. *Journal of Clinical Pathology*, **40**, 1042–1054
27. Mazza, P., Gherlinzoni, F., Kemna, G. et al. (1987) Clinicopathological study on non-Hodgkin's lymphomas. *Haematologica*, **72**, 351–357
28. Melo, J. V. M., Hegde, U., Parreira, A., Thompson, I., Lampert, I. A. and Catovsky, D. (1987) Splenic B-cell lymphoma with circulating 'villous' lymphocytes: differential diagnosis of B-cell leukaemias with a large spleen. *Journal of Clinical Pathology*, **40**, 642–651
29. Melo, J. V., Robinson, D. S. F., de Oliveira, M. P. et al. (1988) Morphology and immunology of circulating cells in the leukaemic phase of follicular lymphoma. *Journal of Clinical Pathology*, **41**, 951–959
29a. Melo, J. V., Robinson, D. S. F., Gregory, C. and Catovsky, D. (1987) Splenic B cell lymphoma with 'villous' lymphocytes in the peripheral blood: a disorder distinct from hairy cell leukemia. *Leukemia*, **1**, 294–299
30. Morra, E., Lazzarino, M., Orlandi, E. et al. (1984) Leukemic phase of non-Hodgkin's lymphomas. Hematological features and prognostic significance. *Haematologica*, **69**, 15–29
31. Nadler, L. M., Takvorian, T., Botnick, L. et al. (1984) Anti-B1 monoclonal antibody and complement treatment in autologous bone-marrow transplantation for relapsed B-cell non-Hodgkin's lymphoma. *Lancet*, **ii**, 427–432
32. Narang, S., Wolf, B. C. and Neiman, R. S. (1985) Malignant lymphoma presenting with prominent splenomegaly. A clinico-pathologic study with special reference to intermediate cell lymphoma. *Cancer*, **55**, 1948–1957
33. Neiman, R. S., Sullivan, A. L. and Jaffe, R. (1979) Malignant lymphoma simulating leukemic reticuloendotheliosis: a clinico-pathologic study of ten cases. *Cancer*, **43**, 329–342
33a. Ngan, B-Y., Nourse, J. and Cleary, M. L. (1989) Detection of chromosomal translocation t(14;18) within the minor cluster region of bcl-2 by polymerase chain reaction and direct genomic sequencing of the enzymatically amplified DNA in follicular lymphomas. *Blood*, **73**, 1759–1762
34. Pangalis, G. A., Roussou, P. A., Kittas, C. et al. (1984) Patterns of bone marrow involvement in chronic lymphocytic leukemia and small lymphocytic (well differentiated) non-Hodgkin's lymphoma. *Cancer*, **54**, 702–708
35. Palutke, M., Eisenberg, L., Mirchandani, I., Tabaczka, P. and Husain, M. (1982) Malignant lymphoma of small cleaved lymphocytes of the follicular mantle zone. *Blood*, **59**, 317–322
35a. Pombo de Oliveira, M. S., Jaffe, E. S. and Catovsky, D. (1989) Leukaemic phase of mantle zone (intermediate) lymphoma: its characterisation in 11 cases. *Journal of Clinical Pathology*, **42**, 962–972
36. Rappaport, H. (1966) Tumors of the hematopoietic system. In *Atlas of Tumor Pathology* (Section 3, Fascicle 8). Washington DC: US Armed Forces Institute of Pathology
37. Ritz, J., Nadler, L. M., Bhan, A. K., Notis-McConarty, J., Pesando, J. M. and Schlossman, S. F. (1981) Expression of common acute lymphoblastic leukemia antigen (cALLA) by lymphomas of B-cell and T-cell lineage. *Blood*, **58**, 648–652
38. Robb-Smith, A. H. T. (1982) US National Cancer Institute Working formulation of non-Hodgkin's lymphomas for clinical use. *Lancet*, **ii**, 432–434
38a. Robinson, D., Lackie, P., Aber, V. and Catovsky, D. (1989) Morphometric analysis of chronic

B-cell leukemias – an aid to the classification of lymphoid cell types. *Leukemia Research,* **13,** 357–365

39. Rosenberg, S. A., Berard, C. W., Brown, B. W. et al. (1982) National Cancer Institute Sponsored study of classification of non-Hodgkin's lymphomas. Summary and description of a working formulation for clinical use. *Cancer,* **49,** 2112–2135

40. Sigaux, F., Berger, R., Bernheim, A., Valensi, F., Daniel, M. T. and Flandrin, G. (1984) Malignant lymphomas with band 8q24 chromosome abnormality: a morphologic continuum extending from Burkitt's to immunoblastic lymphoma. *British Journal of Haematology,* **57,** 393–405

41. Sklar, J., Cleary, M. L., Thielemans, K., Gralow, J., Warnke, R. and Levy, R. (1984) Biclonal B-cell lymphoma. *New England Journal of Medicine,* **311,** 20–27

42. Spiro, S., Galton, D. A. G., Wiltshaw, E. and Lohmann, R. C. (1975) Follicular lymphoma: A survey of 75 cases with special reference to the syndrome resembling chronic lymphocytic leukaemia. *British Journal of Cancer,* **31** (suppl. II), 60–72

43. Spriano, P., Barosi, G., Invernizzi, R. et al. (1986) Splenomegalic immunocytoma with circulating hairy cells. Report of eight cases and revision of the literature. *Haematologica,* **71,** 25–33

44. Stansfeld, A., Diebold, J., Noel, H. et al. (1988) Updated Kiel classification for lymphomas. *Lancet,* **i,** 292–293

45. Stein, H., Lennert, K., Feller, A. C. and Mason, D. Y. (1984) Immunohistological analysis of human lymphoma: correlation of histological and immunological categories. In *Advances in Cancer Research,* edited by G. Klein and S. Weinhouse, vol. 42, pp. 67–147. Orlando: Academic Press

45a. Stetler-Stevenson, M., Raffeld, M., Cohen, P. and Cossman, J. (1988) Detection of occult follicular lymphoma by specific DNA amplification. *Blood,* **72,** 1822–1825

45b. Suchi, T., Lennert, K., Tu, L-Y. et al. (1987) Histopathology and immunohistochemistry of peripheral T cell lymphomas: a proposal for their classification. *Journal of Clinical Pathology,* **40,** 995–1015

46. Swerdlow, S. H., Habeshaw, J. A., Murray, L. J., Dhaliwal, H. S., Lister, T. A. and Stansfeld, A. G. (1983) Centrocytic lymphoma: A distinct clinicopathologic and immunologic entity. A multiparameter study of 18 cases at diagnosis and relapse. *American Journal of Pathology,* **113,** 181–197

47. Swerdlow, S. H., Murray, L. J., Habeshaw, J. A. and Stansfeld, A. G. (1984) Lymphocytic lymphoma/B-chronic lymphocytic leukaemia – an immunohistopathological study of peripheral B lymphocyte neoplasia. *British Journal of Cancer,* **50,** 587–599

48. Tura, S., Mazza, P., Lauria, F. et al. (1985) Non-Hodgkin's lymphomas in leukaemic phase: Incidence, prognosis and therapeutic implications. *Scandinavian Journal of Haematology,* **35,** 123–131

49. Weisenburger, D. D., Sanger, W. G., Armitage, J. O. and Purtilo, D. T. (1987) Intermediate lymphocytic lymphoma: immunophenotypic and cytogenetic findings. *Blood,* **69,** 1617–1621

50. Weiss, L. M., Warnke, R. A., Sklar, J. and Cleary, M. L. (1987) Molecular analysis of the t(14;18) chromosomal translocation in malignant lymphomas. *New England Journal of Medicine,* **317,** 1185–1189

51. WHO memorandum (1969) Histopathological definition of Burkitt's tumour. *Bulletin of the World Health Organisation,* **40,** 601–607

52. Whittle, H. C., Brown, J., Marsh, K. et al. (1984) T-cell control of Epstein–Barr virus-infected B cells is lost during *P. falciparum* malaria. *Nature,* **312,** 449–450

52a. Young, R. C., Longo, D. L., Glatstein, E., Ihde, D. C., Jaffe, E. S. and DeVita, V. T. (1988) The treatment of indolent lymphomas: Watchful waiting versus aggressive combined modality treatment. *Seminars in Hematology,* **25,** 11–16

53. Yunis, J. J., Frizzera, G., Oken, M. M., McKenna, J., Theologides, A. and Arnesen, M. (1987) Multiple recurrent genomic defects in follicular lymphoma. *New England Journal of Medicine,* **316,** 79–84

54. Yunis, J. J., Oken, M. M., Kaplan, M. E., Ensruf, K. M., Howe, R. R. and Theologides, A. (1982) Distinctive chromosomal abnormalities in histologic subtypes of non-Hodgkin's lymphoma. *New England Journal of Medicine,* **307,** 1231–1236

Chapter 8

Adult T-cell leukaemia/lymphoma

Introduction

Adult T-cell leukaemia/lymphoma (ATLL) is, together with Sézary syndrome, a prototype of the lymphoma/leukaemia syndromes involving immunologically mature T-lymphocytes. The disease was first described in Japan as adult T-cell leukaemia[82] but was later recognized in its full clinical heterogeneity as ATLL[15, 77, 91]. In addition to its many remarkable features the great interest in ATLL, which justifies a full chapter in this book, is the casual relationship with the first retrovirus described in humans, HTLV-I[26, 27]. This has opened the way to studies of the epidemiology and mode of transmission of ATLL which have not been possible so far in other leukaemias and lymphomas.

The demonstration of clonality in T-cell disorders is not possible by the use of immunological reagents (as is the case in B-cell malignancies which express a single Ig light chain). In ATLL it is possible to demonstrate clonal integration of HTLV-I proviral DNA and to contrast the findings with those of HTLV-I seropositive healthy carriers[90, 96]. In other T-cell malignancies it is possible to demonstrate clonality by means of DNA analysis (Southern blotting) with probes for the T-cell receptor (TCR) β-, γ- and δ-chain genes[21, 30b, 50, 61, 84]. For this reason a summary of the modern studies showing TCR gene rearrangements in human T-cell leukaemias has also been included in this chapter. This information should complement the description of immunological markers and Ig gene rearrangements discussed in Chapters 1 and 2.

Clinical features

Patients with ATLL always have florid manifestations which vary according to the clinical form of the disease. A history of protracted skin lesions and opportunistic infections is associated with preleukaemic forms and/or the so-called smouldering ATLL (see below). Acute ATLL, however, is associated with symptomatic disease and major physical signs. When hypercalcaemia is severe the presentation could be very acute and dramatic.

Presenting clinical and laboratory features are summarized in Table 8.1. The most common physical sign is superficial lymphadenopathy. Chest X-rays and CT scans will also show enlarged mediastinal and para-aortic lymph nodes. The skin lesions are often nodular and, more rarely, diffuse with erythroderma.

Table 8.1 Clinical and laboratory features of ATLL

Feature	Percentage
Lymphadenopathy	90
Hepatomegaly	50
Splenomegaly	40
Skin deposits	35
Leukaemia phase[a]	90
Hypercalcaemia[a]	70
Abnormal liver function tests	50
Anaemia/thrombocytopenia	30

[a] Not seen in patients with lymphoma-type ATLL.

Erythematous papular and nodular patches are common. Exfoliative erythroderma and large indurated tumours, as seen in the cutaneous T-cell lymphomas (Sézary syndrome and mycosis fungoides) are almost never seen. The degree of hepatosplenomegaly is only moderate. Massive enlargement of these organs is rarely seen.

The authors' experience of this disease is based on Black patients of Caribbean origin (rarely African) resident in the UK. The presenting features in the first 14 patients studied are summarized in Table 8.2; another 16 patients have now been studied with very similar findings to those shown in Table 8.2. Despite the high frequency of hypercalcaemia (Tables 8.1 and 8.2, and see below) osteolytic bone lesions have been exceptional in the authors' series but have been described in some American patients[12]. ATLL affects almost exclusively adults. The median age in Caribbean patients (45 years) is about 10 years younger than in Japanese patients. There are no major differences between the sexes, both men and women being equally affected. Presentation in the paediatric age group is exceptional. The authors have reviewed material from a 2-year-old Brazilian patient with typical HTLV-I+ ATLL; the mother and grandmother were also seropositive (see below under Modes of transmission).

Clinical forms of the disease

Although the acute form of ATLL is by far the most common manifestation of the disease (75% of the authors' series and 55–65% in Japanese studies), advances in seroepidemiological studies and greater awareness of the natural history of ATLL, with its long incubation period, have allowed the recognition of other clinical forms. After acute ATLL, the second most common form is the lymphoma type which is seen in 15–20% of both Caribbean[7, 12] and Japanese[77, 91] patients. In these patients the disease evolves without obvious blood (and little bone marrow) involvement, behaving clinically like other non-Hodgkin's lymphomas. It is not clear why, in some patients, ATLL remains localized to lymph node areas. In this lymphoma type of ATLL the systemic manifestations of hypercalcaemia are often absent. The lymph nodes are hard and often refractory to therapy.

Chronic ATLL is less common in the authors' experience (5% of cases) but in some series in Japan they may constitute up to 15% of cases. This form is characterized by a chronic course with few physical signs, some skin involvement

Table 8.2 Clinical and laboratory features of 14 ATLL patients

Case no.	Age/sex	Race/origin	Lymph nodes	Liver/spleen	Lesions Skin	Lesions Bone	Ca^{2+} (mmol/l)[a]	CNS disease	WBC count ($\times 10^9$/l)[b]	HTLV abs[c]	Survival months
1	47/M	Black/Car	+	–	+	+	4.10	–	37[d]	ND	4
2	51/M	Black/Car	+	–	–	–	2.81	–	15[d]	ND	3
3	55/M	Black/Car	+	–	–	–	3.87	–	27[d]	ND	6
4	32/F	Black/Car	+	+	–	–	4.52	–	40[d]	ND	0.5
5	21/F	Black/Car	+	+	+	–	4.2	–	90[d]	+	7
6	45/F	Black/Car	+	–	+	–	4.13	–	67[d]	+	3
7	32/F	Black/Car	+	+	+	–	2.31	–	40[d]	+	26
8	31/F	Black/Car	+	–	–	±	3.35	–	39.8[d]	+	2
9	50/F	Black/Car	+	–	–	–	2.2	–	8.0	+	10
10	62/M	Black/Car	+	+	–	–	3.62	+	197[d]	+	4
11	52/M	Black/Car	+	+	–	–	3.22	+	103[d]	+	11
12	29/M	Black/Afr	+	+	–	–	3.94	–	14.5[d]	+	5
13	35/F	Black/Car	+	–	–	–	5.40	+	36.7[d]	+	7
14	58/F	Black/Car	–	–	+	–	3.80	–	81[d]	+	2

[a] Levels at presentation or shortly after diagnosis (normal range 2.15–2.65); when investigated PTH levels were always undetectable.
[b] Highest count recorded; in most cases corresponded to values at diagnosis.
[c] Serum antibodies to HTLV-I.
[d] Abnormal lymphoid cells.

Car: Caribbean region; Afr: West Africa.

and a persistent lymphocytosis in which the cells appear to be less bizarre and slightly more mature than those in acute ATLL. The lymphocytosis may persist unchanged for a long period of time. In contrast, the WBC count always rises rapidly in acute ATLL.

Smouldering (see below) refers to patients with non-specific features, often skin rashes, no organomegaly and almost normal blood counts. Only DNA analysis with HTLV-I probes (or TCR gene rearrangement) demonstrates T-cell clonality[90, 96] in patients without the florid manifestations of ATLL. Some of these will evolve through a 'crisis'[77] to acute ATLL.

Laboratory investigations

Specific tests for the study of ATLL patients include full blood counts and bone marrow aspirates, lymph node histology if the presentation includes significant lymphadenopthy, biochemical screening to assess the degree of liver involvement, renal status and the presence of hypercalcaemia, membrane phenotype of the malignant lymphocytes to establish their T-cell nature and some features of the phenotypic profile which are characteristic of ATLL and, finally, serological evidence for antibodies to HTLV-I.

Haematology

Elevated WBC count is a consistent feature of ATLL (Table 8.2); only patients with the lymphoma form of the disease will have normal counts. Anaemia (haemoglobin $< 10\,\text{g/dl}$) and/or thrombocytopenia (platelets $< 100 \times 10^9/\text{l}$) are seen in one-third of cases only, suggesting that bone marrow involvement is not an early event. As seen in the authors' series of Caribbean-born patients, the WBC count could be very high early on in the evolution; in a more recent series of cases the highest WBC count recorded at presentation was $263 \times 10^9/\text{l}$. Characteristically, the WBC count tends to rise rapidly (Figure 8.1) in this disease so that the figures given in Table 8.2 are only a guide. Except for the rare cases with chronic lymphocytosis, the usual trend is for the WBC count to rise exponentially and to double in weeks rather than months. The median WBC count at presentation in the authors' series of 30 ATLL patients was $40 \times 10^9/\text{l}$ (range 3.6–263).

Morphology of ATLL cells (Figures 8.2 and 8.3)

The morphology of the atypical lymphoid cells in peripheral blood films is quite distinctive and could suggest a diagnosis of ATLL even in the absence of other clinical or laboratory data. Two features are constant: marked nuclear irregularities and pleomorphism with cells of variable shapes and sizes. In general, the predominant cells are small or medium in size with condensed nuclear chromatin and they are often accompanied by larger, blast-like cells with marked cytoplasmic basophilia and nuclear irregularity. The circulating lymphocytes have a high nucleo-/cytoplasmic ratio and an irregular nuclear outline. ATLL cells have been described as 'flower-like', hyperlobated or convoluted because two or more (sometimes up to five or six) nuclear lobes are clearly identified (Figure 8.2). The main difference between ATLL and Sézary cells on Romanovsky-stained blood films is that the space between the nuclear lobes is usually visible in ATLL cells but

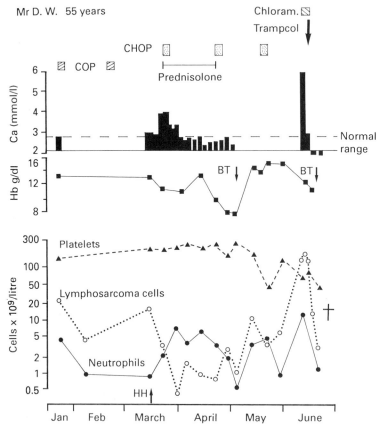

Figure 8.1 Haematology chart illustrating the clinical course of the first Caribbean patient studied by one of the authors[15]. The typical ATLL cells were initially described as 'lymphosarcoma' cells but this term is no longer used because it is too imprecise about the nature of the underlying lymphoma. Note the exacerbation of hypercalcaemia in parallel to clinical deterioration and rising WBC count

is only suggested in Sézary cells at light microscopic examination. This difference is not, however, absolute because the cells in some ATLL cases may resemble Sézary cells (Figure 8.3) even by ultrastructural analysis (see below).

Lymphoid cells with similar appearances are seen in the bone marrow and in imprint preparations of lymph nodes. The morphology of ATLL cells has been extensively described in the literature, particularly by Japanese pathologists[32, 39, 76, 82]. Before the era when marker studies for B- and T-lymphocytes were routinely performed, such cases would have been described as lymphosarcoma-cell leukaemia. This is now inappropriate as this term could encompass a variety of leukaemia/lymphoma syndromes of different cell lineage, natural history, aetiology and prognosis.

Cytochemistry
As described in more detail in Chapter 5, the cytochemical reactions for acid hydrolases are positive in ATLL cells, although with less intensity than in T-PLL.

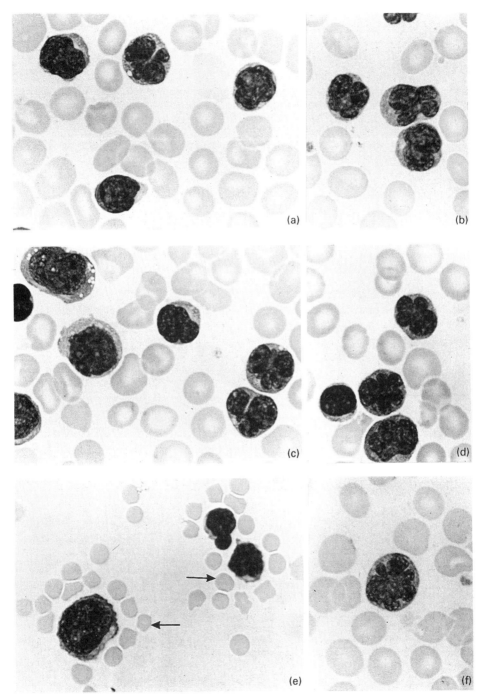

Figure 8.2 Several examples of ATLL cells in peripheral blood films (a–d, f). The main feature is the nuclear irregularities and the pleomorphic appearances with cells of various sizes: small, medium and large (blastic). E-rosette formation in ATLL cells (arrows) is illustrated in e. × 1400, reduced to 68% on reproduction

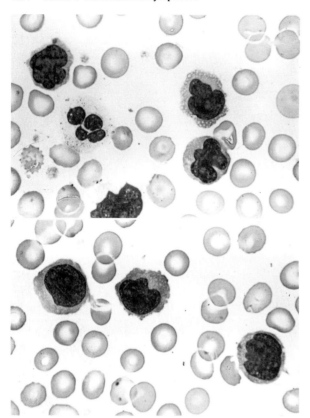

Figure 8.3 Two views of the peripheral blood film of another patient with ATLL in which some of the cells resembled Sézary cells. The main difference at light microscopy between these cell types is the very narrow nuclear indentations in Sézary cells whilst in ATLL cells the nuclear lobes are clearly separated. This is seen in one cell in this figure and in several cells of Figure 8.2a,c,d,f. × 1400, reduced to 65% on reproduction

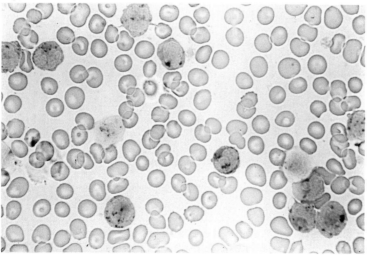

Figure 8.4 Acid phosphatase cytochemical reaction in a blood film from a case of ATLL showing moderately intense positivity with a granular pattern. × 1200, reduced to 81% on reproduction

The acid phosphatase reaction is moderately positive in the majority of cells with a diffuse and/or granular pattern (Figure 8.4). Similarly, other enzymes are usually positive. The periodic acid–Schiff (PAS) reaction is often negative but occasionally it may be positive in the form of granules or, rarely, large blocks.

Hypercalcaemia

Of the biochemical tests, a high serum Ca^{2+} is a common abnormality found in ATLL patients (see Tables 8.1 and 8.2). Levels of parathyroid hormone (PTH) are undetectable but PTH-like peptides have been considered as possible candidates for this effect because of the presence, in some cases, of subperiosteal bone resorption in X-rays of the hands. Such osteoclastic promoting factors may act alone[31] or together with other cytokines, e.g. interleukin-1 (IL-1), on osteoblasts which in turn may transmit signals to osteoclasts which show features of activation in bone marrow trephine biopsies. Levels of 1,25-dihydroxyvitamin D are not increased either. Hypercalcaemia and hypercalciuria, the latter seen even in patients with normal serum Ca^{2+}, are a characteristic almost diagnostic of ATLL. Hypercalcaemia is very rare in other non-Hodgkin's lymphomas[14] when it is seen only as a terminal event. In contrast, in ATLL it is, as a rule, a presenting feature (see Table 8.2). In 30 cases from the authors' series, hypercalcaemia was a major clinical problem in 18 (60%); in only 2 of these were osteolytic lesions demonstrated. This discrepancy between high serum Ca^{2+} levels and the lack of radiological evidence of bone involvement plus the relatively low degree of bone marrow infiltration is typical of ATLL. Ca^{2+} levels are higher in cases with a high WBC count (see Figure 8.1 and Table 8.2) and are normal in most cases of the lymphoma type of ATLL (with normal WBC count).

Membrane phenotype

ATLL lymphocytes have a post-thymic or mature T-cell phenotype, i.e. they do not express the nuclear enzyme terminal deoxynucleotidyl transferase (TdT−) or the cortical thymocyte antigen CD1a (OKT6−) and they express mature T-cell antigens, although with some exceptions. The cells in the majority of cases are CD2+ (and form E-rosettes), CD3+ (membrane and cytoplasmic expression) and CD5+[88]. In the great majority (95%) the T-lymphocytes are CD4+, CD8−, i.e. have a 'helper–inducer' phenotype, although this does not correspond with the functional studies reported (see below). Of interest is the consistent lack of expression on the cell membrane of the p40 glycoprotein demonstrated by monoclonal antibodies of the CD7 group (e.g. 3A1, Leu9, OKT16). The CD7− profile is similar to what has been described in Sézary cells and is different from findings in T-PLL where this antigen is strongly expressed in all cases (see Chapters 1 and 5). A major difference from other mature T-cell disorders (see Table 1.10, Chapter 1) is the consistent expression of CD25 (anti-Tac) on ATLL cells[41, 80, 85] (see below under IL-2 receptors).

A summary of the authors' results in 24 ATLL cases is shown in Table 8.3. It should be noted that as in Sézary syndrome cells, the formation of E-rosettes may be deficient or the percentage is relatively low for the number of T-cells (in 5 of 23 cases). Similarly, membrane staining with the CD3 monoclonal antibody may also be below normal (5 out of 18 cases). A low density of CD3 on the surface of ATLL cells was demonstrated by flow cytometry by Japanese workers[71]. CD4 was

Table 8.3 Membrane markers in ATLL[a]

Case no.	E	CD3	CD4	CD7	CD25
5	+	+	+		
6	+	+/−	+		
7	+	+	+		
8	+	+	−		
9	+	+	+	−	
10	+/−	+	+	−	+
11	+	+	+	−	+
12	+		−	+	+
13	−	+	+	−	−
14	−	−	+	−	+
15	+/−	+/−	+	+/−	+
16		+	+	−	+
17	+	+	+	−	+/−
18	+	+	+	−	+
19	+	+	+	−	+
20	−	−	+	−	+
21	+	+	+	−	+
22	+	+	+	−	+
23	+	+	+	−	+
24	+	+/−	+	−	+

[a] Cases studied by monoclonal antibodies; case numbers 1–4 (not listed) were E+; cells in all 20 cases tested were TdT−, CD1− and CD8−; 8/9 cases were OKT17+.
Percentage positive cells: <20% (−); 20–30% (+/−); >30% (+); blank spaces: test not done.

positive in 17 of our 19 cases tested, whilst reactivity with CD7 was shown in only 2 of 16 cases. The receptor for IL-2 (CD25) was readily demonstrable on 14 of 15 cases (Table 8.3).

The authors have recently carried out subset analysis of CD4+ mature T-cell leukaemias with monoclonal antibodies of the CD45R (2H4; detecting virgin/naive and/or 'suppressor–inducer' T cells) and CD29 (2B4; positive in 'helper–inducer' T cells). According to the studies of Morimoto et al.[56] a 'suppressor–inducer' profile (CD45R+, CD29−) in ATLL lymphocytes should have been expected. However, the cells of none of the five ATLL cases tested showed this phenotype. Instead, two cases were CD45R−, CD29+, two were CD45R−, CD29− and one co-expressed both antigens[87a]. A recent Japanese study[88a] confirmed that ATLL cells were CD4+, CD29+, CD45R− in six cases, but were shown to suppress B-cell differentiation induced in vitro by pokeweed mitogen. Clearly, the explanation for these findings is not yet obvious as the 'helper' phenotype in ATLL cases is not supported by functional studies[48, 56, 88] (see below).

IL-2 receptors

These are expressed on the membrane of the leukaemic T-cells in most cases of ATLL[41, 80, 85]. Normal resting T-lymphocytes do not express these receptors. ATLL cells express IL-2 receptors (CD25+) constitutively (without stimulation) and this may be the result of abnormal regulation. For example, the expression of

IL-2 receptors in normal T-cells after stimulation is down regulated upon the addition of the monoclonal antibody anti-Tac to the culture medium; in contrast, the number of IL-2 receptors in ATLL increases with the addition of anti-Tac[95].

The leukaemic proliferation in ATLL was initially thought to result from autostimulation due to the abnormal expression of IL-2 receptors and evidence that HTVL-I-infected cell lines become independent of the addition of exogenous IL-2. This hypothesis was ruled out when it was established that the level of mRNA for IL-2 is not increased in HTLV-I-infected cell lines and that this lymphokine is not released in culture, and that ATLL cells do not respond with proliferation to the addition of exogenous IL-2 despite the increased binding to its receptor. Nevertheless, some pathogenic role of the IL-2 receptor in one of the multiple steps of the malignant proliferation leading to ATLL has not been completely ruled out[41]. One suggestion is that the *tat* gene may act at a distance by stimulating the transactivation of the IL-2 receptor gene. The continuous expression of this receptor on HTLV-I-infected cells may increase their proliferative potential and the possibility of critical chromosomal changes, which are a prerequisite for a further malignant change.

Functional studies

Independent studies by Yamada[88] in Japanese ATLL patients and by Miedema et al.[48] in three out of five patients of Caribbean origin suggested a suppressor function in vitro by ATLL cells in pokeweed mitogen-induced immunoglobulin synthesis. Both these groups suggested a direct suppressor effect by ATLL cells as CD8+ lymphocytes were specifically excluded from their culture systems. On the other hand, Morimoto suggested that the suppressor effect of ATLL cells was mediated through CD8+ cells ('suppressor–inducer' function). As mentioned above, marker studies with CD45R and CD29 did not confirm in ATLL cells the expected suppressor–inducer phenotype CD45R+, CD29−. Further studies are obviously necessary to establish clearly whether ATLL lymphocytes represent a unique type of suppressor cells. No such observation has been made with other CD4+ leukaemic cells which, if anything, were shown to have 'helper' function in some T-PLL and Sézary syndrome cases.

Diagnostic criteria and differential diagnosis

It is apparent from the above descriptions that ATLL has several features in common with some of the other mature T-cell leukaemias, chiefly Sézary syndrome and T-PLL, and therefore it is difficult to use a single criterion for diagnosis. However, the constellation of some clinical and laboratory findings is probably unique to ATLL, namely: generalized lymphadenopathy, hypercalcaemia, lymphocytosis with pleomorphic morphology and CD4+, CD25+ membrane phenotype, particularly if affecting an individual of Japanese, African or Caribbean origin. The demonstration of antibodies to HTLV-I core proteins, in these circumstances, is useful confirmatory data. Because in endemic areas people suffering from other malignancies may also be seropositive, the demonstration of a high titre of anti-HTLV-I antibodies is not in itself diagnostic. In atypical cases of leukaemia where HTLV-I is suspected as the aetiological agent, confirmatory evidence should be sought by DNA analysis with appropriate probes. Evidence of monoclonal integration of HTLV-I proviral DNA in the malignant cells could, in such cases, be of diagnostic value.

In general, and as discussed above, typical features of ATLL, in particular peripheral blood morphology, lymph node histology and supporting data by monoclonal antibodies, will correlate in over 95% of cases with HTLV-I serology. Even in the absence of antibodies, DNA analysis may demonstrate HTLV-I involvement in the tumour, in a minority of cases[90, 96]. In cases of other T-cell leukaemias which resemble ATLL, short of being typical, the association with HTLV-I may be critical for diagnosis and the authors would support the use of serological or DNA data as confirmatory in borderline cases. One such case was recently studied by the authors in a White patient from a non-endemic area where the diagnosis of the rare disorder Sézary cell leukaemia was initially made, on account of the relatively typical peripheral blood morphology (by both light and electron microscopy) and lack of skin involvement. However, the subsequent evolution of a leukaemia/lymphoma syndrome with an aggressive course and evidence of seropositivity for HTLV-I, brought about the consideration of the more likely diagnosis of ATLL. DNA analysis has not yet been completed and may prove crucial in this particular example.

A different situation has been witnessed in Japan where a case of CD8+ T-cell leukaemia without typical ATLL morphology was shown to have HTLV-I proviral integration in the DNA. In such cases the possibility should be considered that HTLV-I can cause, in endemic areas, other diseases, such as tropical spastic paraparesis, and that it may also be the aetiological agent of other T-cell leukaemias which, nevertheless, could not be designated ATLL on the retroviral evidence alone. The authors are aware, however, that typical ATLL cases with CD4+ cells have also been documented in Japan without serological or molecular evidence of HTLV-I involvement. As in the case of Burkitt's lymphoma, ATLL could be considered a clinicopathological entity which in the majority of cases has a clear-cut association with a virus (Epstein–Barr virus in Burkitt's lymphoma), but which may rarely result from another as yet unknown agent. Experience in Caribbean-born patients with T-PLL and relatively convoluted prolymphocytes has shown that in such cases evidence for HTLV-I was lacking, confirming that when the clinical and laboratory criteria are correct, the likelihood of demonstrating an HTLV-I association is remote. A similar type of observation was made in a serological survey of cutaneous T-cell lymphomas, where antibodies to HTLV-I were found only in ATLL[28].

Histopathology of ATLL

The tissues most commonly affected and which are biopsied as part of diagnostic procedures in ATLL are lymph nodes, skin and bone marrow. In each of them the lesions, although characteristic of the disease, overlap with features of other T-cell disorders. In particular, the lymph node histology may resemble that of other types of peripheral (mature) T-cell lymphoma seen in non-endemic areas for HTLV-I[32, 42, 59, 76]. In addition to conventional histopathological analysis, the affected tissues should be studied by immunohistochemisty which will often demonstrate in ATLL cells the expression of CD25 (anti-Tac) and the lack of the CD7 antigen[42]. Staining with specific monoclonal antibodies against HTLV-I major core proteins should be attempted when serology is negative or inadequate but only cells after culture may give positive results (see below). DNA analysis to document HTLV-I proviral integration may be necessary in rare cases if it is required to establish with certainty that a particular lesion is related to HTLV-I.

Lymph node biopsy

Material from lymph nodes is often available for study as most patients have lymphadenopathy as a presenting feature. There is no unique histological lesion in ATLL although a number of distinct morphological patterns have emerged as being more common. For this reason it has been difficult to include ATLL in the classification of non-Hodgkin's lymphomas. Most cases, for example, will be unclassifiable using the NCI working formulation and more recent classifications have specifically attempted to include HTLV-I-induced T-cell lymphomas with better defined pathological descriptions[76]. The difficulties arise because of the heterogeneity of lymph node lesions in ATLL which may depend on whether the disease has a chronic or an acute course and also reflect the variable appearances of transformed T-cells. Cases have been seen by the authors, for example, in which the blood marrow consisted mainly of small and medium-sized atypical lymphoid cells and lymph node biopsy was characteristic of a large cell non-Hodgkin's lymphoma (NHL) of the immunoblastic type.

The lymph node lesions are always diffuse and the most frequent lesion is that described by Japanese histopathologists as pleomorphic T-NHL seen in at least 50% of cases. There are often a number of keys which suggest a T-cell proliferation, namely involvement of the paracortical zone with preservation of nodal shape and subcapsular sinus, and marked proliferation of postcapillary venules[59].

The cells involved in the malignant proliferation range from small to large. The cells most commonly seen are the medium-sized pleomorphic cells, with marked nuclear irregularities, which resemble those seen in the peripheral blood. The nuclei of the large cells are round or oval with the fine chromatin and prominent vesicular nucleoli[59]. The nuclear outline is slightly irregular and may have one-sided multiple invaginations[76]. These large cells are intensely basophilic with Giemsa stain. Frequently there is an admixture of cells which could then be considered as 'mixed small and large cell types' or as 'large cell, immunoblastic' using the criteria of the working formulation. In the recent proposals by a group of international experts who reviewed a large number of peripheral T-cell non-Hodgkin's lymphomas[76] most cases are included in the high grade pleomorphic, medium and large cell category, but sometimes may have morphological features of pleomorphic small cells (included as low grade) or immunoblastic (high grade). These authors also make the point that not all pleomorphic T-cell lymphomas are HTLV-I positive.

The separation of lymph node lesions of ATLL into low or high grade is justified only if there are clear-cut differences in prognosis. It has been suggested that pleomorphic small cells are usually seen in the rare chronic forms of ATLL[76] but data in this respect are scanty. It is probably wise to classify ATLL on clinical and pathological grounds with due consideration that it corresponds to a single entity with overall poor prognosis. The international panel recommends the classification of cases as ATLL together with the histological type[76].

The authors' observations in cases from the Caribbean were very similar to those described in Japan. One of the cases with a slightly longer clinical course has features resembling those of angioimmunoblastic lymphadenopathy[59], although this is apparently very rare[76]. Cases resembling Lennert's lymphoma or tumours of clear cells are not seen in ATLL[76] and lesions of large anaplastic large cell lymphoma have occasionally been seen[76]. Large (giant) cells with marked nuclear convolutions are seen in the lesions associated with HTLV-I more often than in virus negative T-cell lymphomas[76].

Skin lesions

A major difficulty in the early attempts to recognize ATLL as a distinct entity was the nature of the skin infiltration. Skin involvement is seen in one-third to two-thirds of patients according to the particular series[51]. The patient from whom HTLV-I was first isolated was diagnosed as a cutaneous T-cell lymphoma[64] despite the major peripheral blood involvement, on account of the degree of skin involvement as seen in Sézary syndrome and mycosis fungoides. The authors' experience and that of others suggests that dermal lesions are the most frequent in ATLL. However, epidermal infiltration and even Pautrier's microabcesses have been documented in Japan and elsewhere, in otherwise typical cases[31, 32, 51, 76]. As described above, cells with the typical morphology of Sézary cells are infrequent in ATLL but are sometimes seen as a minority component or, very rarely, as the major cell type. Thus, the presence of Sézary-like cells and/or epidermotropism in skin biopsies does not necessarily exclude a diagnosis of HTLV-I+ ATLL. On the other hand, extensive surveys in typical cases of cutaneous T-cell lymphoma showed that within that group HTLV-I is not encountered as a pathogenic agent[28]. Features common to cutaneous lymphomas such as chronic premycotic lesions, acanthosis and hyperkeratosis are not seen either in ATLL.

Bone marrow

Considering the marked hypercalcaemia and the peripheral blood involvement which may presuppose significant marrow involvement, the degree of bone marrow infiltration by pleomorphic lymphoid cells is only mild to moderate in ATLLs. Aspirates may show variable proportions of the same pleomorphic lymphoid cells as seen in peripheral blood films. Trephine biopsies show a significant degree of osteoclastic activation which is presumed to be the main mechanism of the hypercalcaemia through an osteoclastic activating factor released locally by the tumour cells[31]. The sections often show the osteoclastic proliferation in the trabecular edges with a serrated saw-toothed appearance. Biopsies of lytic lesions may even fail to show involvement by the tumour and show instead osteoclastic activity.

Ultrastructure of ATLL cells

The same cell types as seen in peripheral blood and lymph node samples – small, medium and large cell size – can be defined by ultrastructural analysis. Medium-sized lymphocytes with marked nuclear irregularities are the type most commonly encountered. The nuclear irregularities are the most prominent feature seen under the electron microscope and characterize the ATLL cells. These vary from slight indentations to horseshoe-shaped forms, convolutions and several separated or linked nuclear lobes (Figures 8.5 and 8.6). A minority of cells (about 10%) have a cerebriform nucleus resembling Sézary cells. Most cells show discrete intranuclear clumps of chromatin condensation and a small nucleolus. The cytoplasm shows a small and well-developed Golgi zone and a variable number of

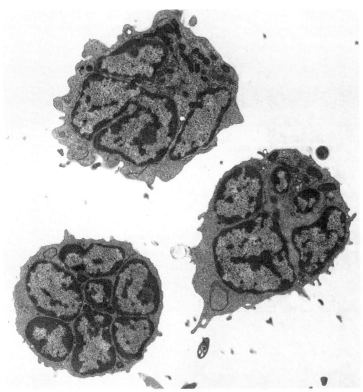

Figure 8.5 Electron micrograph of typical polylobed cells from a Caribbean patient with ATLL. × 7000, reduced to 88% on reproduction

lysosomal granules often seen in clusters (Figure 8.6). In some cases, perinuclear bundles of microfibrils are seen. The authors have observed parallel tubular arrays in cells from one typical case.

Electron microscopy is not necessary for a diagnosis of ATLL but it may be useful, in difficult cases, to recognize the cell morphology and, in particular, to define the nuclear abnormalities. CD4+ lymphocytes resembling, respectively, ATLL and Sézary cells can be recognized in the peripheral blood of normal individuals and may correspond to the normal counterparts of the neoplastic cells (see below). Evidence of HTLV-I infection is seen only after ATLL cells have been cultured in the presence of mitogens for 5–10 days[46, 47] and not on fresh cells.

The association of HTLV-I with ATLL

Work in the 1970s showed that RNA tumour viruses replicate via an intermediate stage of proviral DNA through the existence of the viral enzyme reverse transcriptase which allows the integration of the retrovirus in the cellular DNA. This knowledge, together with the demonstration that T-cell growth factor, or interleukin-2, was essential for the long-term culture of human T-cells facilitated the discovery of HTLV-I by Gallo and co-workers[26–28, 87].

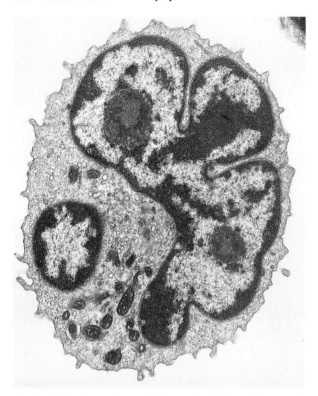

Figure 8.6 Electron micrograph from a circulating cell from another case of ATLL. This cell shows an active Golgi zone with localized electron dense granules in its vicinity. The nuclear features are more immature than those of the cells of Figure 8.5; there are two nucleoli and less chromatin condensation. × 22 000, reduced to 57% on reproduction

In the early 1980s Poiesz et al.[64] isolated HTLV-I from a T-cell line derived from a Black patient with a T-cell malignancy who, at the time, was thought to have Sézary syndrome but was later diagnosed as suffering from the new entity ATLL. This new retrovirus was later characterized by Kalyanaraman et al.[36]. Almost at the same time Hinuma, in Japan, discovered a C-type virus in a cell line established by Miyoshi from a patient with ATLL and coined the term 'ATLV'[34]. By that time it was apparent that this disease, first described as adult T-cell leukaemia (ATL) by Takatsuki et al. at the meeting of the International Society of Haematology in Kyoto in 1976 and later published by Uchiyama et al.[82] from his group, was not uncommon in the south west islands of Japan. Hinuma et al.[34] also demonstrated antibodies in most patients with ATLL which were reactive with cells from ATL-derived lines.

A fortuitous meeting which included one of the authors (DC) with Gallo, Greaves and Blattner in London, convened by the Leukaemia Research Fund, led to the realization that the features of the disease seen in Japan were no different from those of the patient from whom HTLV-I was originally isolated and from those of several patients, also of Black race, born in the Caribbean basin and resident in the UK, which had been diagnosed as T-lymphosarcoma cell leukaemia on account of the pleomorphic morphology of the circulating cells. This meeting was followed by an exchange of samples and the confirmation that the T-cell disorder in the Caribbean patients was, indeed, associated with the newly discovered retrovirus[15]. Subsequently, molecular characterization of this retrovirus and collaborative studies by several groups helped to confirm that ATLV and HTLV-I were, in fact, identical[26, 87]. Definitive proof of the association of HTLV-I and ATLL came from the demonstration by Yoshida et al.[74, 96] of the monoclonal integration of the HTLV-I proviral DNA in the leukaemic cells from these patients, thus comfirming the suspicion that ATLL arises from the malignant transformation of a cell previously infected by HTLV-I. No other types of T-cell leukaemia or lymphoma were found to contain the provirus genome in their tumour cells[96]. Other clinical and laboratory studies confirmed that the disease, ATL or ATLL, is the same in Japan[32, 77–79], in the Caribbean region[4, 7, 8] and in Caribbean immigrants to the UK[15, 30], USA[12] and other European countries[68].

The association between HTLV-I and ATLL has thus been demonstrated by serology (antibodies) (Table 8.4), epidemiology (areas of disease clustering), virology (virus isolation) and molecular analysis (monoclonal integration of proviral sequences).

Table 8.4 Incidence of antibodies to HTLV-I[a]

	Incidence (%)	References
Patients with ATLL	95–100	[4, 7, 8, 15, 18, 34, 36, 78, 79, 90]
Relatives of ATLL patients	10–45	[26, 47, 79]
Healthy carriers in endemic areas (SW Japan, Caribbean basin)	5–15	[26, 72, 94]
Healthy carriers in the UK[b] (of Caribbean origin)	3–8	[30, 47]

[a] Measured by a number of serological assays.
[b] Similar findings in other European countries, e.g. The Netherlands [68].

Recent history has confirmed and highlighted the importance of the discovery of HTLV-I as the causative agent of a CD4+ T-cell leukaemia. A new human retrovirus, now designated HIV (human immunodeficiency virus), also infects preferentially CD4+ T-lymphocytes but does not lead to their proliferation and has been shown to be the causative agent of AIDS (acquired immune deficiency syndrome)[87]. Another related human retrovirus, HTLV-II, has been associated with atypical hairy cell leukaemia[69].

In recent years, HTLV-I has been found to be closely related to a neurological disorder, known in Japan as HTLV-I-associated myelopathy and in the Caribbean as tropical spastic paraparesis. Caribbean-born patients with the disease studied in the UK were all seropositive for HTLV-I. The disorder is characterized by a slowly progressive spastic paraparesis with pyramidal signs and mild sensory and sphincter disturbances.

Mode of transmission of HTLV-I infection

HTLV-I is an exogenous virus which infects certain individuals born in endemic areas, e.g. islands in the south west of Japan (Kyushu, Shikoku and Okinawa)[32,

37, 52, 79], and the Caribbean basin [4, 7, 27, 29]. Observations on the incidence of seropositive individuals in families where one of the members suffers from ATLL have indicated that the incidence of antibodies to HTLV-I in family members is higher than in the general population in endemic areas (see Table 8.4). One consistent finding in family trees, in both Japanese [54] and Caribbean patients (Figure 8.7) is that the mother is nearly always seropositive [79]. This would

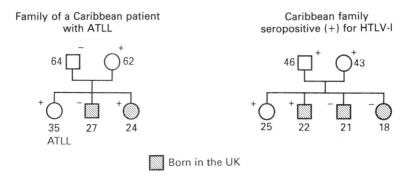

Figure 8.7 Family tree of one of the authors' Caribbean patients resident in the UK showing that the mother, the propositus (ATLL) and one of her sisters (born in the UK) had antibodies to HTLV-I

indicate a mode of vertical transmission from mother to child. In the authors' observations, the majority of seropositive individuals in the UK were first generation born in the Caribbean [47] but a minority were born in the UK and some have never visited the Caribbean. This confirms the importance of the vertical mode of transmission. Epidemiological studies in Japan also seem to indicate the possibility of husband-to-wife transmission. However, no other strong evidence for a role of sexual transmission in HTLV-I infections exists, as is the case for the AIDS virus (HIV).

Recent reports from Japan indicate that the transmission from mother to child may take place mainly through breast-feeding [58]. Observations in seropositive mothers in an endemic area show that maternal antibodies persist in some infants who were breast-fed for about 6 months and lymphocytes bearing HTLV-I are still detected in the infants for up to 18 months. Transmission via the breast milk, rather than via the placenta, is a distinct possibility currently under examination by Japanese investigators [79].

Another form of transmission, suggested by the apparent higher incidence in rural areas, is via a vector, e.g. a mosquito. A parallel has been drawn between the incidence of HTLV-I infection and areas of parasitic infestation. Finally, besides the transmission via natural routes, HTLV-I can be transmitted by blood transfusion. This has been suggested by the incidence of a proportion of seropositive individuals affected by haematological disorders other than ATLL, who are known to have received multiple transfusions, as documented in both Japan and the USA.

Retroviruses causing T-cell malignancy in primates

Following the discovery of HTLV-I in humans, Old World monkeys were found to have cross-reacting antibodies with HTLV-I [35]. Strains of a similar retrovirus were later isolated from such seropositive primates. One such retrovirus, Simian T-cell leukaemia virus type I (STLV-I) has a similar genomic structure and a 95% sequence homology to HTLV-I[81]. STLV-I has a number of biological similarities to HTLV-I including the induction of ATLL in African Green monkeys, which is preceded by a preleukaemic phase with evidence of clonal integration of the STLV-I proviral genome in the cells' DNA. The close similarities of both retroviruses suggest that STLV-I infection in monkeys could be considered as an animal model for ATLL in humans and thus may permit a close study of multiple stages of development of this retroviral induced malignancy. The possibility of transmission of a C-type virus from monkey to humans was raised by experiments by Miyoshi et al.[55].

Stages of HTLV-I infection

Antibodies to HTLV-I are found consistently in the majority of patients with ATLL from Japan, the Caribbean basin and Caribbean immigrants to Europe[8, 29, 30, 34, 36, 68]; clusters in other regions have now been reported[45]. Antibodies to HTLV-I are also found in a proportion of healthy individuals born in the endemic regions for HTLV-I (see Table 8.4). These are usually absent in patients suffering from other forms of post-thymic (mature) T-cell leukaemia (Table 8.5).

Table 8.5 Serum antibodies to HTLV-I in mature T-cell leukaemias[a]

Disease	No. cases	Black	HTLV-I+
ATLL (Caribbean)	22	22	21
T-PLL	16	2	–
Sézary syndrome	11	–	–
Sézary leukaemia	3	–	1[b]
T-CLL (large granular)	6	–	–
T-cell non-Hodgkin's lymphoma	2	–	–

[a] Series studied by Matutes and Catovsky (*Leukaemia*, 1990 in press).
[b] White Greek patient with Sézary cells but no skin involvement and aggressive course (could also be classified as ATLL).

A number of stages of HTLV-I infection can be defined by clinical and laboratory tests and the aid of molecular biology techniques which can demonstrate the integration of HTLV-I proviral DNA in peripheral blood lymphocytes[74, 90, 96]. These range from the seropositive healthy individuals without symptoms through various clinical stages of preleukaemia and florid ATL[38, 77] (Figure 8.8).

Healthy seropositive donors

Normal HTLV-I seropositive donors have a very low proportion (<1%) of lymphocytes with convoluted nucleus and a slightly raised proportion of Tac+ (CD25+) lymphocytes compared to in seronegative subjects[47]. Cultures for 5–28 days in the presence of phytohaemagglutinin (PHA) have shown that these cells

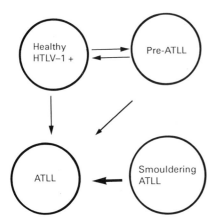

Figure 8.8 Diagram illustrating the patterns of evolution following HTLV-I infection in an individual. The state of healthy carrier may evolve to a preleukaemic state which is rarely reversible. More often a persistent clone is established and this is associated with skin rashes and other non-specific clinical features. This stage of smouldering ATLL is not reversible and will only progress to the florid manifestation of acute ATLL

harbour the retrovirus in their genome both by ultrastructural examination and by the reactivity with monoclonal antibodies against the retroviral proteins p19 and p24[33, 47]. At this stage, study with molecular probes does not allow the detection of integration of HTLV-I proviral DNA in the peripheral blood lymphocytes, probably reflecting the limitation of Southern blot analysis to detect less than 1% of HTLV-I-infected lymphocytes.

A group of these 'normal' seropositive individuals from the endemic areas of Japan have been shown, nevertheless, to have random (polyclonal) integration of HTLV-I in their circulating lymphocytes. These individuals were found to be suffering from a number of complaints, namely infection with *Strongyloides stercoralis*, respiratory problems or carcinomas, all of which were deemed to be unrelated to the manifestations of ATLL. Furthermore, an interesting association of HTLV-I infection and strongyloidiasis has emerged. In Okinawa, 65% of HTLV-I+ individuals had opportunistic infections of which *Strongyloides* is the most frequent[18]. However, up to 40% of such individuals have monoclonal integration of HTLV-I proviral DNA in their lymphocytes[57]. The risk of ATLL in HTLV-I seropositive carriers has been estimated as between 1/1000 and 1/2000 but may be higher (1/500) in older individuals.

ATLL-like cells in normal and HTLV-I-infected individuals

Studies by electron microscopy with the immunogold method have shown that a minority (<1%) of circulating peripheral blood lymphocytes have the morphology and membrane phenotype (CD4+) of ATLL (and Sézary) cells (see also Chapter 9). These normal ATLL-like cells in HTLV-I seronegative controls are, as a rule, Tac−(CD25−). Similar studies by light and electron microscopy in HTLV-I seropositive individuals of Caribbean descent showed also the presence of 1–2% of cells with a polylobed nucleus and some larger cells with basophilic cytoplasm resembling transformed lymphocytes; these cells are CD4+ and Tac+, as are the neoplastic cells in ATLL. An even higher proportion of these cells (2–5%) may be found in patients with smouldering ATLL. The proportion of such Tac+(CD25+) polylobed lymphocytes is higher in individuals with polyclonal integration (0.2%) and those with strongyloidiasis and monoclonal integration of HTLV-I proviral DNA (0.5%) than in asymptomatic healthy carriers[57]. Studies by Matutes et al.[47] have suggested that these convoluted cells correspond to HTLV-I-infected lymphocytes. A relationship between the areas of the cell membrane positive with anti-Tac and the sites where HTLV-I is released from the cell membrane has been documented by means of the immunogold method[46]. It is possible that HTLV-I infects preferentially a population of CD4+ convoluted lymphocytes which increase in number and become Tac+ following activation. This situation may remain unchanged for many years until a new event at the DNA level determines, in a minority of HTLV-I+ individuals, a further malignant change and the expansion of a clone of convoluted, HTLV-I infected, Tac+(CD25+) lymphocytes.

Smouldering ATLL

This condition has been defined in individuals with a series of clinical problems, chiefly skin lesions[77, 90], mild lymphocytosis and antibodies to HTLV-I[39]. As distinct from the healthy carriers, monoclonal integration of HTLV-I proviral DNA is often demonstrated. Although insufficient follow-up data are available, several cases of smouldering ATLL have been shown to evolve to acute ATLL after variable periods of time. Thus, smouldering ATLL could be considered a true preleukaemic condition, in which a clonal population of HTLV-I-infected cells has already been established. If infection with HTLV-I is the first stage in the development of ATLL[40], the second stage seems to be the establishment of a clone, which initially may not be clinically aggressive but may cause a degree of immunodeficiency with a variety of symptoms. The third and final event(s) presumably associated with chromosomal changes[72] and/or other irreversible changes in the genome will result in acute ATLL. Rare patients with reactive, non-clonal, lymphocytosis associated with HTLV-I may sometimes regress to the normal state. These stages of HTLV-I infection represent the best example of multistage leukaemogenesis associated with a retrovirus infection in humans[72]. Detailed studies of these patients may provide clues about the mechanism of leukaemogenesis which may operate also in other tumours whose causative agent is unknown.

Pathogenesis of the HTLV-I-induced malignancy

One of the early clues about the pathogenesis of this unique T-cell malignancy derives from the knowledge that, although each tumour is clonal (shown by the integration of the proviral DNA by Southern blotting analysis with the digestion endonuclease *pts*)[90, 96], HTLV-I is found randomly integrated in the cellular genome[74]. This combination of clonality with random integration in each tumour suggested that HTLV-I was acting by a new mechanism, different from that known for other leukaemia-causing retroviruses[26]. Like the chronic and acute leukaemia viruses, HTLV-I has the basic DNA sequences *gag*, *pol* and *env* which encode respectively for the core proteins, the enzyme reverse transcriptase (an unusual type of DNA polymerase) and the viral envelope proteins. In addition, and in common with HTLV-II and HIV, HTLV-I has a fourth region, designated as *px* or *lor* (long open reading frame) that encodes four proteins[75]. One of them, designated *tat*, may be crucial for the action at a distance (*trans*-acting activation) of HTLV-I[26, 27, 87]. There are at least two targets for the action of the *tat* protein. One is on the production of IL-2 and its receptor (abundant on the surface of ATLL cells)[41] and another on the long terminal repeats of HTLV-I which contain the regulatory sequences for viral replication[26]. There is little doubt that ATLL provides an ideal model for the elucidation of one of the mechanisms of human malignancy caused by a retrovirus. Further studies at a molecular level may clarify further the steps necessary for HTLV-I to induce T-cell leukaemia after 30 or more years from the initial infection in 1 in 2000 of the infected individuals.

Epidemiology of ATLL

One of the aspects of greatest interest in ATLL is the distinct distribution of the disease which is prevalent in the areas where HTLV-I is endemic. Advances in this field resulted from improved serological assays which are the main tool for these studies. Because HTLV-I is also associated with a neurological disorder, tropical spastic paraparesis, in addition to ATLL, the discovery of groups of patients with either disorder should stimulate further serological surveys in areas of the world apparently not yet associated with this retrovirus. For example, HTLV-I has not been recognized in temperate climates but recent evidence would suggest that occasional patients with ATLL (E. Matutes, personal communication) and others with spastic paraparesis[14a] with positive serology for HTLV-I can be found in Chile or in Chilean residents abroad. A group of 12 patients with ATLL has recently been identified in Brazil by the authors, in collaboration with Dr M. P. de Oliveira.

In addition to Japan and the Caribbean, ATLL has been diagnosed in Europe but almost exclusively in patients born in the Caribbean or, rarely, in Africa[15, 48, 68]. In the USA some clusters of the disease have been demonstrated but most patients are of Black race[12, 31, 64] and often of Caribbean descent. Serological surveys are currently being carried out in a number of countries and it is hoped that these will provide a more accurate picture of the epidemiology of the HTLV-I-associated diseases.

Serological assays

Serum antibodies against HTLV-I have been investigated by a number of assay systems of variable sensitivity and specificity. Many studies have relied on ELISA (enzyme-linked immunosorbent assay) and strip radioimmunoassay with radiolabelled antibody, both of which are highly sensitive but may give some false positive results in samples of patients with high concentrations of polyclonal immunoglobulins or with autoimmune disorders. For the ELISA special equipment is required. Indirect immunofluorescence has been carried out in the early studies by Hinuma et al. [34] and requires ATL cells (e.g. the MT-I cell line) to be fixed on a slide and tested with sera at various dilutions. This method may sometimes give equivocal results in patients with a high titre of antibodies, not necessarily against HTLV-I[17]. The gelatin particle agglutination test is quick and easy and it is probably a good method for general population screening. A modification of the immunofluorescence method, but using immunoperoxidase staining instead of the fluorescein-conjugated reagents, has been used by the authors with good specificity in samples from autoimmune disorders[89]. The authors have used the C91/PL cell line (established from cord blood lymphocytes co-cultivated with HTLV-I+ T-cells in Gallo's laboratory)[27] and fixed these cells on cytospin slides with acetone. Sera at various dilutions are incubated covering the slides on a moist chamber and, after washing, a peroxidase-conjugated rabbit anti-human immunoglobulin is used. It is important, in any epidemiological study when new or atypical findings are described, that a positive screening test for HTLV-I should be confirmed by the method considered as the gold standard for antibody analysis: Western blotting. The reliability of the latter depends on the quality of the antigen which is purified HTLV-I derived from lysates from infected cell lines. Western blot positivity is usually defined by the presence of bands indicating antibodies to the p24 and p19 major core proteins of HTLV-I. The need for confirming claims of HTLV-I positivity in new areas is important for a precise knowledge of the spread of this retrovirus. For example, data of high antibody titres in Papua New Guinea reported by gelatin agglutination and ELISA were not confirmed by the specific Western blotting assay.

South west of Japan

As described in other parts of this chapter, both the discovery and the first serological survey originated from Japan where the disease is prevalent, particularly in the south western islands of Kyushu and Shikoku. Nation-wide surveys in Japan showed that 70% of ATLL cases cluster in rural and coastal areas of Kyushu, whilst 24% are observed in northern areas, e.g. Hokkaido and Tohoku[79]. In south western Japan the incidence of ATLL and T-cell non-Hodgkin's lymphoma is of the order of 18–20% among the lymphoid malignancies, much higher than in other areas of the country, western Europe and North America.

It is not clear for how long the disease has been present in Japan or whether the actual incidence is increasing. Two surveys, with a 13–15 year interval between them, on the island of Okinawa showed no changes in the incidence of seropositivity for HTLV-I[37]. Before lymphoid malignancies were classified separately as B or T, the only earlier account of the disease may have emerged from morphological descriptions. However, even with these there is no precise knowledge as to whether ATLL is a new disease or, more probably, existed in that region for many years. The rate of antibody positive individuals in the south western islands is as high as 15% of the whole population which suggests that the infection with HTLV-I may have been present for a long period of time. Rates are also high in Japanese immigrants to Hawaii. It is apparent that some of the key questions about epidemiology and transmission of HTLV-I and ATLL will come from studies based in Japan.

The Caribbean basin

Surveys in Trinidad[4], Jamaica[7] and Martinique[29] have shown that a high proportion, close to 75%, of non-Hodgkin's lymphomas in adults have a T-cell phenotype and the majority have clinical and laboratory features compatible with ATLL (generalized lymphadenopathy, skin infiltration and leukaemic blood picture) and are seropositive for HTLV-I. This suggests that ATLL is the most common form of non-Hodgkin's lymphoma in Jamaica and that it is closely associated with HTLV-I[7]. This confirms the impression from the incidence of ATLL in Caribbean immigrants to the UK[30] and other European countries[68].

As in Japan, there is a spectrum of clinicopathological manifestations of ATLL, from smouldering to acute disease, the latter being the most common. The birth places of the patients of Caribbean origin with ATLL in the authors' series were Jamaica, St Vincent, Trinidad, Grenada, Guyana and Dominique. They have all been resident in the UK for many years (range 6–22, median 20 years) which suggests a very long incubation time for the disease.

There are no detailed studies of the incidence of ATLL in other islands of the Caribbean. In Cuba, a neighbour state of Jamaica, the incidence appears to be much lower and it may be of interest to establish the reason for this difference. It is not due to a lack of recognition of the disease by Cuban haematologists with whom the authors have discussed this issue on several occasions. Unfortunately, there are no published seroepidemiological data on the incidence of antibodies to HTLV-I in the Cuban population.

A better understanding of the factors which account for the apparently different incidence of ATLL in Cuba and Jamaica may help to clarify the origin of the HTLV-I infection in the Caribbean region. It is unlikely that geography and climatic factors could make a significant difference in these two neighbouring islands. The origin of the main population in both countries may provide some clues. Jamaica was colonized by the British in 1655 and has a predominant population of African and Afro-European origin resulting from the large scale introduction of African slaves to work in the sugar plantations. Cuba has a more heterogeneous population with only 15% being Blacks of African origin and at least 20% being Mulattos, resulting from mixed marriages between Africans and Spaniards. The remaining population is White of European origin, mainly from Spain. Although the Spaniards brought slaves from Senegal and Guinea coast, the African population never became predominant, as in Jamaica.

Data from Bartholomew et al.[4] would support the importance of racial factors. Cases of T-cell non-Hodgkin's lymphoma and ATLL in Trinidad were all of African origin and none was of East Indian descent which constitutes 40% of the population. Considering the suggestion, and the circumstantial evidence, that HTLV-I originates from the African continent, in both Japan and the Caribbean[27], the stated differences in the population may indicate that genetic and related epidemiological factors could account for the different incidence of HTLV-I infection.

HTLV-I in Africa

Serological surveys in Africa by Saxinger from Gallo's group[27] have shown an incidence of seropositive individuals of 5% in urban areas and 10% in rural ones. However, some of the data are contradictory because of possible cross-reactivity in some of the assays with the proteins of HIV, and the problem of non-specific reactivity in people with high levels of serum immunoglobulins. However, in some of the studies the findings were confirmed by the specific Western blot assay. There are few reports of ATLL in Africa but cases of ATLL in Africans who have been living in Europe have been found. One of the patients in the authors' ATLL series was born in Sierra Leone (West Africa) and has been living in the UK for 7 years.

Prognosis and treatment

There is some correlation between the clinical forms of the disease and patients' survival, e.g. the lymphoma type of ATLL may have a slightly better prognosis than the acute (or frankly leukaemic) form of ATLL. Almost by definition, too, smouldering ATLL and chronic lymphocytosis have a long protracted clinical course. The overall prognosis of ATLL is poor and both the series of Caribbean patients and those from Japan show median survivals of between 6 and 8 months. In general, patients with a good response to treatment may do better but this is not always the case as relapse may occur very rapidly and without much warning.

The poor prognosis of ATLL almost pre-empts the issue that no satisfactory treatment has yet emerged for this T-cell malignancy. Most patients have been treated with combination chemotherapy regimens used for high-grade non-Hodgkin's lymphoma, e.g. CHOP, M-BACOD etc. and, in some, good partial remissions or, rarely, complete remissions, have been obtained, but of short duration (1–4 months).

In recent years the authors and others[92] have employed the adenosine deaminase inhibitor 2'-deoxycoformycin (DCF) to treat ATLL with variable results. Two-thirds of patients are poor responders or resistant to DCF[38, 92]. However, relatively prolonged remission may occasionally be observed in the remainder. So far the authors have treated 10 Caribbean-born ATLL patients, with a median age of 37 years (range 20–53), with DCF given at $4\,mg/m^2$ a week for the first 4–6 weeks. Others have used higher doses, e.g. $5\,mg/m^2$ for 3 consecutive days[92], but these are usually too toxic. For the treatment with DCF a normal creatinine clearance is required and it is advisable to give antibacterial, antiviral and antifungal prophylaxis, e.g. with co-trimoxazole, acyclovir and amphotericin, all given orally, because DCF has immunosuppressive and myelotoxic properties. Eight of these ten ATLL patients had relapsed or were resistant following prior chemotherapy. Three had good responses to DCF (two complete and one partial). One of the complete responders died, whilst still in remission, of an opportunistic infection; the other is still alive and off therapy for over 1 year. The partial responder survived only 3 months. In the seven remaining patients there was either no response or a minimal improvement short of partial remission.

The response to DCF in other mature T-cell malignancies has not been much better than in ATLL, but seems to be correlated with the membrane phenotype. In ATLL, the three responders were from a group of eight with a CD4+, CD8− phenotype; two patients with different markers (which is a rare event; see above) did not respond. Overall, 50% of cases of CD4+, CD8− (TdT−, CD1a−) T-cell leukaemias responded to DCF whilst only 15% of cases with a different phenotype (e.g. CD4+, CD8+ or CD4−, CD8− etc.) showed responses which were never complete. The authors also observed in ATLL that bulky disease was nearly always non-responsive (C. Dearden and D. Catovsky, unpublished observation).

In both treated and untreated ATLL patients the main factors responsible for morbidity and mortality are opportunistic infections with atypical or uncommon organisms. In some respects, patients with HTLV-I+ ATLL behave like HIV+ AIDS patients. Pulmonary complications, e.g. interstitial pneumonitis and *Pneumocystis carinii* pneumonia are common. In the authors' series cryptococcal infections, systemic candidiasis, salmonella and campylobacter infections were observed. These may occur even in patients in remission. Therefore the prophylaxis with co-trimoxazole, acyclovir and amphotericin suggested above for DCF-treated patients may need to be extended on a long-term basis.

There are insufficient molecular data on ATLL to answer the question of whether relapses occur in the same malignant clone or if they occur in new clones of HTLV-I-infected lymphocytes. Both possibilities are likely. The few attempts at bone marrow transplantation have so far failed, presumably because it is probably impossible to eradicate all HTLV-I-infected T-lymphocytes.

Chromosome abnormalities in ATLL

Most of the reports on chromosome abnormalities in ATLL have originated in Japan[53, 73, 83] but the results are no different in the small series published from the UK, in Caribbean-born patients[10,11], and in the USA[70]. Some of the karyotypic changes demonstrated in ATLL are similar to those of other lymphoid malignancies, e.g. a terminal deletion of chromosome 6, 6q−, which has also been documented in T-PLL and cutaneous T-cell lymphoma[11]. Others, like trisomy 7 and 7q[11, 73] are rarely seen in other leukaemias.

The most frequent clonal changes reported in ATLL are: trisomy 7/7q (22.5%; Table 8.6); trisomy or partial trisomy 3[53, 70, 73] in 23% of cases; 6q−[10, 11, 53] in 25%; and abnormalities of chromosome 14[10, 53, 73] in 17%. The changes in chromosome 14 always affect the long (q) arm with a breakpoint at 14q32 in 12%, site of the Ig heavy chain gene[2] but also of a candidate oncogene tcl-1[19] and, less frequently, at 14q11 (5% of cases), where the gene for the α-chain of the human T-cell receptor is localized[19].

Table 8.6 Trisomy 7/7q in ATLL

Authors	Year	Number of cases		Country of origin
		Studied	Positive	
Ueshima et al. [83]	1981	15	5	Japan
Miyamoto et al. [53]	1984	30	2	Japan
Rowley et al. [70]	1984	6	2	USA
Sanada et al. [73]	1985	18	5	Japan
Brito-Babapulle et al. [10, 11]	1986	2	2	Caribbean
Total		71	16	

The distinct rearrangement inv(14) (q11;q32), seen in two-thirds of T-PLL patients (see Chapter 5), has been reported rarely in ATLL. Studies on the molecular basis of this abnormality are currently keenly pursued by several groups. Only in a T-cell lymphoma cell line the inversion of chromosome 14 was found to involve both the T-cell receptor α-chain gene at 14q11 and the immunoglobulin heavy chain gene variable segment at 14q32, resulting in a productive rearrangement[19]. Breakpoints at 14q11 are also a feature of other translocations in T-cell leukaemias[43], including T-ALL and the preleukaemic disorder ataxia telangiectasia. The abnormalities of chromosome 14 in ATLL are most frequently described as 14q+[10, 53, 73] with the breakpoint nearly always at the level of band q32.

The possible significance of the abnormalities in ATLL has been examined by several groups. With respect to trisomy +7/7q a correlation was noticed with the expression of the IL-2 receptor, not just in ATLL[11]. As the IL-2 (Tac) receptor is induced in ATLL cells by HTLV-I, the finding of a correlation may be coincidental, although the exact mechanism leading to IL-2 expression is not completely clear[41]. The gene for the Tac antigen has been mapped to chromosome 10 at p14–15. Perhaps more significant in relation to abnormalities of the long arm of chromosome 7 is the mapping of the T-cell receptor β-chain gene at 7q35[13]. By analogy with rearrangements involving other functional genes it is possible that events during normal T-cell differentiation may trigger, or be the target of, malignant change.

The bulk of evidence suggests that chromosome abnormalities are not a primary event in the pathogenesis of ATLL but may be responsible for clinical progression. In this respect, the study of Sanada et al.[73] elegantly makes this point. Of nine patients with the acute form of ATLL, they demonstrated trisomy 3 and/or trisomy 7 in eight, whereas these abnormalities were not found in eight patients with chronic or smouldering ATLL[73]. Further evidence that HTLV-I infection (and not a chromosome change) is the first event in the multistep pathogenesis of ATLL is provided by another report by Sanada et al.[72] in a patient in whom four different clones with abnormal chromosomes were found on circulating ATLL cells whilst Southern blot analysis showed that HTLV-I proviral DNA was monoclonal. These findings suggest that the original cells infected by HTLV-I had a normal karyotype. In the first case of Caribbean ATLL that the authors have reported[10], two distinct chromosome clones were demonstrated without any abnormality in common. Thus, the chromosome changes in ATLL may bear some analogy to the secondary changes of chronic granulocytic leukaemia, in both diseases having a direct relationship to clinical progression. Nevertheless, the fact that in most cases the changes observed are circumscribed to particular chromosomes and chromosome bands (nos 3, 6, 7, 14) suggests some degree of specificity which may relate to the aetiological agent, HTLV-I, as well as to the T-cell nature of the cells.

T-cell antigen receptor

In the last few years it has been established that T-lymphocytes display specific antigen recognition structures analogous to the immunoglobulins (Ig) or antigen receptors on B-cells. There are now two recognized types of T-cell antigen receptor (TCR). Both consist of heterodimer molecules: αβ- and γδ-chains. The TCR αβ was first recognized and consists of two disulphide-linked chains encoded in different gene segments, V, D, J and C, which rearrange, as the Ig genes, during T-cell differentiation[16, 20, 50, 71, 93]. Both types of TCR are linked to the CD3 (T3) complex which is required for their membrane expression. The TCR γδ, identified recently [20], rearranges earlier than the TCR αβ gene during T-cell ontogenesis and may not require, as the TCR αβ, recognition through major histocompatibility complex molecules. In adults, the majority of T-cells with a CD3+, CD4+ or CD8+ phenotype bear the TCR αβ, whilst less than 5% of peripheral blood T-lymphocytes, which are CD3+, CD4– and CD8+ or CD8–, bear the TCR γδ[20].

The availability of probes for the TCR complex has introduced a new laboratory tool for the characterization of T-lymphoproliferative disorders. Although the exploitation of these techniques has so far lagged behind those used for the study of the Ig heavy and light chain genes (see also Chapter 2), the evaluation of the configuration of the TCR chain genes has, nevertheless, enabled useful contributions in the classification of lymphoid leukaemias. This development has been particularly welcomed considering that no consistent marker of clonality was previously available for the T-cell lineage. Thus, gene rearrangement patterns, in addition to confirming the T-cell nature of a given malignancy, may be used to distinguish between polyclonal and monoclonal T-cell proliferations[1, 5, 21, 24, 30a, 30b, 50, 65, 67].

Findings in leukaemia

As expected, in the majority of cases of T-ALL the leukaemic cells show a monoclonal rearrangment of the TCR β-chain gene[23, 66, 84] (Table 8.7). However, in a minority the TCR β-chain gene may be in germ-line configuration[23, 63]. In 40 cases of T-ALL studied by the authors, 5 were germ line. When the DNA configuration was correlated with the subclassification based

Table 8.7 Ig heavy (H) and light (L) chain genes, TCR β-, γ- and δ-genes in acute and chronic T- and B-cell leukaemias

Disease	H	L	TCRβ	TCRγ	TCRδ
Null-ALL	R	G R	G R	G R	R D (G)
cALL	R	G R	G R	G R	R D (G)
Pre-T-ALL	G	G	G	G	R D
T-ALL	G (R)	G	R	R	R D
TdT− AML	G (R)	G	G	G	G
TdT+ AML	R G	G	G R	G R	
B-CLL	R	R	G	G	G
B-PLL	R	R	G	G	G
HCL	R	R	G	G	G
T-CLL[a]	G	G	R P[b]	R P[b]	D
T-PLL	G	G	R	R	D
Sézary syndrome	G	G	R	R	D
ATLL	G	G	R	R	D

G: germ-line; R: rearranged; P: polyclonal; AML = acute myeloid leukaemia; HCL = hairy cell leukaemia.

[a] Full details in Table 8.8.
[b] Rare CD3+, CD8+ cases, best designated as T-lymphocytosis.

on the immunotype of the T-blasts, it was observed that the germ-line configuration was confined to the more immature, pre-thymic cases, which express only the CD7 antigen (and usually also CD5) and are TdT+. According to the authors' data, a similar pattern is observed also with the Tγ-gene, confirming that the TCR β-chain and Tγ-genes are closely correlated in T-cell ontogeny. Thus, it appears that in T-ALL the CD7 antigen precedes the rearrangement of both the TCR β-chain and Tγ-genes. The apparently conflicting evidence of a rearrangement of the TCR gene in the absence of the T3/CD3 complex, may be explained by evidence that the CD3 antigen is found first in the cytoplasm of T-cells and that the transcription of CD3 occurs at the mRNA level[25, 44]. Nevertheless, the lack of surface expression of the T3/CD3 antigen in the presence of a TCR rearrangement is not completely understood. It has, however, been recently demonstrated that the T3 complex assembly on the cell membrane requires the concomitant expression of a TCR αβ heterodimer or the more recently recognized TCR γδ gene[3, 9]. The rearrangement of the genes encoding for the γδ heterodimer precedes that of the TCR αβ genes during ontogeny and it is therefore not surprising to detect the rearrangement of the TCR γδ genes before that of the αβ-chain genes. Studies in T-ALL indicate that the TCR δ-gene is involved (either rearranged or deleted) in almost all cases[6b, 24a, 30a]. In the authors' experience, based on 35 T-ALL cases, a rearrangement or deletion of the δ-gene was documented, including three pre-T-ALL cases which were germ-line for the β- and γ-genes (Foa, unpublished data).

Chronic T-cell leukaemias

All cases of chronic T-lymphoproliferative disorders which express the T4/CD4 antigen, i.e. T-PLL, mycosis fungoides, Sézary syndrome, ATLL and peripheral T-cell lymphomas, appear to be rearranged with a monoclonal pattern at both TCR β- and TCR γ- genes[1, 6, 24, 60–62, 66, 84, 86] (Table 8.8). These findings correlate well with the unequivocal neoplastic origin of these disorders.

Table 8.8 Configuration of the TCR β-, γ- and δ-genes in acute and chronic T-lymphoproliferative disorders

Disorder	Phenotype[a]	TCRβ	TCRγ	TCRδ
Pre-T-ALL	CD2/3−, CD5+/−, CD7+	G	G	R D
T-ALL	CD1/5/7+, CD4/8+/−	R	R	R D
T-PLL	CD4+, CD8−	R	R	D
Sézary syndrome	CD4+, CD8−	R	R	D
ATLL	CD4+, CD8−	R	R	D
T-lymphoma	CD4+, CD8−	R	R	D
T-CLL/T-lymphocytosis[b]	CD4−, CD8+	R	R	D
		G	R[c]	
		P[d]	P[d]	
	CD3/4/8−, CD16+	G	G	G

G: germ-line; R: rearranged; P: polyclonal.

[a] CD2(T11 or E-rosettes)+ and CD3(T3)+ (membrane staining) unless indicated as negative.
[b] Expansion of large granular lymphocytes.
[c] One case studied at Hammersmith Hospital. A γ mRNA transcript was also demonstrated in this case and rearrangement of TCR γδ[24a].
[d] Rare in cases defined by persistent T-lymphocytosis (≥3 months) of over 5 × 10^9/l.

Molecular analyses have been extremely useful in clarifying the nature of the expansions of granular lymphocytes (T-CLL/T-cell lymphocytosis) which, for a long time, had remained uncertain, particularly in view of the relatively benign and stable clinical course. Details of this disorder and of the arguments about its neoplastic or clonal origin are discussed in Chapter 4. In the majority of T-CLL cases that display the common CD3+, CD4−, CD8+ phenotype, the cells show a monoclonal rearrangement of the TCR β-chain gene[5, 24, 67]. These findings, which have been confirmed also with the TCR γ-gene, point to the neoplastic origin of these cases. However, it should be noted that some cases which appear to have haematological and immunological similarities to monoclonal cases (true T-CLL) may display a polyclonal of both the TCR β- and Tγ-genes. These findings underline the relevant diagnostic and prognostic implications that DNA analyses may have in the study of haematological malignancies. It should be borne in mind that these studies should not be limited to the probes for the β-chain gene as the cells of some cases of CD3+, CD4−, CD8+ T-CLL may show the rearrangement of the TCR γ- and δ-genes but not of the TCR β-gene[24a]. Finally, the rare forms of CD3−, CD4−, CD8−, CD2+, CD16+ granular expansions with strong natural killer activity show a germ-line configuration of the TCR β-, γ- and δ-genes, suggesting a possible separate differentiation lineage for these natural killer-derived proliferations[6a, 24].

The relatively extensive characterization of human leukaemias carried out with the TCR genes, coupled with the information previously obtained with the probes for the Ig heavy and light chain genes, allows a more comprehensive view of the findings obtained with these techniques and permits a 'mapping' of the various disorders and identification of the relevance and limitations of these assays. Table 8.7 summarizes the results of the configuration of the TCR and Ig genes in the acute and chronic lymphoproliferative disorders of both T- and B-cell origin, as well as in acute myeloid leukaemia (AML).

Unexpected TCR rearrangements

In the authors' experience, in non-B-disorders, acute and chronic T-cell leukaemias and TdT− AMLs, the demonstration of Ig gene rearrangement is rare. In 35 cases of T-ALL this was observed in 3 (8.6%); furthermore, this was not observed in 27 chronic T-cell disorders and in only 2 of the 42 cases (4.7%) of TdT− AMLs analysed[22]. A different picture is observed instead in B-cell leukaemias, in which rearrangements of both Ig and TCR genes may occur[63]. In the authors' series of over 50 cases, the possibility of a rearrangement of the TCR β- and/or TCR γ-gene in B-lineage ALL (common- and null-ALL) was in the range of 30–40% of cases[23]. Interestingly, in leukaemias of mature B-lymphocytes, i.e. B-CLL and hairy cell leukaemia, the demonstration of a TCR rearrangement is exceptional[49]. Furthermore, TCR rearrangement has not been found in 42 cases of TdT− AMLs[22]. Recent studies have documented a high frequency of TCR δ-gene rearrangement or deletion in non-T-ALL[30a, 44a]. In the authors' experience, based on 75 cases, this occurred in 87%[6c]. These data indicate that the TCR δ-gene is, therefore, a marker of clonality rather than of lineage.

The cases classified as TdT+ AMLs, which account for 10–20% of all AMLs, deserve special mention. In a recent study the authors observed evidence of Ig gene rearrangement in 8 out of 10 cases of TdT+ AMLs[22]. In addition, in several of them a rearrangement of the TCR β-chain gene or, more frequently, of the TCR γ-gene, was also documented. These results, which differ from those of TdT− AMLs, confirm the important role of the enzyme terminal deoxynucleotidyl transferase in the insertion of extra nucleotides (N regions) on the one hand and suggest that, on the other, despite the expression of myeloid-related markers, the neoplastic clone shows a molecular configuration which closely resembles that observed in B-lineage ALL. This suggestion gains further support by the evidence of at least two cases, one child and one adult, diagnosed as TdT+ AML, who, at the time of relapse, lost the myeloid features and acquired a phenotype typical of B-lineage ALL (null- or common-ALL). Molecular analysis of one of these cases showed that the leukaemic cells, both at diagnosis and at relapse, had an identical pattern of rearrangement of the Ig heavy chain and TCR γ-gene. This observation indicates that the clone had remained structurally the same, despite the switch of the blast cells from a myeloid to a lymphoid phenotype.

TCR and Ig rearrangements as clonal markers

With the advent of these new techniques of DNA analysis there now exists a clonal tool, the utility of which may well extend beyond the characterization of the neoplastic lymphoid populations at diagnosis and may be of great relevance in monitoring the course of the disease and the response to treatment. All patients with acute and chronic lymphoid leukaemias have, in fact, an individual marker of clonality characterized by the rearranged configuration of the Ig or TCR genes. These markers gain particular relevance in view of the well-known difficulties in evaluating small numbers of leukaemic cells by conventional morphological and immunological methods. In the authors' experience these molecular analyses appear to be sufficiently sensitive to allow the recognition of a clonal population which accounts for only 0.5–1% of the total cell sample. Thus, these techniques have valuable clinical implications in assessing the response to treatment, the presence of minimal residual disease and thus the true significance of a complete remission. For example, using probes for the Ig genes, the authors have recently documented the disappearance of the neoplastic clone in hairy cell leukaemia patients treated with α-interferon, suggesting that this lymphokine has a cytostatic, rather than a differentiating, effect on hairy cells. Furthermore, in common-ALL and in T-cell lymphomas the complete disappearance of leukaemic cells from the bone marrow following induction therapy has been documented by the authors, as well as early relapse in patients considered to be in complete remission. DNA analysis, by Southern blotting or by the newly developed technique of polymerase chain reaction (PCR), represents a most promising approach towards identifying the presence of residual leukaemic cells in cryopreserved bone marrow samples stored with a view to autografting procedures, and towards defining the true remission state of a patient scheduled to undergo allogeneic bone marrow transplantation.

References

1. Aisenberg, A. C., Krontiris, T. G., Mak, T. W. and Wilkes, B. M. (1985) Rearrangement of the gene for the beta chain of the T-cell receptor in T-cell chronic lymphocytic leukemia and related disorders. *New England Journal of Medicine,* **313,** 529–533
2. Baer, R., Chen, K-C., Smith, S. D. and Rabbitts, T. H. (1985) Fusion of an immunoglobin variable gene and a T-cell receptor constant gene in the chromosome 14 inversion associated with T-cell tumours. *Cell,* **43,** 705–713
3. Bank, I., DePinho, R. A., Brenner, M. B., Cassimeris, J., Alt, F. W. and Chess, L. (1986) A functional T3 molecule associated with a novel heterodimer on the surface of immature human thymocytes. *Nature,* **322,** 179–181
4. Bartholomew, C., Charles, W., Saxinger, C. et al. (1985) Racial and other characteristics of human T cell leukaemia/lymphoma (HTLV-I) and AIDS (HTLV-III) in Trinidad. *British Medical Journal,* **290,** 1243–1246
5. Berliner, N., Duby, A. D., Linch, D. C. et al. (1986) T cell receptor gene rearrangements define a monoclonal T cell proliferation in patients with T cell lymphocytosis and cytopenia. *Blood,* **67,** 914–918
6. Bertness, V., Kirsch, I., Hollis, G., Johnson, B. and Bunn, P. A. Jr (1985) T-cell receptor gene rearrangements as clinical markers of human T-cell lymphomas. *New England Journal of Medicine,* **313,** 534–538
6a. Biondi, A., Allavena, P., Rossi, V. et al. (1989) T-cell receptor δ-gene organization and expression in normal and leukemic natural killer cells. *Journal of Immunology,* **143,** 1009–1014
6b. Biondi, A., Champagne, E., Rossi, V. et al. (1989) T-cell receptor delta gene rearrangement in childhood T-cell acute lymphoblastic leukemia. *Blood,* **73,** 2133–2138

6c. Biondi, A., Franci di Celle, P., Rossi, V. et al. (1990) High prevalence of T-cell receptor δ V2-(D)-D3 or D2-D3 rearrangements in B-precursor acute lymphoblastic leukemias. *Blood*, in press

7. Blattner, W. A., Gibbs, W. N., Saxinger, C. et al. (1983) Human T-cell leukaemia/lymphoma virus associated lymphoreticular neoplasia in Jamaica. *Lancet*, **ii**, 61–64

8. Blattner, W. A., Kalyanaraman, V. S., Robert-Guroff, M. et al. (1982) The human type-C retrovirus, HTLV, in blacks from the Caribbean region, and relationship to adult T-cell leukemia/lymphoma. *International Journal of Cancer*, **30**, 257–264

9. Brenner, M. B., McLean, J., Dialynas, D. P. et al. (1986) Identification of a putative second T-cell receptor. *Nature*, **322**, 145–149

10. Brito-Babapulle, V., Matutes, E., Hegde, U. and Catovsky, D. (1984) Adult T-cell lymphoma/leukemia in a Caribbean patient: cytogenetic, immunologic and ultrastructural findings. *Cancer Genetics and Cytogenetics*, **12**, 343–357

11. Brito-Babapulle, V., Matutes, E., Parreira, L. and Catovsky, D. (1986) Abnormalities of chromosome 7q and Tac expression in T cell leukemias. *Blood*, **67**, 516–521

12. Bunn, P. A., Jr, Schechter, G. P., Jaffe, E. et al. (1983) Clinical course of retrovirus-associated adult T-cell lymphoma in the United States. *New England Journal of Medicine*, **309**, 257–264

13. Caccia, N., Kronenberg, M., Saxe, D. et al. (1984) The T cell receptor B chain genes are located on chromosome 6 in mice and chromosome 7 in humans. *Cell*, **37**, 1091–1099

14. Canellos, G. P. (1974) Hypercalcemia in malignant lymphoma and leukemia. *Annals of the New York Academy of Science*, **230**, 240–246

14a. Cartier-Rovirosa, L., Mora, C., Araya, F. et al. (1989) HTLV-I positive spastic paraparesis in a temperate zone. *Lancet*, **i**, 556–567

15. Catovsky, D., Greaves, M. F., Rose, M. et al. (1982) Adult T-cell lymphoma-leukaemia in blacks from the West Indies. *Lancet*, **i**, 639–643

16. Chien, U., Becker, D. M., Lindsten, T., Okamura, M., Cohen, D. I. and Davis, M. M. (1984) A third type of murine T-cell receptor gene. *Nature*, **312**, 31–35

17. Chosa, T., Hattori, T., Matsuoka, M., Yamaguchi, K., Yamamoto, S. and Takatsuki, G. (1986) Analysis of anti-HTLV-I antibody by strip radioimmunoassay – comparison with indirect immunofluorescence assay, enzyme-linked immunosorbent assay and membrane immunofluorescence assay. *Leukemia Research*, **10**, 605–610

18. Clark, J. W., Robert-Guroff, M., Ikehara, O., Henzan, E. and Blattner, W. A. (1985) Human T-cell leukemia-lymphoma virus Type 1 and adult T-cell leukemia-lymphoma in Okinawa. *Cancer Research*, **45**, 2849–2852

19. Croce, C. M., Isobe, M., Palumbo, A. et al. (1985) Gene for a-chain of human T-cell receptor: location on chromosome 14 region involved in T-cell neoplasms. *Science*, **227**, 1044–1047

20. Davis, M. M. and Bjorkman, P. J. (1988) T-cell antigen receptor genes and T-cell recognition. *Nature*, **334**, 395–402

21. Flug, F., Pelicci, P-G., Bonetti, F., Knowles, D. M. II and Dalla-Favera, R. (1985) T-cell receptor gene rearrangements as markers of lineage and clonality in T-cell neoplasms. *Proceedings of the National Academy of Sciences of the USA*, **82**, 3460–3464

22. Foa, R., Casorati, G., Giubellino, M. C. et al. (1987) Rearrangements of immunoglobulin and T cell receptor β and γ genes are associated with terminal deoxynucleotidyl transferase expression in acute myeloid leukemia. *Journal of Experimental Medicine*, **165**, 879–890

23. Foa, R., Migone, N. and Gavosto, F. (1986) Immunological and molecular classification of acute lymphoblastic leukaemia. *Haematologica*, **71**, 277–286

24. Foa, R., Pelicci, P-G., Migone, N. et al. (1986) Analysis of T-cell receptor beta chain ($T_β$) gene rearrangements demonstrates the monoclonal nature of T-cell chronic lymphoproliferative disorders. *Blood*, **67**, 247–250

24a. Foroni, L., Laffan, M., Boehm, T., Rabbitts, T. H., Catovsky, D. and Luzzatto, L. (1989) Rearrangement of the T-cell receptor δ genes in human T-cell leukemias. *Blood*, **73**, 559–565

25. Furley, A. J., Mizutani, S., Weilbaecher, K. et al. (1986) Developmentally regulated rearrangement and expression of genes encoding the T-cell receptor-T3 complex. *Cell*, **46**, 75–87

26. Gallo, R. C. (1986) The first human retrovirus. *Scientific American*, **255**, 78–88

27. Gallo, R. C., Essex, M. E. and Gross, L. (Eds) (1984) *Human T-cell Leukemia-Lymphoma Viruses*. New York: Cold Spring Harbor Laboratory
28. Gallo, R. C., Kalyanaraman, V. S., Sarngadharan, M. G. et al. (1983) Association of the human type C retrovirus with a subset of adult T-cell cancers. *Cancer Research*, **43**, 3892–3899
29. Gessain, A., Jouannelle, A., Escarmant, P., Calender, A., Schaffar-Deshayes, L. and De-The, G. (1984) HTLV antibodies in patients with non-Hodgkin lymphomas in Martinique. *Lancet*, **i**, 1183–1184
30. Greaves, M. F., Verbi, W., Tilley, R. et al. (1984) Human T-cell leukaemia virus (HTLV) in the United Kingdom. *International Journal of Cancer*, **33**, 795–806
30a. Griesinger, F., Greenberg, J. M. and Kersey, J. H. (1989) T-cell receptor gamma and delta rearrangement in hematologic malignancies. Relationship to lymphoid differentiation. *Journal of Clinical Investigations*, **84**, 506–516
30b. Griesser, H., Tkachuk, D., Reis, M. D. and Mak, T. W. (1989) Gene rearrangements and translocations in lymphoproliferative diseases. *Blood*, **73**, 1402–1415
31. Grossman, B., Schechter, G. P., Horton, J. H., Pierce, L., Jaffe, E. and Wahl, L. (1981) Hypercalcemia associated with T-cell lymphoma-leukemia. *American Journal of Clinical Pathology*, **75**, 149–155
32. Hanaoka, M., Takatsuki, K. and Shimoyama, M. A. (Eds) (1982) Adult T-cell leukemia and related diseases. *Gann Monograph on Cancer Research*, No. 29. New York: Plenum Press
32a. Hansen-Hagge, T. E., Yokota, S. and Bartram, C. R. (1989) Detection of minimal residual disease in acute lymphoblastic leukemia by in vitro amplification of rearranged T-cell receptor δ-chain sequences. *Blood*, **74**, 1762–1767
33. Haynes, B. F., Palker, T. J., Robert-Guroff, M. et al. (1984) Monoclonal antibodies against human T-cell leukemia/lymphoma virus p19 and p24 internal core proteins: spectrum of normal tissue reactivity and use as diagnostic probes. In *Human T-cell Leukemia/Lymphoma Virus*, edited by R. C. Gallo, M. E. Essex and L. Gross, pp. 197–203. New York: Cold Spring Harbor Laboratory
34. Hinuma, Y., Nagata, K., Hanaoka, M. et al. (1981) Adult T-cell leukemia antigen in an ATL cell line and detection of antibodies to the antigen in human sera. *Proceedings of the National Academy of Sciences of the USA*, **78**, 6476–6480
35. Hunsmann, G., Schneider, J., Schmitt, J. and Yamamoto, N. (1983) Detection of serum antibodies to adult T-cell leukemia virus in non-human primates and in people from Africa. *International Journal of Cancer*, **32**, 329–332
36. Kalyanaraman, V. S., Sarngadharan, M. G., Bunn, P. A., Minna, J. D. and Gallo, R. C. (1981) Antibodies in human sera reactive against an internal structural protein of human T-cell lymphoma virus. *Nature*, **294**, 271–273
37. Kashiwagi, S., Kajiyama, W., Hayashi, J., Nomura, H. and Ikematsu, H. (1986) No significant changes in adult T-cell leukemia virus infection in Okinawa after intervals of 13 and 15 years. *Japanese Journal of Cancer Research (Gann)*, **77**, 452–455
38. Kawano, F., Yamaguchi, K., Nishimura, H., Tsuda, H. and Takatsuki, K. (1985) Variation in the clinical courses of adult T-cell leukemia. *Cancer*, **55**, 851–856
39. Kinoshita, K., Amagasaki, T., Ikeda, S. et al. (1985) Preleukemic state of adult T cell leukemia: abnormal T lymphocytosis induced by human adult T cell leukemia-lymphoma virus. *Blood*, **66**, 120–127
40. Kinoshita, K., Hino, S., Amagasaki, T. et al. (1982) Development of adult T-cell leukemia-lymphoma (ATL) in two anti-ATL-associated antigen-positive healthy adults. *Japanese Journal of Cancer Research (Gann)*, **73**, 684–685
41. Lando, Z., Sarin, P., Megson, M. et al. (1983) Association of human T-cell leukaemia/lymphoma virus with the Tac antigen marker for the human T-cell growth factor receptor. *Nature*, **305**, 733–736
42. Lennert, K., Kikuchi, M., Sato, E. et al. (1985) HTLV-positive and negative T-cell lymphomas. Morphological and immunohistochemical differences between European and HTLV-positive Japanese T-cell lymphomas. *International Journal of Cancer*, **35**, 65–72
43. Lewis, W. H., Michalopoulos, E. E., Williams, D. L., Minden, M. D. and Mak, T. W. (1985) Breakpoints in the human T-cell antigen receptor α-chain locus in two T-cell leukaemia patients with chromosomal translocations. *Nature*, **317**, 544–546

44. Link, M. P., Stewart, S. J., Warnke, R. A. and Levy, R. (1985) Discordance between surface and cytoplasmic expression of the Leu-4 (T3) antigen in thymocytes and in blast cells from childhood T lymphoblastic malignancies. *Journal of Clinical Investigation,* **76**, 248–253

44a. Loiseau, P., Guglielmi, P., Le Paslier, D. et al. (1989) Rearrangements of the T-cell receptor δ-gene in T acute lymphoblastic leukemia cells are distinct from those occurring in B-lineage acute lymphoblastic leukemia and preferentially involve one Vδ gene segment. *Journal of Immunology,* **142**, 3305–3311

45. Manzari, V., Gradilone, A., Barillari, G. et al. (1985) HTLV-I is endemic in Southern Italy: detection of the first infectious cluster in a white population. *International Journal of Cancer,* **36**, 557–559

46. Matutes, E., Brito-Babapulle, V. and Catovsky, D. (1985) Clinical, immunological, ultrastructural and cytogenetic studies in black patients with adult T-cell leukemia/lymphoma. In *Retroviruses in Human Lymphoma/Leukemia,* edited by M. Miwa, H. Sugano, T. Sugimura and R. Weiss, pp. 59–70. Tokyo: Japan Scientific Societies Press

47. Matutes, E., Dalgleish, A. G., Weiss, R. A., Joseph, A. P. and Catovsky, D. (1986) Studies in healthy human T-cell leukaemia lymphoma virus (HTLV-I) carriers from the Caribbean. *International Journal of Cancer,* **38**, 41–45

48. Miedema, F., Terpstra, F. G., Smit, J. W. et al. (1984) Functional properties of neoplastic T cells in adult T cell lymphoma/leukemia patients from the Caribbean. *Blood,* **63**, 477–481

49. Migone, N., Giubellino, M. C., Casorati, G., Tassinari, A., Lauria, F. and Foa, R. (1987) Configuration of the immunoglobulin and T-cell receptor gene regions in hairy cell leukemia and B-chronic lymphocytic leukemia. *Leukemia,* **1**, 393–394

50. Minden, M. D. and Mak, T. W. (1986) The structure of the T cell antigen receptor genes in normal and malignant T cells. *Blood,* **68**, 327–336

51. Mitsui, T., Suchi, T. and Kikuchi, M. (1982) Macroscopical and histopathological analysis on cutaneous lymphomatous lesions of peripheral T cell nature. *Gann Monograph on Cancer Research,* **28**, 135–145

52. Miwa, M., Sugano, H., Sugimura, T. and Weiss, R. A. (Eds) (1985) *Retroviruses in Human Lymphoma/Leukemia.* Tokyo: Japan Scientific Societies Press

53. Miyamoto, K., Tomita, N., Ishii, A. et al. (1984) Chromosome abnormalities of leukemia cells in adult patients with T-cell leukemia. *Journal of the National Cancer Institute,* **73**, 353–362

54. Miyamoto, Y., Yamaguchi, K., Nishimura, H. et al. (1985) Familial adult-T-cell leukemia. *Cancer,* **55**, 181–185

55. Miyoshi, I., Taguchi, H., Yoshimoto et al. (1983) Transmission of Japanese monkey type C virus to human lymphocytes. *Lancet,* **ii**, 166–167

56. Morimoto, C., Matsuyama, T., Oshige, C. et al. (1985) Functional and phenotypic studies of Japanese adult T-cell leukemia cells. *Journal of Clinical Investigation,* **75**, 836–843

57. Nakada, K., Yamaguchi, K., Furugen, S. et al. (1987) Monoclonal integration of HTLV-I proviral DNA in patients with strongyloidiasis. *International Journal of Cancer,* **40**, 145–148

58. Nakano, S., Ando, Y., Saito, K. et al. (1986) Primary infection of Japanese infants with adult T-cell leukaemia-associated retrovirus (ATLV): evidence for viral transmission from mothers to children. *Journal of Infection,* **12**, 205–212

59. O'Brien, C. J., Lampert, I. A. and Catovsky, D. (1983) The histopathology of adult T-cell lymphoma; leukaemia in blacks from the Caribbean. *Histopathology,* **7**, 349–364

60. O'Connor, N. T. J., Feller, A. C., Wainscoat, J. S. et al. (1986) T-cell origin of Lennert's lymphoma. *British Journal of Haematology,* **64**, 521–528

61. O'Connor, N. T. J., Wainscoat, J. S., Weatherall, D. J. et al. (1985) Rearrangement of the T-cell-receptor β-chain gene in the diagnosis of lymphoproliferative disorders. *Lancet,* **i**, 1295–1296

62. Pelicci, P-G., Knowles, D. M., II and Dalla-Favera, R. (1985) Lymphoid tumors displaying rearrangements of both immunoglobulin and T cell receptor genes. *Journal of Experimental Medicine,* **162**, 1015–1024

63. Pittaluga, S., Raffeld, M., Lipford, E. H. and Cossman, J. (1986) 3A1 (CD7) expression precedes T β gene rearrangements in precursor T (lymphoblastic) neoplasms. *Blood,* **68**, 134–139

64. Poiesz, B. J., Ruscetti, F. W., Gazdar, A. F., Bunn, P. A., Minna, J. D. and Gallo, R. C. (1980) Detection and isolation of type-C retrovirus particles from fresh and cultured lymphocytes of a

patient with cutaneous T-cell lymphoma. *Proceedings of the National Academy of Sciences of the USA,* **77**, 7415–7419

65. Rabbitts, T. H., Lefranc, M. P., Stinson, M. A. et al. (1985) The chromosomal location of T-cell receptor genes and a T cell rearranging gene: possible correlation with specific translocations in human T cell leukaemia. *EMBO Journal,* **4**, 1461–1465

66. Rabbitts, T. H., Stinson, A., Forster, A. et al. (1985) Heterogeneity of T-cell β-chain gene rearrangements in human leukaemias and lymphomas. *EMBO Journal,* **4**, 2217–2224

67. Rambaldi, A., Pelicci, P-G., Allavena, P. et al. (1985) T-cell receptor β chain gene rearrangements in lymphoproliferative disorders of large granular lymphocytes/natural killer cells. *Journal of Experimental Medicine,* **162**, 2156–2162

68. Robert-Guroff, M., Coutinho, R. A., Zadelhoff, A. W., Vyth-Dreese, F. A. and Rumke, P. (1984) Prevalence of HTLV-specific antibodies in Surinam emigrants to the Netherlands. *Leukemia Research,* **8**, 501–504

69. Rosenblatt, J. D., Golde, D. W., Wachsman, W. et al. (1986) A second isolate of HTLV-II associated with atypical hairy-cell leukaemia. *New England Journal of Medicine,* **315**, 372–377

70. Rowley, J. D., Haren, J. M., Wong-Staal, F., Franchini, G., Gallo, R. C. and Blattner, W. (1984) Chromosome pattern in cells from patients positive for human T-cell leukemia/lymphoma virus. In *Human T-cell Leukemia/Lymphoma Viruses*, edited by R. C. Gallo, M. E. Essex and L. Gross, pp. 85–89. New York: Cold Spring Harbor Laboratory

71. Saito, H., Kranz, D. M., Takagaki, Y., Hayday, A. C., Eisen, H. N. and Tonegawa, S. (1984) Complete primary structure of a heterodimeric T-cell receptor deduced from cDNA sequence. *Nature,* **309**, 757–762

72. Sanada, I., Nakada, K., Furugen, S. et al. (1986) Chromosomal abnormalities in a patient with smoldering adult T-cell leukemia: evidence for a multistep pathogenesis. *Leukemia Research,* **10**, 1377–1382

73. Sanada, I., Tanaka, R., Kumagai, E. et al. (1985) Chromosomal aberrations in adult T cell leukemia: relationship to the clinical severity. *Blood,* **65**, 649–654

74. Seiki, M., Eddy, R., Shows, T. B. and Yoshida, M. (1984) Nonspecific integration of the HTLV provirus genome into adult T-cell leukaemia cells. *Nature,* **309**, 640–642

75. Seiki, M., Hattori, S., Hirayama, Y. and Yoshida, M. (1983) Human adult T-cell leukemia virus: complete nucleotide sequence of the provirus genome integrated in leukemia cell DNA. *Proceedings of the National Academy of Sciences of the USA,* **80**, 3618–3622

76. Suchi, T., Lennert, K., Tu, L-Y. et al. (1987) Histopathology and immunohistochemistry of peripheral T cell lymphomas: a proposal for their classification. *Journal of Clinical Pathology,* **40**, 995–1015

77. Takatsuki, K., Yamaguchi, K., Kawano, F. et al. (1985) Clinical diversity in adult T-cell leukemia-lymphoma. *Cancer Research,* **45** (suppl), 4644s–4645s

78. Tamura, K., Nagamine, N., Araki, Y. et al. (1986) Clinical analysis of 33 patients with adult T-cell leukemia (ATL)-diagnostic criteria and significance of high- and low-risk ATL. *International Journal of Cancer,* **37**, 335–341

79. The T- and B-cell Malignancy Study Group (1988) The third nation-wide study on adult T-cell leukemia/lymphoma (ATL) in Japan: characteristic patterns of HLA antigen and HTLV-I infection in ATL patients and their relatives. *International Journal of Cancer,* **41**, 505–512

80. Tsudo, M., Uchiyama, T., Uchino, H. and Yodoi, J. (1983) Failure of regulation of Tac antigen/TGCF receptor on adult T-cell leukemia cells by anti-Tac monoclonal antibody. *Blood,* **61**, 1014–1016

81. Tsujimoto, H., Noda, Y., Ishikawa, K. et al. (1987) Development of adult T-cell leukemia-like disease in African Green monkey associated with clonal integration of simian T-cell leukemia virus Type I. *Cancer Research,* **47**, 269–274

82. Uchiyama, T., Yodoi, J., Sagawa, K., Takatsuki, K. and Uchino, H. (1977) Adult T-cell leukemia: clinical and hematologic features of 16 cases. *Blood,* **50**, 481–491

83. Ueshima, Y., Fukuhara, S., Hattori, T., Uchiyama, T., Takatsuki, K. and Uchino, H. (1981) Chromosome studies in adult T cell leukaemia in Japan. Significance of trisomy 7. *Blood,* **58**, 420–425

84. Waldmann, T. A., Davis, M. M., Bongiovanni, K. F. and Korsmeyer, S. J. (1985) Rearrangements

of genes for the antigen receptor on T cells as markers of lineage and clonality in human lymphoid neoplasms. *New England Journal of Medicine*, **313**, 776–783

85. Waldmann, T. A., Greene, W. C., Sarin, P. S. et al. (1984) Functional and phenotypic comparison of human T cell leukemia/lymphoma virus positive adult T cell leukemia with human T cell leukemia/lymphoma virus negative Sézary leukemia and their distinction using anti-Tac monoclonal antibody identifying the human receptor for T cell growth factor. *Journal of Clinical Investigation*, **73**, 1711–1718

86. Weiss, L. M., Hu, E., Wood, G. S. et al. (1985) Clonal rearrangements of T-cell receptor genes in mycosis fungoides and dermatopathic lymphadenopathy. *New England Journal of Medicine*, **313**, 539–544

87. Wong-Staal, F. and Gallo, R. C. (1985) The family of human T-lymphotropic leukemia viruses: HTLV-I as the cause of adult T cell leukemia and HTLV-III as the cause of acquired immunodeficiency syndrome. *Blood*, **65**, 253–263

87a. Worner, I., Matutes, E. and Catovsky, D. (1990) *British Journal of Haematology* (in press)

88. Yamada, Y. (1983) Phenotypic and functional analysis of leukemic cells from 16 patients with adult T-cell leukemia/lymphoma. *Blood*, **61**, 192–199

88a. Yamada, Y., Ichimaru, M. and Shiku, H. (1989) Adult T cell leukemia cells are of CD4+, CDw29+ T cell origin and secrete a B cell differentiation factor. *British Journal of Haematology*, **72**, 370–377

89. Yamaguchi, K., Matutes, Kiyokawa, T. et al. (1988) Comparison of immunoperoxidase staining with indirect immunofluorescence, ELISA and Western blotting assays for detecting anti-HTLV-I antibodies in systemic lupus erythematosus. *Journal of Clinical Pathology*, **41**, 57–61

90. Yamaguchi, K., Seiki, M., Yoshida, M., Nishimura, H., Kawano, F. and Takatsuki, K. (1984) The detection of human T cell leukemia virus proviral DNA and its application for classification and diagnosis of T cell malignancy. *Blood*, **63**, 1235–1240

91. Yamaguchi, K., Yoshioka, R., Kiyokawa, T., Seiki, M., Yoshida, M. and Takatsuki, K. (1986) Lymphoma type adult T-cell leukemia – a clinicopathologic study of HTLV related T-cell type malignant lymphoma. *Haematological Oncology*, **4**, 59–65

92. Yamagushi, K., Yul, L. S., Oda, T. et al. (1986) Clinical consequences of 2'-deoxycoformycin treatment in patients with refractory adult T-cell leukaemia. *Leukemia Research*, **10**, 989–993

93. Yanagi, Y., Yoshikai, Y., Leggett, K., Clark, S. P., Aleksander, I. and Mak, T. W. (1984) A human T-cell specific cDNA clone encodes a protein having extensive homology to immunoglobulin chains. *Nature*, **308**, 145–149

94. Yasuda, K., Sei, Y., Yokoyama, M. M., Tanaka, K. and Hara, A. (1986) Healthy HTLV-I carriers in Japan: the haematological and immunological characteristics. *British Journal of Haematology*, **64**, 195–203

95. Yodoi, J. and Uchiyama, T. (1986) IL-2 receptor dysfunction and adult T-cell leukemia. *Immunological Reviews*, **92**, 135–156

96. Yoshida, M., Seiki, M., Yamaguchi, K. and Takatsuki, K. (1984) Monoclonal integration of human T-cell leukemia provirus in all primary tumors of adult T-cell leukemia suggests causative role of human T-cell leukemia virus in the disease. *Proceedings of the National Academy of Sciences of the USA*, **81**, 2534–2537

Chapter 9

Cutaneous T-cell lymphomas

Introduction

The term 'cutaneous T-cell lymphomas' (CTCLs) encompasses two clinical entities: mycosis fungoides and Sézary syndrome. Although some authors have considered these two disorders as being distinct[124], others believe that Sézary syndrome represents the leukaemic manifestation of mycosis fungoides and that they are both different expressions of the same biological entity[11, 69]. Despite some controversy on the neoplastic nature of all cases of CTCL[76], there is now general agreement that the clinical evolution of most patients is strongly indicative of a true malignancy.

Both diseases result from the malignant proliferation of mature post-thymic T-lymphocytes with helper features which show a characteristic tropism for the epidermis. The term 'mycosis fungoides' was suggested over 100 years ago, because of the mushroom-like appearance of tumours. Thereafter, the characteristic progression of mycosis fungoides, over a period of time which may stretch for many years, from non-specific skin lesions to tumour involvement was recognized. Sézary cells were first described by Sézary and Bouvrain[102] who reported the presence of unusual mononuclear cells in the epidermis and in the peripheral blood of patients with generalized exfoliative erythroderma. Baccaredda[3] also described a pigmented cutaneous erythroderma considering it as a benign histiocytic reticulosis. Only in the early 1970s was the lymphocytic origin of the abnormal cell suggested[25]. This was later confirmed by membrane marker studies which demonstrated the T-cell origin of the Sézary cells (see below).

Clinical features

Both forms of CTCL (Sézary syndrome and mycosis fungoides) are relatively uncommon; the incidence in the USA has been estimated to be of the order of two cases per 1×10^6 individuals[43]. This figure appears to be increasing, possibly as a consequence of more accurate diagnostic procedures. The average age at presentation is 50 years; these disorders are rare under 30 years of age[125]. A male predominance is usually found with a male:female ratio of about 2:1.

The main complaint at presentation is the skin lesions which may lead to extreme itching; these are the hallmarks of CTCLs and will be discussed in detail below; no other characteristic clinical features occur in the early stages of the illness. Lymphadenopathy is rare in the initial phases of mycosis fungoides but is frequently present as the disease progresses and it is seen in most cases of Sézary syndrome (Table 9.1). If biopsied (see below) the lymph nodes show infiltration by abnormal T-lymphocytes. Both splenomegaly and hepatomegaly are rare in mycosis fungoides whilst they are more frequent in Sézary syndrome.

Table 9.1 Clinical and laboratory findings in CTCLs

Disease	Feature	Stage	Percentage
Mycosis fungoides	Lymphadenopathy[a]	Premycotic	0
		Plaques	15
		Tumour	50
	Hepatosplenomegaly[b]	Premycotic	0
		Plaques	15
		Tumour	35
	Hb, WBC count, platelets	*Normal findings*	
Sézary syndrome	Lymphadenopathy		80
	Hepatosplenomegaly[b]		40
	Hb, platelets	*Normal findings*	
	WBC count	$>15 \times 10^9/l$	

[a] Special studies suggest a greater degree of lymph node involvement.
[b] Staging laparotomy and autopsy findings indicate that visceral involvement is more frequent.

Although often unrecognized in life, autopsy studies have demonstrated that in CTCLs almost every organ may be invaded by the malignant cells[16, 31, 68, 95 125]. These include pulmonary infiltrates which may or may not give rise to clinical manifestations. Skeletal involvement is rare, although osteolytic lesions, which may result in pathological fractures, do occur. These lesions are a consequence of progressive medullary invasion followed by cortical destruction without evidence of new bone formation. The nervous system is only rarely affected, whilst the gastrointestinal tract frequently shows T-cell infiltration, but without significant clinical manifestations. Cardiac and renal involvement have been documented in one-third of the cases.

Eye involvement has also been reported, including infiltration of the conjunctiva, cornea, sclera and lacrimal glands. The upper respiratory tract and the oral cavity may be affected in 20% of patients; the pattern of infiltration usually follows the typical progression from erythema to plaques and finally to tumour lesions (see below).

Patients presenting with advanced disease are often febrile and may suffer from infective episodes, commonly due to Gram-negative organisms[49].

Laboratory findings

With the exception of the blood changes in Sézary syndrome, laboratory studies are usually of limited diagnostic value in CTCLs. The haemoglobin level, WBC count and platelet counts are as a rule normal. Abnormal lymphocytes may be seen on films stained with May–Grünwald–Giemsa[99], but this occurs chiefly in Sézary syndrome in which the WBC count is often elevated with a predominance of typical Sézary cells. Neutropenia and thrombocytopenia may also occur in Sézary syndrome patients. Not rarely the peripheral blood shows eosinophilia and circulating plasma cells.

Bone marrow aspirates are usually unhelpful as the degree of lymphocyte infiltration is limited, if at all present[29]. An analysis of 443 bone marrow aspirates showed that bone involvement could be documented only in 11 (2.5%) cases[11,

16]. This incidence is only marginally higher in postmortem bone marrow biopsies[68, 95]. The degree of infiltration is remarkably low even in the presence of marked peripheral leucocytosis. This bone marrow sparing property represents a distinguishing feature between Sézary syndrome and other chronic T-cell leukaemias and is probably the result of a specific homing pattern by the T-lymphocytes involved in the disease.

Blood chemistry is usually normal, with the exception of hyperuricaemia. A polyclonal increase of the serum immunoglobulins, particularly IgA or IgE[7] is often present. In a few cases, an associated monoclonal gammapathy has been reported[57, 60, 117]. Increased serum levels of lactic acid dehydrogenases have also been described in CTCLs and this has been associated with poor prognosis[69].

Chest X-rays may show pulmonary infiltrates which occur with advanced disease in the form of either nodular or diffuse interstitial involvement.

Skin lesions

The skin changes in CTCLs are well known (for reviews see the literature[11, 125]). For many decades, it has been suggested that the evolution of mycosis fungoides is characterized by a three-stage progression, which includes (1) a 'premycotic' stage with erythematous or eczemoid lesions, (2) an infiltrative 'plaque' stage, and finally (3) the tumour stage. Although it is generally agreed that mycosis fungoides patients usually evolve through these stages, the timing of this process may be extremely variable. The premycotic stage is characterized by localized or diffuse areas of erythema or dry eczema. This phase is non-specific and the lesions may mimic those of psoriasis, seborrhoeic dermatitis, neurodermatitis, parapsoriasis in plaques or poikiloderma; in some cases it may be difficult to establish a definite diagnosis.

The likelihood of progression to a true malignant disorder, i.e. mycosis fungoides, is greater in patients with the so-called 'large plaque' form of parapsoriasis[64], particularly those who also show areas of poikiloderma. The premycotic stage, often associated with severe itching, may last several months or years before progressing eventually to the plaque stage. The latter is characterized by oval or round lesions which become gradually more indurated. Plaques may be flat or raised, according to the degree of lymphocyte infiltration above the skin surface and may occur both in previously erythematous areas as well as in unaffected sites. A diagnosis of mycosis fungoides or Sézary syndrome is most often established in this phase of the disease, which, as the premycotic stage, may last for a long period before proceeding to the final stage of tumour lesions. The latter may develop in premycotic sites, in the plaques or, less frequently, in previously uninvolved areas. The tumours may be limited in number or may be very numerous (even more than 100), sometimes reaching a diameter of 10 cm. These tumours may be found anywhere although the face and body folds are the most frequent sites, and are usually painless. They may regress leaving no visible lesions or may tend to ulcerate.

Some patients may present with a tumour d'emblée in which the tumour lesions appear without being preceded by the premycotic and plaque stages. Another variant is represented by the erythrodermic form of mycosis fungoides which is characterized by generalized erythroderma and may be complicated by the development of tumour lesions. The clinical manifestation of this form encompasses exfoliative erythroderma characterized by intense scaling and the so-called 'homme rouge' in which redness is more frequent. These forms are generally associated with very intense itching and are often complicated by infections.

In typical Sézary syndrome, the cutaneous lesions are represented by generalized erythroderma, often with hyperpigmentation and exfoliation. The skin may sometimes be infiltrated and give rise to plaque formation. This occurs most often in the face giving rise to the 'leonine' facies. Ocular inflammation due to ectropion may also take place, as well as scaling and splitting of the palms and soles and dystrophy of the nail plates.

Diagnosis

Morphology

A diagnosis of Sézary syndrome can be suspected upon examination of peripheral blood films stained with May–Grünwald–Giemsa showing the presence of abnormal cells. The circulating cell of Sézary syndrome was defined in early reports[102] as monstrous with a large, irregularly shaped nucleus and scanty cytoplasm, and was considered to be a giant histiomonocyte derived from the skin. A description of the morphological features, which are still used today, was made by Taswell and Winkelmann in 1961[108]. Ten years later Crossen et al.[25] suggested that this abnormal cell belonged to the lymphocyte series. Immunological studies demonstrated shortly afterwards the T-cell origin of these pathological cells (see below).

Two morphological subtypes of Sézary cells, large and small, can be seen in the peripheral blood of CTCL patients. The large Sézary cell measures 15–20 μm in diameter; the smaller cells or Lutzner cells[70] are 8–10 μm in diameter and may predominate in some cases (Figure 9.1). The cytoplasm is scanty in both cell

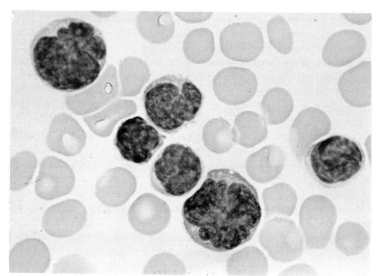

Figure 9.1 Peripheral blood film from a patient with Sézary syndrome and a WBC count of 45 × 10⁹/l. Note four small and two large Sézary cells. × 1400, reduced to 76% on reproduction

variants. In the large cells the nucleus is large and hyperchromatic with a markedly infolded grooved appearance; in the small cell variant, the nucleus is also hyperchromatic but is often slightly less convoluted. In the advanced stages of the disease, more lymphoblastic looking cells may also be found. The morphological recognition of the abnormal cells as Sézary cells is difficult by light microscopic examination but can be suspected by the irregular folding of the nucleus. Analysis with a Coulter S linked to a Channelizer may occasionally demonstrate the presence of small and large Sézary cells (Figure 9.2).

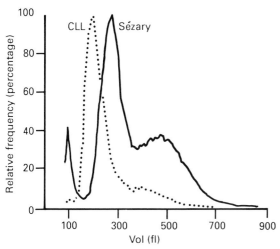

Figure 9.2 Cell volume curve from the Sézary syndrome case illustrated in Figure 9.1 obtained with a Coulter Model ZBI linked to a Coulter Channelizer. Note the bimodal volume distribution corresponding to the small and large Sézary cells. The dotted line illustrates the smaller volume of B-CLL lymphocytes

Electron microscopy

Ultrastructural analysis has greatly contributed to define the morphology of the Sézary cells. These are characterized by a high nuclear to cytoplasmic (N/C) ratio and a markedly convoluted nucleus with a cerebriform appearance; the heterochromatin is condensed in the periphery of the nucleus[23, 71, 72] (Figures 9.3 and 9.4). The nuclear convolutions are often more evident in the large cell variant[70]. The depth of the nuclear indentations and the narrow space between the nuclear lobes help distinguish Sézary cells from ATLL cells[78].

The nuclear irregularities of Sézary cells have been quantified using a nuclear contour index system[100] which expresses the ratio between the nuclear circumference and the square root of the nuclear cross-sectional area; the measurements for this ratio are obtained from electron micrographs. The nuclear contour indices in CTCL cells is two- to three-fold greater than in normal lymphocytes[67, 69]. Several reports have suggested that this index represents a valuable diagnostic tool[74, 114] and this has also been demonstrated recently in biopsies stained with anti-T monoclonal antibodies[56].

Although ultrastructural features similar to those found in CTCLs have been reported in other conditions[36] and may also be seen in normal resting

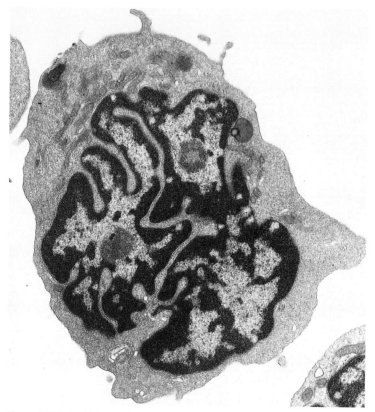

Figure 9.3 Typical Sézary cell from the peripheral blood of a case of Sézary syndrome. The cerebriform nucleus with deep and narrow indentations is unique to this cell type. × 17 500, reduced to 65% on reproduction

lymphocytes or after mitogenic stimulation[78, 79, 112, 128], the importance of identifying cells with typical cerebriform serpentine nuclei for the diagnosis of CTCLs cannot be overemphasized. This is particularly relevant in the presence of clusters or high numbers of these cells in affected tissues and of a high degree of nuclear convolution[48, 74, 95, 98]. The morphology of the infiltrating Sézary cells in skin and lymph nodes is identical to that of the circulating cells[15, 71].

Cytochemistry

As in most T-cell leukaemias, Sézary cells are positive with the reactions for acid phosphatase, α-naphthylacetate esterase (ANAE) and β-glucuronidase[23, 24, 35]. Interestingly, the enzyme DAP IV (dipeptidylaminopeptidase IV), which reacts mainly with the helper/inducer T-lymphocyte subset, is often negative in Sézary cells[24, 126]. Whether the latter is related to the level of T-differentiation or to the proliferation of a distinct subset of CD4+ cells (see below) with low DAP IV expression is at present uncertain. The pattern reactivity with several acid hydrolases in CTCLs and other T-cell leukaemias is summarized in Table 5.5 (Chapter 5).

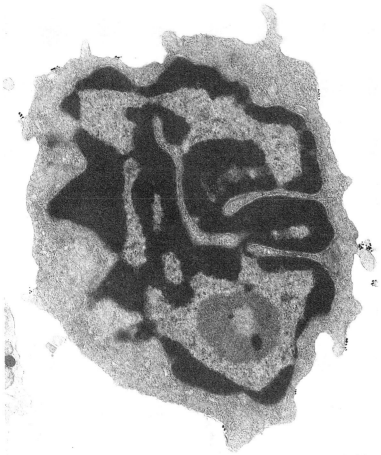

Figure 9.4 Small cerebriform cell from the mononuclear fraction of a normal subject. This Sézary-like cell can be identified as a T-cell by the labelling with the pan-T monoclonal antibody OKT17 visualized by colloidal gold particles, 30 nm in size, conjugated to the goat anti-mouse Ig used as second layer (× 24 000, reduced to 72% on reproduction). For technical details of this immunogold method see Matutes et al. [78]

Histopathology

Skin lesions

The initial diagnosis is often established by means of a skin biopsy. Whilst this is easy in advanced stages of the disease, it could be difficult in the initial phases. For this reason it is often necessary to perform multiple biopsies from different sites and/or to repeat them at regular intervals if the skin lesions do not recede and the diagnosis is still not clear.

In CTCLs the infiltrate is characteristically epidermotropic with the presence of clusters of abnormal lymphoid cells known as Pautrier's microabscesses. The epidermis is also often affected by keratosis, hyperkeratosis, acanthosis etc. The upper dermis in the proximity to the epidermis is infiltrated with band-like aggregates of different cell populations, including neutrophils, lymphocytes, eosinophils and plasma cells. Atypical, convoluted lymphocytes with the features described in Sézary cells are consistently found. The absence of Pautrier's microabscesses does not rule out a diagnosis of CTCL; conversely it has been reported that lymphocyte clusters resembling Pautrier's microabscesses may be found in the epidermis of patients with benign eczematous disease[2]. In the presence of abnormal lymphocytes, the diagnosis of CTCL becomes most likely.

The histology of the skin lesions varies according to the phases of the disease. In the earliest stages the histological pattern may be that of a non-specific lymphocyte infiltration. As the disease progresses, the dermal infiltrate becomes gradually less pleomorphic and the degree of infiltration with abnormal cerebriform elements becomes more apparent, extending deeper into the subdermis.

The histological material could be processed for light and electron microscopy and immunological studies can also be performed (see below).

Lymph nodes

In the majority of cases, lymph node biopsies do not show typical features. Only in advanced disease a partial or complete derangement of the node architecture due to the infiltration with Sézary cells may occur[18]. This is indicative of widespread disease and is usually associated with poor prognosis[18, 113]. In many cases, the architecture of the lymph node is not affected, although dermatopathic changes with abnormal lymphocytes may be found in the T-cell paracortical areas. The prognostic significance of this type of infiltration is controversial[22]. It is worth noting, however, that whilst in benign dermatoses these dermatopathic features are often considered to be non-specific, cytogenetic studies suggest that this picture may represent the first evidence of lymph node involvement in patients with mycosis fungoides[32].

Membrane markers

The use of immunological markers has clearly demonstrated that Sézary cells, both the large and small types, are thymus-derived lymphocytes[13, 14]. This has been shown on the basis of their capacity to form E-rosettes and to react with anti-T sera. It should be noted that the percentage of E-rosettes may be low in blood samples of Sézary syndrome. The optimal way of performing this test in such cases is to pre-treat the lymphoid cells with neuraminidase; without this step very low percentages of E-rosettes have been observed by the authors in 15% of Sézary syndrome cases. Conversely, the cells lack B-cell characteristics. Monoclonal antibodies have confirmed the T-cell nature of the Sézary cells and have documented their mature, post-thymic origin and in particular the expression of the helper/inducer antigen CD4[8, 42, 52, 61, 101, 110], although rare CD8+ cases of Sézary syndrome have also been described[121]. The majority of cases reported in the literature are CD1a−, CD2+, CD3+, CD4+, CD8−. The enzyme terminal deoxynucleotidyl transferase (TdT) which is present in immature T-cells is always negative in CTCL cells. Expression of class II major histocompatibility complex (MHC) antigens is usually absent, although exceptions have been observed particularly in skin biopsies[51, 97, 127]. As discussed below, the phenotypic expression of the cells correlates well with the helper function demonstrated in many of the cases studied.

It is of interest that most Sézary cells, unlike normal CD4+ T-lymphocytes, do not express the p40 antigen recognized by the monoclonal antibody 3A1 (CD7)[50]. The reason for this lack of reactivity is not clear but it represents, nevertheless, an important difference between CTCL and CD4+ T-PLL (see Table

1.10, Chapter 1). By using as immunogens T-cells from a patient with CTCL, two monoclonal antibodies (BE1 and BE2) have been raised and these appear to recognize cells from most cases of CTCL[5]. The authors' experience with BE2 in T-cell disorders is summarized in Table 9.2. The only other T-cell disorder with CD4+, BE2+ cells was a case of adult T-cell leukaemia/lymphoma (ATLL) which was HTLV-I+.

Table 9.2 Monoclonal antibody BE2 in chronic T-cell leukaemias[a]

Disease	No. tested	Positive
Sézary (CD4+)	8	4
ATLL (CD4+)	3	1
T-PLL (CD4+)	4	–
T-CLL (CD8+)	4	–
T-CLL (CD4+)	2	–

[a] Mature (post-thymic) membrane phenotype: CD3+, CD1d−, TdT−; BE2 [5] was a gift of Drs A. Chu and C. L. Berger.

Immunological analyses can also be performed on tissue sections from skin or lymph node biopsies from CTCL patients. The membrane expression in these biopsies is similar to that found on the abnormal circulating T-cells (CD3+, CD4+, CD8−), except for the presence of HLA-DR+ macrophages and HLA-DR+, CD1a+ dendritic cells[127] which corresponds to the presence of Langerhans' cells in the infiltrates. Furthermore, unlike circulating Sézary cells, cells of the skin infiltrates frequently express CD7[51]. The monoclonal antibody anti-Tac (CD25) which reacts with the interleukin-2 (IL-2) receptor and is frequently positive in ATLL, is, as a rule, negative in Sézary cells[121], but with a few exceptions (see Table 1.7, Chapter 1). An immunocytochemical study with several anti-T monoclonal antibodies on skin biopsies from 91 patients with CTCL and 19 with benign dermatosis[20] showed that, although no single pattern of reactivity was specific for CTCL, the following features were helpful for the diagnosis of this disease:

1. The even, as opposed to nodular, distribution of the T-cell population.
2. The selective loss of some antigens, i.e. CD5 and BE3 (pan-T).
3. The co-expression of CD4 and CD8 on the same cells.
4. The presence of CD38+ cells[20].

Only one case of typical Sézary syndrome studied by the authors had the phenotype of natural killer cells, CD4−, CD8−, Leu11+ (CD16+).

In addition to typical cases of Sézary syndrome, the authors have studied four patients without skin involvement and high WBC count – designated Sézary cell leukaemia. One of them was CD4+, CD8−, one was CD4−, CD8+, one CD4−, CD8− and the fourth expressed CD4 and CD8 weakly; morphologically two of them had typical Sézary cells[78a].

Differential diagnosis

This must take into account primarily other forms of benign dermatosis, i.e. psoriaris, atopic dermatitis, neurodermatitis etc., and the skin lesions which may occur in some leukaemias and lymphomas. The diagnosis of CTCL should be suspected and skin biopsies performed in dermatoses which do not regress upon appropriate treatment or in the presence of evolving lesions. Often in those cases several samples may be necessary to make a diagnosis. Furthermore, if a concomitant lymphadenopathy is present, a lymph node biopsy should always be performed. On morphological grounds, the nuclear contour index has been reported as useful to differentiate between CTCLs and other benign dermatological disorders[56]. If indices greater than 6.5 are seen in 25% of infiltrating T-cells a diagnosis of CTCL is likely.

Detailed analysis of peripheral blood films may be useful for diagnosis as well as for prognosis. A large study by Vonderheid et al.[119] examined blood films from 124 CTCLs and 70 from other skin disorders. Large lymphocytes with cerebriform nucleus were seen only in films from CTCL cases. The presence of more than 15% cerebriform (Sézary) lymphocytes correlated with erythroderma and the presence of a chromosomally abnormal clone. The presence of increased proportions of large Sézary cells on blood films was one of the features that correlated with poor survival on multivariate analysis in that study[119].

The main difficulties for a correct diagnosis are experienced in the premycotic stage of mycosis fungoides which shows erythematous or eczemoid lesions and in patients with generalized erythroderma. In the presence of infiltrated plaques the diagnosis of mycosis fungoides should be suspected but histological confirmation is always required. This may also be difficult, particularly in order to distinguish mycosis fungoides from other malignant lymphomas. Additional analyses, including ultrastructural and immunohistochemical studies, should be performed in order to define the T-cell features of the infiltrating cells and to demonstrate the characteristic morphology of CTCL cells. Recent progress includes DNA analysis of T-cell receptor (TCR) genes. Clonal rearrangement of the TCR β-chain gene was shown in typical mycosis fungoides cases and in some lymph nodes of cases thought to have dermatopathic lymphadenopathy[122]. These techniques are likely to be extremely valuable to confirm a diagnosis of CTCL in skin biopsies and other involved tissues in cases where histological criteria are uncertain (see also Chapter 8).

Any differential diagnosis should always take into account a condition designated as lymphomatoid papulosis, a T-cell disorder with a benign clinical course despite the malignant histological appearance of the papular lesions[9, 75]. Its clinical course, and the self-healing but recurrent nature of the skin lesions, are usually sufficient to distinguish this disease from mycosis fungoides. Again here the analysis of TCR β- and γ-chain genes has recently shown that this disease is clonal despite its benign clinical course[123].

The difference between Sézary syndrome and other T-cell leukaemias may not always be straightforward. In addition to bone marrow and skin biopsy studies, a detailed analysis of the surface markers, cytochemistry and, in particular, the electron microscopy of the malignant cells, may also be required.

Natural history and prognosis

The course of the CTLCs may be extremely variable. In the presence of minimal skin lesions without other organ involvement, the disease may remain stable for many years and, in some cases, it may even regress spontaneously although this is frequently followed by relapse. Other cases progress rapidly from minimally infiltrating lesions to the plaque and tumour stages. Consequently, the survival will vary ranging from patients who die within the first year to patients who are alive and well 10 or more years after diagnosis. The overall median survival for CTCLs is approximately 5 years. Patients under the age of 50 years appear to survive twice as long as those over the age of 60 years[31, 38]. Sometimes the onset of symptoms may precede the diagnosis of CTCL by several years. This is mainly contributed by diagnostic difficulties encountered with the early erythematous lesions.

The most frequent cause of death is infection[31, 68] often originating from the cutaneous lesions themselves. *Staphylococcus* and *Pseudomonas* spp. are the most frequently involved organisms resulting in pneumonia or septicaemia[91]. Herpetic infections (herpes simplex and varicella-zoster) have also been described, particularly in advanced disease[118]. High levels of macrophage inhibition factor documented in the serum of CTCL patients[129] may contribute to the defective host's immune defences. The second most common cause of death is progressive visceral involvement by the disease leading to organ failure.

Although several features have been reported to bear prognostic significance, i.e. age, lymphocyte count, symptoms etc., the only factor which has been consistently shown to be important is the extent of the disease at diagnosis[31, 38, 95]. Based on the various parameters which influence the extent of the disease, namely skin lesions, lymphadenopathy, visceral involvement and peripheral blood picture, e.g. the percentage of large Sézary cells[119], several staging systems have been proposed[21, 38, 69]. At a workshop on CTCL held at the National Cancer Institute, it was proposed to adopt the TNM system[109] slightly modified by adding a category which took into account blood involvement[19] (Table 9.3). In this staging system, T represents the skin, N the lymph nodes and M the visceral organs. Each of these parameters bears prognostic value and will be discussed below.

Table 9.3 TNM classification of CTCLs[a]

Classification	Description
T: skin	
T0	Clinically and/or histopathologically suspicious lesions
T1	Limited plaques, papules, or eczematous patches covering <10% of the skin surface
T2	Generalized plaques, papules or erythematous patches covering ≥10% of the skin surface
T3	Tumours (≥1)
T4	Generalized erythroderma
N: lymph nodes	
N0	No clinically abnormal peripheral lymph nodes, pathology negative for CTCL
N1	Clinically abnormal peripheral lymph nodes, pathology negative for CTCL
N2	No clinically abnormal peripheral lymph nodes, pathology positive for CTCL
N3	Clinically abnormal peripheral lymph nodes, pathology positive for CTCL
B: peripheral blood	
B0	Atypical circulating cells not present (<5%)
B1	Atypical circulating cells present (>5%)
M: visceral organs	
M0	No visceral organ involvement
M1	Visceral involvement (must have pathology confirmation)

[a] From Bunn and Lamberg [19].

Skin lesions

The extent of the skin lesions is a very important prognostic feature[18, 62, 63, 120]. Patients with limited plaque disease (T1) have the most favourable prognosis, those with generalized plaques (T2) show an intermediate prognosis, and those with either tumour lesions (T3) or generalized erythroderma (T4) have the worst outcome. A poor prognosis is also contributed by the increased incidence of extracutaneous involvement which occurs as the disease progresses.

Lymph nodes

Lymph node enlargement occurs in about 45% of cases of CTCL; this incidence increases with disease progression and it is as high as 90% in patients with erythroderma. As expected patients with lymphadenopathy have a worse prognosis compared with those with skin lesions only[18, 31, 63, 120]. Controversy as to whether the degree of lymph node involvement bears prognostic significance is probably related to difficulties in the histological assessment of CTCL lesions. The number of involved lymph nodes is also of prognostic relevance[62]; an 85% 3-year survival was observed in patients without palpable lymph nodes; this decreased to 68% in the presence of one involved nodal site and to 60% in patients with two or more enlarged lymph nodes.

Visceral organs

This is the single most important prognostic factor. CTCLs with liver and spleen involvement have a median survival of less than 1 year[31, 38]. The incidence of visceral involvement increases with disease progression. According to autopsy data, it probably occurs to some extent in most patients, despite being clinically inapparent[31, 68, 95]. Staging laparotomy performed in 14 patients showed unexpected splenic involvement in 4 and hepatic involvement in 2[45, 116]. By performing peritoneoscopy and percutaneous multiple liver biopsies, visceral involvement was documented in 18% of cases[55]; these were mainly those with lymph node and/or blood involvement.

Peripheral blood

Abnormal lymphocytes (Sézary cells) can be found in the peripheral blood of 25% of patients with mycosis fungoides and in over 90% of those with Sézary syndrome. Ultrastructural and immunological analyses may help to detect these abnormal cells in a higher proportion of cases. Peripheral blood involvement is often associated with lymph node and visceral dissemination; furthermore, it has been shown that the percentage of circulating Sézary cells, particularly large ones, correlates inversely with prognosis[119, 120].

Treatment

Although there is no definite evidence that treatment prolongs the survival of patients with CTCLs, it is apparent that it improves the quality of life and that disease-free intervals may be obtained.

Several forms of treatment can be considered in the management of this group of disorders. The choice will greatly depend upon the stage of the disease. The approaches frequently employed include: topical chemotherapy, photochemotherapy, radiotherapy and systemic chemotherapy. Other forms of treatment which also appear to be beneficial are: leucapheresis, 2'-deoxycoformycin, retinoid acid, anti-thymocyte globulin and monoclonal antibodies.

Topical chemotherapy

Whole-body topical applications of aqueous solution of mechlorethamine (nitrogen mustard) have been used for many years to effectively control the cutaneous manifestations of mycosis fungoides[115]. This form of treatment may be beneficial in the early phases of the disease but it is inadequate in patients with extracutaneous localizations in whom it must be substituted or supplemented by other forms of therapy[120]. In treating patients with topical mechlorethamine, the risk of allergic reactions and of skin cancers must be taken into account[26]. Mechlorethamine has also been prepared in the form of an ointment which appears to be similarly effective[93].

Favourable results have been described with other chemotherapeutic agents used topically including cytosine arabinoside and BCNU[1,3-bis(2-chloroethyl)-1-nitrosourea] (carmustine)[1, 130]. These drugs may be considered in patients in the early stages of mycosis fungoides and in those who are allergic to mechlorethamine.

Phototherapy

On the basis of beneficial effects reported in the treatment of psoriasis and other dermatoses[84, 88], phototherapy has been attempted also in mycosis fungoides with promising results. Methoxsalen, or 8-methoxypsoralen, is a phototoxic compound and as such can be activated by low-wave ultraviolet light and thus bind covalently and reversibly to DNA. This effect is exerted only in the epidermis and papillary dermis as only less than 1% of the energy produced penetrates to the subcutaneous fat. Methoxsalen is given orally 2 hours prior to ultraviolet light exposure. Treatment can be repeated three or four times weekly. After resolution of the lesions a maintenance regimen may be continued. This form of treatment is ineffective for involved lymph nodes or visceral organs. A complete clearing or a marked improvement of the skin lesions has been reported in small series of mycosis fungoides patients, some of whom were refractory to other forms of treatment[40, 96]. This effect is less beneficial in patients with tumours or generalized erythroderma. The best way of administering this therapy and its long-term effects need still to be defined. It should be borne in mind that skin cancers have been reported in patients with psoriasis treated with photochemotherapy[107].

An innovative approach to the use of photochemotherapy was recently reported by Edelson et al.[28]. The procedure involves the extracorporeal photoactivation by ultraviolet A energy. A lymphocyte-rich fraction separated from the patient by discontinuous leucapheresis 2 hours after ingestion of methoxsalen is then returned to the patient. Twenty-seven out of 37 patients with resistant CTCL responded to this treatment with little or no side effect. It is apparent that this technique is only the first in a new line of attack for these refractory tumours.

Radiotherapy

The malignant cells of CTCL are very sensitive to radiotherapy. This has been exploited since the advent of electron-beam energy based on the knowledge that electrons, unlike photons, penetrate only into the upper dermis, thus sparing the deeper tissues, i.e. mucous membranes, bone marrow, gastrointestinal tract etc. This form of therapy, particularly with total doses greater than 30 Gy, appears to be effective[53, 86]. In the Stanford series[53] 84% of patients achieved a complete remission and this correlated inversely with the extent of the skin lesions. At 10 years the overall survival was 46%. Unfortunately, no controlled trials have been carried out to establish whether there is an increased life expectancy following radiotherapy, although the subjective benefits of this treatment are widely recognized.

In patients unresponsive or only moderately responsive to radiotherapy other forms of adjuvant therapy may be necessary[94]. The treatments described above can only produce a beneficial local effect and thus be potentially curative only in patients with disease confined to the skin. This approach may also be of value as a palliative tool.

The development of more precise diagnostic techniques coupled to the knowledge that organ involvement in CTCLs occurs more frequently than previously recognized, points to the systemic nature of these disorders and provides a rationale for a more aggressive management of patients with minimal extracutaneous involvement. Whilst topical chemotherapy and phototherapy may in this context be inadequate, a role for local or total lymph node irradiation has been advocated. Furthermore, if nodal disease can be documented it is likely that visceral involvement has already occurred and thus systemic therapy may be preferable.

Systemic chemotherapy

This is necessary for patients with advanced disease, or when radiotherapy is no longer effective or the tolerance limits have been reached, or still when other forms of treatment have not been beneficial. As for radiotherapy, no randomized controlled trials have so far been reported for single-agent chemotherapy and the published series refer to small numbers of cases. Several drugs have been employed, but the greatest experience is with the alkylating agents. Objective responses have been documented in over 60% of patients with single alkylating agents[31] and with methotrexate[31]. High doses of methotrexate followed by rescue with folinic acid showed beneficial effects in a series of 11 patients with advanced disease[73]. Doxorubicin and bleomycin alone also appear effective with results similar to those obtained with alkylating agents and methotrexate[66, 106]. The results of combination chemotherapy are encouraging. In a series of 24 patients with advanced mycosis fungoides treated with CHOP, including cyclophosphamide (C), hydroxydaunorubicin (doxorubicin) (H), oncovin (O) and prednisolone (P), COP plus bleomycin and HOP, an objective response was seen in 95% with 7 achieving a complete remission[47]. More recently a higher complete remission rate (44%) has been reported using repeated courses of COP in advanced stage mycosis fungoides[111].

Combined treatment

All forms of treatment have shown some beneficial effect in the management of CTCLs, particularly in patients with limited disease. Although in most cases regression of the lesions has been documented the duration of these remissions has been variable. Excluding chemotherapy, for which few data are at present available, only radiotherapy and, in a few cases, topical nitrogen mustard have achieved long-lasting remissions. The knowledge that radiotherapy may be curative in more than 40% of patients with limited disease and the evidence of good responses with chemotherapy in advanced disease suggest that there may be an additive effect when combining these two modalities. Data on a few cases with short follow-up periods seem to confirm this view and underline the need of randomized trials comparing conservative treatments with this combined approach in CTCLs[17, 46, 83]. One such trial, comparing the combination of electron-beam radiation and chemotherapy with topical therapy, for the initial treatment of mycosis fungoides, failed to show an improvement in prognosis for the more aggressive approach[58a].

Leucapheresis

This procedure may be useful to reduce rapidly the abnormal circulating cells in patients with high lymphocyte counts. Sézary syndrome patients with low WBC counts may also benefit from leucapheresis[89]. This treatment can be repeated regularly and may result in disease control for long periods of time. The beneficial effect of leucapheresis in improving skin lesions strengthens the concept of a recirculation of neoplastic cells between the skin and the blood stream[81].

2′-Deoxycoformycin

This compound is an inhibitor of the enzyme adenosine deaminase, which is present at higher concentrations in T-lymphocytes than in other cell types. The genetic deficiency of this enzyme causes a severe impairment of cellular immunity[39]. The high levels of adenosine deaminase in T-lymphoblasts[104] prompted the clinical utilization of this agent in T-ALL and this resulted in significant anti-leukaemic effects[92]. Recent evidence suggests that 2′-deoxycoformycin (DCF) may be effective in the management of CTCLs.

Grever et al.[44] treated four patients with advanced disease (extensive plaque lesions in the skin, lymph node involvement or hepatosplenomegaly) with DCF 4–10 mg/m^2 daily for 3 consecutive days on a 28-day schedule for a total of one to three courses. Two patients experienced complete remission for 7+ and 9+ months and the other two achieved partial remission, i.e. complete regression of the lymphadenopathy and a greater than 80% clearing of the skin lesions. At the doses used in this study the side effects of DCF – myelosuppression, nausea, vomiting, conjunctivitis and nephrotoxicity (all patients had normal renal function before therapy) – were reversible. Promising results have also been reported by Spiers[105] who observed complete and partial remissions. A number of serious infections were reported in this study[105] which may have been contributed by the immunosuppressive effect of DCF. In a patient with an aggressive form of Sézary syndrome resistant to CHOP, treatment with DCF 4 mg/m^2 weekly for a total of 12 weeks resulted in prolonged complete remission lasting longer than 4 years (Dr H. J. Williams, personal communication). As stated in other chapters, in the authors' experience mainly CD4+ malignancies respond to DCF. One case of Sézary syndrome with an unusual phenotype, CD16+, and another of Sézary cell leukaemia and CD8+ cells did not respond to DCF.

Retinoid acid

Kessler et al.[59] treated four patients with advanced CTCLs with daily oral administration of 13-*cis*-retinoic acid. Almost complete clearing of extensive tumours and plaques was observed in one patient, who was still in partial remission after 15 months. In two patients a 50% reduction in the skin lesions was documented after 4–6 weeks' treatment. All patients suffered from variable degrees of skin dryness and scaling and, as a result, therapy had to be stopped in one and reduced in another. The authors are aware of another patient with Sézary syndrome resistant to CHOP therapy, who achieved a prolonged complete remission with retinoid acid (Dr S. Amin, personal communication).

Anti-thymocyte globulin

Some beneficial effects, albeit short lived, have been reported following repeated intravenous administration of horse anti-lymphocyte globulin[4, 30, 34]. Anti-lymphocyte globulin may cause serious allergic or serum-sickness-like reactions and profound immunosuppression which in a patient treated by one of the authors (RF) was associated with a fatal varicella pneumonia.

Monoclonal antibodies

Miller and Levy[82] treated one patient with CTCL using the monoclonal antibody Leu1 directed against the p67 (CD5) antigen. Complete remission was not reached but marked improvement of the skin, lymph nodes and blood was documented. This effect was short lived as the patient relapsed a few months later with progressive lymph node involvement and subsequently died.

Special studies

T-lymphocyte function

In agreement with the expression of the CD4 antigen (see above), the tumour cells from most cases of CTCL possess in vitro helper function towards Ig production in a pokeweed mitogen driven system[6, 12, 49, 121]. However, in rare cases the cells have been shown to exert suppressor activity despite the presence of the CD4 antigen[33, 54, 58, 80]; in others neither helper nor suppressor function could be demonstrated[12, 80, 121].

Although these findings may reflect functional heterogeneity within the CD4+ T-cell subset, attention must be focused on the possible admixture of the neoplastic cells tested with non-malignant cells which may contribute to the helper function reported in most cases. In normal peripheral blood practically all the helper activity resides in the small CD4+, CD8−, Leu8−, T-cell subset; there is not enough information regarding the reactivity of Sézary cells with the monoclonal antibody Leu8. Purification experiments by cell sorting will help to clarify this point. It is of interest that despite the similarity in membrane phenotype of Sézary cells with ATLL cells (both CD4+), the latter cells act as suppressor cells in functional assays (see Chapter 8) whilst Sézary cells act as helpers.

The delayed cutaneous hypersensitivity reactions, the response to T-cell mitogens and the capacity to form T-cell colonies are usually depressed in the majority of CTCLs tested[37, 69, 80, 85]. These functional deficiencies by the neoplastic CD4+ cells may contribute to the infections which are the main cause of death in this disease. A low natural killer cell activity has also been described[65].

The nature of the Sézary cell

The history of the Sézary cell is reminiscent of that of the hairy cell. Both these cells have attracted attention because of their unique morphology and recognized association with distinct clinicopathological entities: CTCL, in particular Sézary syndrome and hairy cell leukaemia. Both cells were originally thought to be derived from the 'reticuloendothelial system' and have now, with the advent of modern immunological and molecular techniques, been shown to correspond to discrete and well-defined T- or B-lymphocyte subpopulations. Sézary cells were first recognized in 1938[102] and their cerebriform appearance was described by electron microscopy 30 years later[72]. The response of these cells to the mitogen phytohaemagglutinin (PHA) led to the demonstration of their lymphocytic nature in 1971[25] and their T-cell origin was shown later by their ability to form rosettes with sheep red blood cells (RBCs)[13, 14]. Molecular studies have confirmed the T-cell nature of Sézary cells[122, 123].

The presence of Sézary-like cells in the mononuclear fraction from cord blood and blood from healthy donors was demonstrated in 1977[79]. A few years later the same group[112] showed that these cerebriform cells were found mainly within T-lymphocytes with Fcμ receptors which are also characterized by a dot positivity with the ANAE reaction. Recently, the combined use of the immunogold method with monoclonal antibodies at the ultrastructural level has allowed the authors' group to define more precisely the phenotype of the putative normal counterpart of the Sézary cell[78]. These studies have shown that the cerebriform cell found in normal blood has, in fact, the same membrane phenotype as the neoplastic Sézary cell[78] (see Figure 9.4). Several other aspects of the biology of these cells have not been completely elucidated yet. The typical skin infiltration of CTCL suggests that the Sézary cell is an epidermotropic helper T-cell with a physiological affinity for the skin[20], but it is still not known whether the cell recirculates between blood and skin and/or whether it is a particular form of activated T-cell[79]. Again, the analogy with hairy cells, which appear to be activated B-cells with an affinity for the spleen (see Chapter 6), becomes apparent. The frequent absence of the receptor for IL-2 (shown by the monoclonal antibody anti-Tac) and the lack of expression of the antigen demonstrated by OKT10 (CD38) argues against T-cell activation in the case of Sézary cells.

The relationship between small and large Sézary cells is also a matter of great interest. The size difference relates to ploidy and DNA content. Small Sézary cells resemble those found in normal blood and it is possible that the large Sézary cell may result from the antigenic stimulation in vivo of the small cells and their subsequent failure to divide.

Chromosome abnormalities in CTCLs

The karyotypic abnormalities observed in CTCLs are often complex with variation in ploidy being a frequent finding. Of the five cases of Sézary syndrome studied in the authors' laboratory one had hypotetraploid cells and another both hypodiploid and hypotetraploid cells. In the latter case both small and large Sézary cells were observed which corresponded to cells with 44 and 88 chromosomes, respectively.

In two reports[27, 87] 8 out of 13 cases had available metaphases from more than one involved tissue and the same aberrant clones were observed in all the tissues examined from individual patients, although the chromosome abnormalities varied from case to case. These findings further support the monoclonal nature of the cell proliferation in CTCLs which can also be demonstrated now by the rearrangement of the TCR genes[122].

Structural abnormalities involving chromosomes 2, 6, 7, 14 and 17 have frequently been described[10]. Abnormalities of chromosome 2 include deletions of the short and long arms (2p−, 2q−)[27, 41, 77] and are similar to those described in other chronic T-leukaemias[90]. A deletion of the long arm of chromosome 6 with breakpoints ranging from 6q21 to q23 was observed in three of five cases of Sézary syndrome studied by the authors and has also been reported by others[87]. A marker 6q− is also a frequent feature of both T- and B-cell malignancies although in the latter conditions the breakpoint is more often at 6q23–24.

Trisomy for 7q, a frequent abnormality in ATLL[10] has also been observed by the authors in two CTCLs[77]. A tandem translocation t(14;14)(q12;q31) similar to the abnormality found in ataxia telangiectasia has also been described in one case of CTCL[103]. Within the T-cell disorders an isochromosome 17q[i(17q)] has been observed with some frequency in Sézary syndrome[10]; this abnormality has been observed in two of the five cases studied in the authors' laboratory.

References

1. Argyropoulos, C. L., Lamberg, S. I., Clendenning, W. E. et al. (1979) Preliminary evaluation of 15 chemotherapeutic agents applied topically in the treatment of mycosis fungoides. *Cancer Treatment Reports*, **63**, 619–621

2. Ackerman, A. B., Breza, T. S. and Capland, L. (1974) Spongiotic simulants of mycosis fungoides. *Archives of Dermatology*, **109**, 218–220

3. Baccaredda, A. (1939) Reticulohistiocytosis cutanea hyperblastica benigna cum melanodermia. *Archiv für Dermatologische Forschung*, **179**, 209–256

4. Barrett, A. J., Staughton, R. C. D., Brigden, D., Byrom, N., Roberts, J. T. and Hobbs, J. R. (1975) Antilymphocyte globulin in the treatment of advanced Sézary syndrome. *Lancet*, **i**, 940–941

5. Berger, C. L., Morrison, S., Chu, A. et al. (1982) Diagnosis of cutaneous T cell lymphoma by use of monoclonal antibodies reactive with tumor-associated antigens. *Journal of Clinical Investigation*, **70**, 1205–1215

6. Berger, C. L., Warburton, D., Raafat, J., Logerfo, P. and Edelson, R. L. (1979) Cutaneous T-cell lymphoma: neoplasm of T cells with helper activity. *Blood*, **53**, 642–651

7. Blaylock, W. K., Clendenning, W. E., Carbone, P. P. and Van Scott, E. J. (1966) Normal immunologic reactivity in patients with the lymphoma mycosis fungoides. *Cancer*, **19**, 233–236

8. Boumsell, L., Bernard, A., Reinherz, E. L. et al. (1981) Surface antigens on malignant Sézary and T-CLL cells correspond to those of mature T cells. *Blood*, **57**, 526–530

9. Brehmer-Andersson, E. (1976) Mycosis fungoides and its relation to Sézary's syndrome, lymphomatoid papulosis, and primary cutaneous Hodgkin's disease. A clinical, histopathologic and cytologic study of fourteen cases and a critial review of the literature. *Acta Dermato-venereologica Supplementum (Stockholm)*, **56**, 3–142

10. Brito-Babapulle, V., Matutes, E., Hegde, U. and Catovsky, D. (1984) Adult T-cell lymphoma/leukemia in a Caribbean patient: cytogenetic, immunologic and ultrastructural findings. *Cancer Genetics and Cytogenetics*, **12**, 343–357

11. Broder, S. and Bunn, P. A. Jr (1980) Cutaneous T-cell lymphomas. *Seminars in Oncology,* **7,** 310–331
12. Broder, S., Edelson, R. L., Lutzner, M. A. et al. (1976) The Sézary syndrome: A malignant proliferation of helper T cells. *Journal of Clinical Investigation,* **58,** 1297–1306
13. Broome, J. D., Zucker-Franklin, D., Weiner, M. S., Bianco, C. and Nussenzweig, V. (1973) Leukemic cells with membrane properties of thymus-derived (T) lymphocytes in a case of Sézary syndrome morphologic and immunologic studies. *Clinical Immunology and Immunopathology,* **1,** 319–329
14. Brouet, J. C., Flandrin, G. and Seligmann, M. (1973) Indications of the thymus-derived nature of the proliferating cells in six patients with Sézary's syndrome. *New England Journal of Medicine,* **289,** 341–344
15. Brownlee, T. R. and Murad, T. M. (1970) Ultrastructure of mycosis fungoides. *Cancer,* **26,** 686–698
16. Bunn, P. A. Jr and Carney, D. N. (1980) Manifestations of cutaneous T-cell lymphoma. *Journal of Dermatologic Surgery and Oncology,* **6,** 369–377
17. Bunn, P. A. Jr, Fischmann, A. B., Schechter, G. P. et al. (1979) Combined modality therapy with electron-beam irradiation and systemic chemotherapy for cutaneous T-cell lymphomas. *Cancer Treatment Reports,* **63,** 713–717
18. Bunn, P. A. Jr, Huberman, M. S., Whang-Peng, J. et al. (1980) Prospective staging evaluation of patients with cutaneous T-cell lymphomas. Demonstration of a high frequency of extracutaneous dissemination. *Annals of Internal Medicine,* **93,** 223–230
19. Bunn, P. A. Jr and Lamberg, S. I. (1979) Report of the committee on staging and classification of cutaneous T-cell lymphomas. *Cancer Treatment Reports,* **63,** 725–728
20. Chu, A., Patterson, J., Berger, C., Vonderheid, E. and Edelson, R. (1984) In situ study of T-cell subpopulations in cutaneous T-cell lymphoma. Diagnostic criteria. *Cancer,* **54,** 2414–2422
21. Cohen, S. R., Stenn, K. S., Braverman, I. M. and Beck, G. J. (1980) Mycosis fungoides: clinicopathologic relationships, survival, and therapy in 59 patients with observations on occupation as a new prognostic factor. *Cancer,* **46,** 2654–2666
22. Colby, T. V., Burke, J. S. and Hoppe, R. T. (1981) Lymph node biopsy in mycosis fungoides. *Cancer,* **47,** 351–359
23. Costello, C., Catovsky, D., O'Brien, M., Morilla, R. and Varadi, S. (1980) Chronic T-cell leukemias – I. Morphology, cytochemistry and ultrastructure. *Leukemia Research,* **4,** 463–476
24. Crockard, A. D., Macfarlane, E., Andrews, C., Bridges, J. M. and Catovsky, D. (1984) Dipeptidylaminopeptidase IV activity in normal and leukemic T-cell subpopulations. *American Journal of Clinical Pathology,* **82,** 294–299
25. Crossen, P. E., Mellor, J. E. L., Finley, A. G., Ravich, R. B. M., Vincent, P. C. and Gunz, F. W. (1971) The Sézary syndrome. Cytogenetic studies and identification of the Sézary cell as an abnormal lymphocyte. *American Journal of Medicine,* **50,** 24–34
26. DuVivier, A., Vonderheid, E. C., Van Scott, E. J. and Urbach, F. (1978). Mycosis fungoides, nitrogen mustard and skin cancer. *British Journal of Dermatology,* **99,** 61–63
27. Edelson, R. L., Berger, C. L., Raafat, J. and Warburton, D. (1979) Karyotype studies of cutaneous T cell lymphoma: evidence for clonal origin. *Journal of Investigative Dermatology,* **73,** 548–550
28. Edelson, R., Berger, C., Gasparro, F. et al. (1987) Treatment of cutaneous T-cell lymphoma by extracorporeal photochemotherapy. Preliminary results. *New England Journal of Medicine,* **316,** 297–303
29. Edelson, R. L., Kirkpatrick, C. H., Sherach, E. M. et al. (1974) Preferential cutaneous infiltration by neoplastic thymus-derived lymphocytes. Morphologic and functional studies. *Annals of Internal Medicine,* **80,** 685–692
30. Edelson, R. L., Raafat, J., Berger, C. L., Grossman, M., Troyer, C. and Hardy, M. (1979) Antithymocyte globulin in the management of cutaneous T cell lymphoma. *Cancer Treatment Reports,* **63,** 675–680
31. Epstein, E. H. Jr, Levine, D. L., Croft, J. D. Jr and Lutzner, M. A. (1972) Mycosis fungoides: Survival, prognostic features, response to therapy, and autopsy findings. *Medicine (Baltimore),* **51,** 61–72

32. Erkman-Balis, B. and Rappaport, H. (1974) Cytogenetic studies in mycosis fungoides. *Cancer*, **34**, 626–633

33. Farnarier-Seidel, C., Kaplanski, S., Golstein, M-M., Jancovici, E., Sayag, J. and Depieds, R. (1983) An OKT4+ T-cell population with suppressor activity in Sézary syndrome. *Scandinavian Journal of Immunology*, **18**, 389–398

34. Fisher, R. I., Silver, B. A., Vanhaelen, C. P., Jaffe, E. S. and Cossman, J. (1982) Objective regressions of T- and B-cell lymphomas in patients following treatment with anti-thymocyte globulin. *Cancer Research*, **42**, 2465–2469

35. Flandrin, G. and Daniel, M. T. (1974) β-Glucuronidase activity in Sézary cells. *Scandinavian Journal of Haematology*, **12**, 23–31

36. Flaxman, B. A., Zelazny, G. and Van Scott, E. J. (1971) Non-specificity of characteristic cells in mycosis fungoides. *Archives of Dermatology*, **104**, 141–147

37. Foa, R., Catovsky, D., Incarbone, E. et al. (1982) Chronic T-cell leukemias. III. T-colonies, PHA response and correlation with membrane phenotype. *Leukemia Research*, **6**, 809–814

38. Fuks, Z. Y., Bagshaw, M. A. and Farber, E. M. (1973) Prognostic signs and the management of the mycosis fungoides. *Cancer*, **32**, 1385–1395

39. Giblett, E. R., Anderson, J. E., Cohen, F., Pollara, B. and Meuwissen, H. J. (1972) Adenosine-deaminase deficiency in two patients with severely impaired cellular immunity. *Lancet*, **ii**, 1067–1069

40. Gilchrest, B. A. (1979) Methoxsalen photochemotherapy for mycosis fungoides. *Cancer Treatment Reports*, **63**, 663–667

41. Goh, K-O., Reddy, M. M. and Joishy, S. K. (1978) Chromosomes and B and T cells in mycosis fungoides. *American Journal of Medical Sciences*, **276**, 197–204

42. Greaves, M. F., Rao, J., Hariri, G. et al. (1981) Phenotypic heterogeneity and cellular origins of T cell malignancies. *Leukemia Research*, **5**, 281–299

43. Greene, M. H., Dalager, N. A., Lamberg, S. I., Argyropoulos, C. E. and Fraumeni, J. F. Jr (1979) Mycosis fungoides: epidemiologic observations. *Cancer Treatment Reports*, **63**, 597–606

44. Grever, M. R., Bisaccia, E., Scarborough, D. A., Metz, E. N. and Neidhart, J. A. (1983) An investigation of 2'-deoxycoformycin in the treatment of cutaneous T-cell lymphoma. *Blood*, **61**, 279–282

45. Griem, M. L., Moran, E. M., Ferguson, D. J., Mettler, F. A. and Griem, S. F. (1975) Staging procedures in mycosis fungoides. *British Journal of Cancer*, **32** (suppl. II), 362–367

46. Griem, M. L., Tokars, R. P., Petras, V., Variakojis, D., Baron, J. M. and Griem, S. F. (1979) Combined therapy for patients with mycosis fungoides. *Cancer Treatment Reports*, **63**, 655–657

47. Grozea, P. N., Jones, S. E., McKelvey, E. M., Coltman, C. Jr, Fisher, R. and Haskins, C. L. (1979) Combination chemotherapy for mycosis fungoides: a Southwest Oncology Group Study. *Cancer Treatment Reports*, **63**, 647–653

48. Guccion, J. G., Fischmann, A. B., Bunn, P. A. Jr, Schechter, G. P., Patterson, R. H. and Matthews, M. J. (1979) Ultrastructural appearance of cutaneous T cell lymphomas in skin, lymph nodes, and peripheral blood. *Cancer Treatment Reports*, **63**, 565–570

49. Haynes, H. A. (1979) Mycosis fungoides. *Clinics in Haematology*, **8**, 685–698

50. Haynes, B. F., Bunn, P., Mann, D. et al. (1981) Cell surface differentiation antigens of the malignant T cell in Sézary syndrome and mycosis fungoides. *Journal of Clinical Investigation*, **67**, 523–530

51. Haynes, B. F., Hensley, L. L. and Jegasothy, B. V. (1982) Phenotypic characterization of skin-infiltrating T cells in cutaneous T-cell lymphoma: comparison with benign cutaneous T-cell infiltrates. *Blood*, **60**, 463–473

52. Haynes, B. F., Metzgar, R. S., Minna, J. D. and Bunn, P. A. (1981) Phenotypic characterization of cutaneous T-cell lymphoma. *New England Journal of Medicine*, **304**, 1319–1323

53. Hoppe, R. T., Cox, R. S., Fuks, Z., Price, N. M., Bagshaw, M. A. and Farber, E. M. (1979) Electron-beam therapy for mycosis fungoides: the Stanford University experience. *Cancer Treatment Reports*, **63**, 691–700

54. Hopper, J. E. and Haren, J. M. (1980) Studies on a Sézary lymphocyte population with T-suppressor activity. Suppression of Ig synthesis of normal peripheral blood lymphocytes. *Clinical Immunology and Immunopathology*, **17**, 43–54

55. Huberman, M. S., Bunn, P. A., Jr, Matthews, M. J. et al. (1980) Hepatic involvement in the cutaneous T-cell lymphomas. Results of percutaneous biopsy and peritoneoscopy. *Cancer, 45*, 1683–1688

56. Iwahara, K. and Hashimoto, K. (1984) T-cell subsets and nuclear contour index of skin-infiltrating T-cells in cutaneous T-cell lymphoma. *Cancer, 54*, 440–446

57. Joyner, M. V., Cassuto, J-P., Dujardin, P., Barety, M., Duplay, H. and Audoly, P. (1979) Cutaneous T-cell lymphoma in association with a monoclonal gammopathy. *Archives of Dermatology, 115*, 326–328

58. Kansu, E. and Hauptman, S. P. (1979) Suppressor cell population in Sézary syndrome. *Clinical Immunology and Immunopathology, 12*, 341–350

58a. Kaye, F. J., Bunn, P. A. Jr, Steinberg, S. M. et al. (1989) A randomized trial comparing combination electron-beam radiation and chemotherapy with topical therapy in the initial treatment of mycosis fungoides. *New England Journal of Medicine, 321*, 1784–1790

59. Kessler, J. F., Meyskens, F. L. Jr, Levine, N., Lynch, P. J. and Jones, S. E. (1983) Treatment of cutaneous T-cell lymphoma (mycosis fungoides) with 13-*cis*-retinoid acid. *Lancet, i*, 1345–1347

60. Kovary, P. M., Suter, L., Macher, E. et al. (1981) Monoclonal gammopathies in Sézary syndrome: a report of four new cases and a review of the literature. *Cancer, 48*, 788–792

61. Kung, P. C., Berger, C. L., Goldstein, G., Logerfo, P. and Edelson, R. L. (1981) Cutaneous T cell lymphoma: characterization by monoclonal antibodies. *Blood, 57*, 261–266

62. Lamberg, S. I., Green, S. B., Byar, D. P. et al. (1984) Clinical staging for cutaneous T-cell lymphoma. *Annals of Internal Medicine, 100*, 187–192

63. Lamberg, S. I., Green, S. B., Byar, D. P. et al. (1979) Status report of 376 mycosis fungoides patients at 4 years: mycosis fungoides cooperative group. *Cancer Treatment Reports, 63*, 701–707

64. Lambert, W. C. (1979) Parapsoriasis. In *Dermatology in General Medicine*, 2nd edn, edited by T. B. Fitzpatrick, A. Z. Eisen, K. Wolff, I. M. Freedberg and K. F. Austen, pp. 808–817. New York: McGraw-Hill

65. Laroche, L. and Kaiserlian, D. (1983) Decreased natural-killer-cell activity in cutaneous T-cell lymphomas. *New England Journal of Medicine, 308*, 101–102

66. Levi, J. A., Diggs, C. H. and Wiernik, P. H. (1977) Adriamycin therapy in advanced mycosis fungoides. *Cancer, 39*, 1967–1970

67. Litovitz, T. L. and Lutzner, M. A. (1974) Quantitative measurements of blood lymphocytes from patients with chronic lymphocytic leukemia and the Sézary syndrome. *Journal of the National Cancer Institute, 53*, 75–77

68. Long, J. C. and Mihm, M. C. (1974) Mycosis fungoides with extracutaneous dissemination: a distinct clinicopathologic entity. *Cancer, 34*, 1745–1755

69. Lutzner, M., Edelson, R., Schein, P., Green, I., Kirkpatrick, C. and Ahmed, A. (1975) Cutaneous T-cell lymphomas: the Sézary syndrome, mycosis fungoides, and related disorders. NIH conference. *Annals of Internal Medicine, 83*, 534–552

70. Lutzner, M. A., Emerit, I., Durepaire, R., Flandrin, G., Grupper, Ch. and Prunieras, M. (1973) Cytogenetic, cytophotometric, and ultrastructural study of large cerebriform cells of the Sézary syndrome and description of a small-cell variant. *Journal of the National Cancer Institute, 50*, 1145–1162

71. Lutzner, M. A., Hobbs, J. W. and Horvath, P. (1971) Ultrastructure of abnormal cells in Sézary syndrome, mycosis fungoides, and parapsoriasis en plaque. *Archives of Dermatology, 103*, 375–386

72. Lutzner, M. A. and Jordan, H. W. (1968) The ultrastructure of an abnormal cell in Sézary syndrome. *Blood, 31*, 719–726

73. McDonald, C. J. and Bertino, J. R. (1979) Treatment of mycosis fungoides lymphoma: effectiveness of infusions of methotrexate followed by oral citrovorum factor. *Cancer Treatment Reports, 62*, 1009–1014

74. McNutt, N. S. and Crain, W. R. (1981) Quantitative electron microscopic comparison of lymphocyte nuclear contours in mycosis fungoides and in benign infiltrates in the skin. *Cancer, 47*, 698–709

75. Macaulay, W. L. (1968) Lymphomatoid papulosis. A continuing self-healing eruption, clinically benign – histologically malignant. *Archives of Dermatology, 97*, 23–30

76. Mackie, R. M. (1981) Initial event in mycosis fungoides of the skin is viral infection of epidermal Langerhans' cells. *Lancet*, **ii**, 283–285

77. Matutes, E., Brito-Babapulle, V. and Catovsky, D. (1985) Clinical, immunological, ultrastructural and cytogenetic studies in black patients with adult T-cell leukemia/lymphoma. In *Retroviruses in Human Lymphoma/Leukemia*, edited by M. Miwa et al., pp. 59–70. Tokyo: Japan Scientific Society Press

78. Matutes, E., Robinson, D., O'Brien, M., Haynes, B. F., Zola, H. and Catovsky, D. (1983) Candidate counterparts of Sézary cells and adult T-cell lymphoma-leukaemia cells in normal peripheral blood: an ultrastructural study with the immunogold method and monoclonal antibodies. *Leukemia Research*, **7**, 787–801

78a. Matutes, E., Worner, I., Sainati, L., de Oliveira, M. P. and Catovsky, D. (1989) Advances in the lymphoproliferative disorders. Review of our experience in the study of over 1000 cases. *Biologia y Clinica Hematologica*, **11**, 53–62

79. Meyer, C. J. L. M., van Leeuwen, A. W. F. M., van der Loo, E. M., van de Putte, L. B. A. and van Vloten, W. A. (1977) Cerebriform (Sézary-like) mononuclear cells in healthy individuals: a morphologically distinct population of T cells. Relationship with mycosis fungoides and Sézary's syndrome. *Virchows Archiv Abteilung B Zellpathologie*, **25**, 95–104

80. Miedema, F., Willemze, R., Terpstra, F. G., Van Vloten, W. A., Meijer, C. J. L. M. and Melief, C. J. M. (1984) Regulatory activity of neoplastic T cells in Sézary syndrome on *in vitro* immunoglobulin production. *Leukemia Research*, **8**, 873–884

81. Miller, R. A., Coleman, C. N., Fawcett, H. D., Hoppe, R. T. and McDougall, I. R. (1980) Sézary syndrome: a model for migration of T lymphocytes to skin. *New England Journal of Medicine*, **303**, 89–92

82. Miller, R. A. and Levy, R. (1981) Response of cutaneous T-cell lymphoma to therapy with hybridoma monoclonal antibody. *Lancet*, **ii**, 226–230

83. Minna, J. D., Roenign, H. H. Jr and Glatstein, E. (1979) Report of the committee on therapy for mycosis fungoides and Sézary syndrome. *Cancer Treatment Reports*, **63**, 729–736

84. Morison, W. L., Parrish, J. A. and Fitzpatrick, T. B. (1978) Oral methoxsalen photochemotherapy of recalcitrant dermatoses of the palms and soles. *British Journal of Dermatology*, **99**, 297–302

85. Musiani, P., Lauriola, L., Maggiano, N., Ranelletti, F. O. and Piantelli, M. (1983) Dissociation between coupled lymphocyte phenotypic and functional properties in Sézary cells. *Clinical Immunology and Immunopathology*, **29**, 103–110

86. Nisce, L. Z. and Safai, B. (1979) Once weekly total-skin electron-beam therapy for mycosis fungoides: 7 years' experience. *Cancer Treatment Reports*, **63**, 633–638

87. Nowell, P. C., Finan, J. P. and Vonderheid, E. C. (1982) Clonal characteristics of cutaneous T cell lymphomas: cytogenetic evidence from blood, lymph nodes and skin. *Journal of Investigative Dermatology*, **78**, 64–75

88. Parrish, J. A., Fitzpatrick, T. B., Tananbaum, L. and Pathak, M. A. (1974) Photochemotherapy of psoriasis with oral methoxsalen and longwave ultraviolet light. *New England Journal of Medicine*, **291**, 1207–1211

89. Pineda, A. A. and Winkelmann, R. K. (1981) Leukapheresis in the treatment of Sézary syndrome. *Journal of the American Academy of Dermatology*, **5**, 544–549

90. Pittman, S., Morilla, R. and Catovsky, D. (1982) Chronic T-cell leukemias II. Cytogenetic studies. *Leukemia Research*, **6**, 33–42

91. Posner, L. E., Fossieck, B. E. Jr, Eddy, J. L. and Bunn, P. A. Jr (1981) Septicemic complications of the cutaneous T-cell lymphomas. *American Journal of Medicine*, **71**, 210–216

92. Prentice, H. G., Smyth, J. F., Ganeshaguru, K. et al. (1980) Remission induction with adenosine-deaminase inhibitor 2'-deoxycoformycin in Thy-lymphoblastic leukaemia. *Lancet*, **ii**, 170–172

93. Price, N. M., Deneau, D. G. and Hoppe, R. T. (1982) The treatment of mycosis fungoides with ointment-based mechlorethamine. *Archives of Dermatology*, **118**, 234–237

94. Price, N. M., Hoppe, R. T., Constantine, V. S., Fuks, Z. Y. and Farber, E. M. (1977) The treatment of mycosis fungoides. Adjuvant topical mechlorethamine after electron beam therapy. *Cancer*, **40**, 2851–2853

95. Rappaport, H. and Thomas, L. B. (1974) Mycosis fungoides: the pathology of extracutaneous involvement. *Cancer,* **34**, 1198–1229

96. Roenigk, H. H. J. (1979) Photochemotherapy for mycosis fungoides: long-term follow up study. *Cancer Treatment Reports,* **63**, 669–673

97. Romagnani, S., Del Prete, G. F., Maggi, E. et al. (1982) Phenotypic and functional characterization of a Sézary cell. *Journal of Clinical Immunology,* **2**, 343–349

98. Sandbank, M. and Ben-Bassat, M. (1972) Mycosis fungoides and Sézary's syndrome. Light and electron microscopic study before and after treatment. *Israel Journal of Medical Sciences,* **7**, 1262–1270

99. Schechter, G. P., Bunn, P. A., Fischmann, A. B. et al. (1979) Blood and lymph node T lymphocytes in cutaneous T-cell lymphoma: evaluation by light microscopy. *Cancer Treatment Reports,* **63**, 571–574

100. Schrek, R. (1972) Ultrastructure of blood lymphocytes from chronic lymphocytic and lymphosarcoma cell leukemia. *Journal of the National Cancer Institute,* **48**, 51–64

101. Schroff, R. W., Foon, K. A., Billing, R. J. and Fahey, J. L. (1982) Immunologic classification of lymphocytic leukemias based on monoclonal antibody-defined cell surface antigens. *Blood,* **59**, 207–215

102. Sézary, A. and Bouvrain, Y. (1938) Erythrodermie avec presence des cellules monstreuses dans le derm et dans le sang circulant. *Bulletin de la Société française de dermatologie et de syphiligraphie,* **45**, 254–260

103. Shah-Reddy, S. I., Mayeda, K., Mirchandani, I. and Koppitch, F. C. (1982) Sézary syndrome with a 14;14 (q12;q31) translocation. *Cancer,* **49**, 75–79

104. Smyth, J. F. and Harrap, K. R. (1975) Adenosine deaminase activity in leukaemia. *British Journal of Cancer,* **31**, 544–549

105. Spiers, A. S. D. (1984) Experience with 2'-deoxycoformycin in treatment of refractory leukemias and lymphomas. *Cancer Treatment Symposia,* **2**, 51–54

106. Spigel, S. C. and Coltman, C. A. Jr (1975) Therapy of mycosis fungoides with bleomycin. *Cancer,* **32**, 767–770

107. Stern, R. S., Thibodeau, L. A., Kleinerman, R. A., Parrish, J. A., Fitzpatrick, T. B. and 22 Participating Investigators (1979) Risk of cutaneous carcinoma in patients treated with oral methoxsalen photochemotherapy for psoriasis. *New England Journal of Medicine,* **300**, 809–813

108. Taswell, H. F. and Winkelmann, R. K. (1961) Sézary syndrome – a malignant reticulemic erythroderma. *Journal of the American Medical Association,* **177**, 465–472

109. The Mycosis Fungoides Cooperative Study Group Steering Committee (1975) Mycosis fungoides cooperative study. *Archives of Dermatology,* **111**, 457–459

110. Thomas, J. A., Janossy, G., Graham-Brown, R. A. C., Kung, P. C. and Goldstein, G. (1982) The relationship between T lymphocyte subsets and Ia-like antigen positive non-lymphoid cells in early stages of cutaneous T cell lymphoma. *Journal of Investigative Dermatology,* **78**, 169–176

111. Tirelli, U., Carbone, A., Veronesi, A. et al. (1982) Combination chemotherapy with cyclophosphamide, vincristine, and prednisone (CVP) in TNM – classified stage IV mycosis fungoides. *Cancer Treatment Reports,* **66**, 167–169

112. Van Der Loo, E. M., Cnossen, J. and Meijer, C. J. L. M. (1981) Morphological aspects of T cell subpopulations in human blood: characterization of the cerebriform mononuclear cells in healthy individuals. *Clinical and Experimental Immunology,* **43**, 506–516

113. Van der Loo, E. M., Meijer, C. J. L. M., Scheffer, E. and Van Vloten, W. A. (1981) The prognostic value of membrane markers and morphometric characteristics of lymphoid cells in blood and lymph nodes from patients with mycosis fungoides. *Cancer,* **48**, 738–744

114. Van der Loo, E. M., Van Vloten, W. A., Cornelisse, C. J., Scheffer, E. and Mcijer, C. J. L. M. (1981) The relevance of morphometry in the differential diagnosis of cutaneous T cell lymphomas. *British Journal of Dermatology,* **104**, 257–269

115. Van Scott, E. J. and Kalmanson, J. D. (1973) Complete remissions of mycosis fungoides lymphoma induced by topical nitrogen mustard (HN2). Control of delayed hypersensitivity to HN2 by desensitization and by induction of specific immunologic tolerance. *Cancer,* **32**, 18–30

116. Variakojis, D., Rosas-Uribe, A. and Rappaport, H. (1974) Mycosis fungoides: pathologic findings in staging laparotomies. *Cancer,* **33**, 1589–1600

117. Venencie, P. Y., Winkelmann, R. K., Puissant, A. and Kyle, R. A. (1984) Monoclonal gammopathy in Sézary syndrome. Report of three cases and review of the literature. *Archives of Dermatology*, **120**, 605–608

118. Vonderheid, E. C., Milstein, H. J., Thompson, K. D. and Wu, B. C. (1980) Chronic herpes simplex infection in cutaneous T-cell lymphomas. *Archives of Dermatology*, **116**, 1018–1022

119. Vonderheid, E. C., Sobel, E. L., Nowell, P. C., Finan, J. B., Helfrich, M. K. and Whipple, D. S. (1985) Diagnostic and prognostic significance of Sézary cells in peripheral blood smears from patients with cutaneous T cell lymphoma. *Blood*, **66**, 358–366

120. Vonderheid, E. C., Van Scott, E. J., Wallner, P. E. and Johnson, W. C. (1979) A 10-year experience with topical mechlorethamine for mycosis fungoides: comparison with patients treated by total-skin electron-beam radiation therapy. *Cancer Treatment Reports*, **63**, 681–689

121. Waldmann, T. A., Greene, W. C., Sarin, P. S. et al. (1984) Functional and phenotypic comparison of human T cell leukemia/lymphoma virus positive adult T cell leukemia with human T cell leukemia/lymphoma virus negative Sézary leukemia, and their distinction using anti-Tac. *Journal of Clinical Investigation*, **73**, 1711–1718

122. Weiss, L. M., Hu, E., Wood, G. S. et al. (1985) Clonal rearrangements of T-cell receptor genes in mycosis fungoides and dermatopathic lymphadenopathy. *New England Journal of Medicine*, **313**, 539–544

123. Weiss, L. M., Wood, G. S., Trela, M., Warnke, R. A. and Sklar, J. (1986) Clonal T-cell populations in lymphomatoid papulosis. Evidence of a lymphoproliferative origin for a clinically benign disease. *New England Journal of Medicine*, **315**, 475–479

124. Winkelmann, R. K. and Caro, W. A. (1977) Current problems in mycosis fungoides and Sézary syndrome. *Annual Review of Medicine*, **28**, 251–269

125. Winkler, C. F. and Bunn, P. A. Jr (1983) Cutaneous T-cell lymphoma: a review. *Critical Reviews in Oncology/Hematology*, **1**, 49–92

126. Wirthmuller, R., Denning, D., Oertel, J. and Gerhartz, H. (1983) Dipeptidylaminopeptidase IV (DAP IV) activity in normal and malignant T-cell subsets as defined by monoclonal antibodies. *Scandinavian Journal of Haematology*, **31**, 197–205

127. Wood, G. S., Deneau, D. G., Miller, R. A., Levy, R., Hoppe, R. T. and Warnke, R. A. (1982) Subtypes of cutaneous T-cell lymphoma defined by expression of Leu-1 and 1a. *Blood*, **59**, 876–882

128. Yeckley, J. A., Weston, W. L., Thorne, G. and Krueger, G. G. (1975) Production of Sézary-like cells from normal human lymphocytes. *Archives of Dermatology*, **111**, 29–32

129. Yoshida, T., Edelson, R., Cohen, S. and Green, I. (1975) Migration inhibitory activity in serum and cell supernatants in patients with Sézary syndrome. *Journal of Immunology*, **114**, 915–918

130. Zackheim, H. S., Epstein, E. H. Jr and Grekin, D. A. (1979) Treatment of mycosis fungoides with topical BCNU. *Cancer Treatment Reports*, **63**, 623

Chapter 10

Plasma cell neoplasias

This group of disorders is characterized by the malignant proliferation of a clone of plasma cells capable of producing excessive amounts of monoclonal (M) immunoglobulins (Ig). According to the class or to the part of Ig secreted, different types of plasma cell dyscrasia have been recognized. These are listed in Table 10.1 and each of them will be dealt with separately.

Table 10.1 Plasma cell disorderrs

Myelomatosis (multiple myeloma)
Benign monoclonal gammopathy
Solitary myeloma
Extramedullary plasmacytoma
Plasma cell leukaemia
Heavy chain disease (γ, α, μ)
Lymphoplasmacytic lymphoma
Waldenström's macroglobulinaemia

Myelomatosis

Myelomatosis is the most common of the plasma cell disorders. It is a tumour characterized by a progressive proliferation of plasma cells within the bone marrow, which secrete paraproteins or M components in the serum and/or in the urine, with an associated decrease in the normal serum Ig. The disease is characterized by typical bone lesions and by a number of events resulting from the circulating excess of myeloma proteins and the bone marrow involvement by pathological plasma cells.

The incidence of multiple myeloma is of the order of 0.02–0.04% in adults with no clear sex predominance and with a progressive increase in incidence with age, reaching a maximum peak in the seventh decade of life[59]. The disease is exceedingly rare under the age of 40 years and accounts for about 10% of all haematological neoplasias[59].

In the majority of patients the paraprotein is a complete Ig molecule with both heavy and light chains[8, 52]. In 15% of cases only light chains can be detected[8]. The rare heavy chain forms represent distinct clinical variants and will be described separately. The most frequent heavy chain class involved in myeloma is IgG, followed by IgA and IgD, whilst both IgE and IgM myelomatosis are very rare. The relative incidence according to two large series[8, 59] is as follows: 70% IgG, 25–30% IgA and 1–2% IgD. Cases with free light chains (Bence-Jones proteinuria) and no 'M' band are well documented. The κ:λ ratio is usually 2:1. Rare cases with more than one paraprotein have also been described[8]. A minority of myelomas have been described as non-secretory, as they do not produce M protein or light chains. These cases should be distinguished from those in which the paraprotein is synthesized but not released from the plasma cells and can, therefore, be detected by immunocytochemical methods.

A comprehensive review of the biology and treatment trends in this disease has recently been published[9].

Clinical manifestations

The clinical manifestations of myelomatosis are polymorphic with a variable long presymptomatic period. Bone pain is the most frequent presenting complaint and pathological fractures are also common. Another frequent presentation is with pneumonia.

Osteolytic lesions

Skeletal abnormalities, in the form of diffuse osteoporosis and osteolytic bone lesions, result from the production of the so-called osteoclast-activating factor (OAF) which causes bone reabsorption and destruction[84]. The existence of OAF has been demonstrated by the production of this lymphokine in myeloma cell cultures[84] and also in the serum of patients with myelomatosis. It is generally assumed that OAF may be involved in the pathogenesis of the hypercalcaemia seen in 10–30% of patients[33, 59]. Recent studies have disclosed the role of some bone-resorbing cytokines, in particular lymphotoxin (also known as tumour necrosis factor B) in the pathogenesis of hypercalcaemia in myeloma[45]. This substance, which is probably one of the main sources of OAF activity in this disease (the other being interleukin-1), may also act as a tumour growth factor, as suggested also in other B-cell malignancies[9].

Osteolytic lesions occur mainly in the red marrow throughout the skeleton and are generally multiple, thus giving rise to bone pain, most frequently in the spine and in the ribs; these are often the presenting symptoms of the disease. Although up to 50–60% of patients with myeloma may show, at presentation, radiographic evidence of osteolytic lesions, the latter are not always accompanied by pain and it is also not infrequent that asymptomatic patients may reveal marked skeletal abnormalities. During the course of the disease osteolytic lesions may lead to pathological fractures, particularly in the spine, femur and ribs. The loss of bone structure and thus the mobilization of calcium contributes towards hypercalcaemia and to the frequent occurrence of 'loss of height' due to the compression of vertebral bodies. The symptoms of hypercalcaemia in myeloma – anorexia, constipation, polydipsia, weakness, nausea and vomiting – are similar to those seen in hypercalcaemia due to other causes.

Haematological findings

At the time of diagnosis, the most frequent abnormality is anaemia which is seen in 60% of cases. The levels of haemoglobin represent an important prognostic factor (see below). In general, the degree of anaemia is moderate but in some cases it may be more severe, with haemoglobin values below 8 g/dl. The anaemia is usually normochromic and normocytic and in most cases is caused by bone marrow infiltration with abnormal plasma cells. However, other causes may be responsible for the anaemia, i.e. decreased red cell survival, iron and/or folate deficiency and, rarely, bleeding. Due to the weight of anaemia as a prognostic factor, it may be important to define its cause in each patient. In cases with severe renal failure, refractory anaemia may be secondary to low levels of erythropoietin.

The leucocyte count is generally normal; leucopenia may be present in 15% of patients at presentation. In half of them a mild neutropenia accompanied by a relative lymphocytosis occurs. Although 20% of patients with myelomatosis present with either thrombocytopenia or thrombocytosis, the majority have a normal platelet count.

Infections
Myeloma patients have an increased susceptibility to infections due to Gram-negative and Gram-positive organisms, particularly *Streptococcus pneumoniae*. A primary role in these complications is played by the hypogammaglobulinaemia which is a constant finding in untreated myelomatosis. The pathogenesis of the hypogammaglobulinaemia is not entirely clear. Several mechanisms have been postulated, including a macrophage-related factor capable of suppressing normal B-cell function. Granulocytopenia, when present, is also a predisposing factor towards infection and most often follows the early phases of treatment; in these circumstances, it may contribute to early morbidity and mortality. In the MRC fifth myelomatosis trial 14% of patients had infections documented before entry and infections were a major cause of morbidity and mortality in the first 3 months of treatment[69a]. Currently a new trial is testing the value of intravenous γ-globulin infusions for the prophylaxis of infections during the early phases of treatment.

Renal function
Renal insufficiency is common in myeloma and is chiefly related to the filtration of large quantities of free light chain proteins through the kidney which results in a lesion known as 'myeloma kidney'. This results from the obstruction of both the proximal and distal convoluted tubules with hyaline casts. A raised serum creatinine concentration may be found in over 50% of patients at presentation[59], often in association with hypercalcaemia, hypercalciuria, cast formation and dehydration. The renal function may further deteriorate by the occurrence of hyperuricaemia following chemotherapy. Together with anaemia, elevated concentrations of blood urea represent an important prognostic factor in myelomatosis (see below).

Other features
The hyperviscosity syndrome due to excessive paraprotein production, although more frequent in Waldenström's macroglobulinaemia, can also be seen in myeloma, particularly in the IgA type (5% of cases) and rarely in IgG myelomatosis[97]. The typical features of this syndrome include: purpura, rectal bleeding, epistaxes, dilated and often tortuous fundal veins, as well as haemorrhages and exudates leading to visual disturbances and Raynaud's phenomenon. Occasionally, painful areas of necrosis due to localized microinfarctions may occur.

Neurological manifestations due to compression of the spinal cord nerves as a result of collapsed vertebrae or of an extramedullary myeloma mass are not uncommon. This can result in paraplegia which may be seen at presentation or, less frequently, during the evolution of the disease.

Diagnosis

The diagnosis of myelomatosis is based on laboratory findings, morphological and radiological criteria. Most patients are symptomatic at the time of diagnosis but in 10% the diagnosis is made by chance. As a rule, two of the following criteria suffice: evidence of an M-component or Bence-Jones protein, abnormal plasma cells in the bone marrow or the presence of osteolytic lesions. In most patients, all these three features are present. When only one of them is demonstrated, the diagnosis may be difficult. An exception could be a non-secretory myeloma with typical bone marrow findings and no bone lesions. In such rare cases immunostaining may be useful to prove the monoclonality of the process.

M-component

Protein electrophoresis on cellulose acetate often shows a narrow spike in the γ-globulin region corresponding to IgG M-components; IgA M-components are usually suspected by a broader spike in the γ-globulin region. Bence-Jones proteinuria (free light chains) is demonstrated in the urine of about 50–60% of patients. Light chains are generally not demonstrated in the serum due to their rapid catabolism by the kidney. Quantitation of the M-component is important both for diagnosis and for patients' follow-up. It is always advisable to store the first serum specimens to use later on as controls to quantitate more precisely subsequent protein estimations. Serum and urine immunoelectrophoresis are necessary in order to identify the class of heavy and/or light chain of the M-component. Serum concentrations of the remaining Ig, other than the M-component, are as a rule decreased (immunoparesis). This may be useful in the differential diagnosis with the benign monoclonal gammopathies, in which these levels are usually normal.

Bone marrow

The bone marrow aspirate and/or the trephine biopsy show more than 10% immature or atypical plasma cells. In 70% of cases more than 30% plasma cells are found in the bone marrow[11]. These cells, although in general bizarre and larger than normal, could be extremely monomorphic (Figure 10.1). Two problems can be encountered in the cytological or histological diagnosis of a suspected case: first, the distinction between myelomatosis and reactive plasmacytosis[23]. Only rarely can a bone marrow with excess of plasma cells be regarded as sufficient for a diagnosis in the absence of either serological or radiological evidence of myelomatosis. One of the morphological features of the plasma cells in myeloma is nuclear cytoplasmic asynchrony as well as the presence of numerous binucleated and trinucleated forms[11]. These features are rare in a reactive process.

Secondly, when aspirates are unsuccessful, the bone marrow involvement of myeloma tissue could be demonstrated by a trephine biopsy. Because the pattern of infiltration may be patchy and restricted to nodules of plasma cells, more than one bone marrow specimen may occasionally be required[11]. Assessment of bone

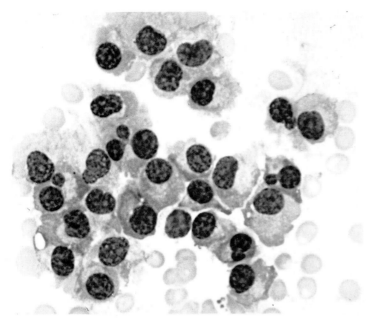

Figure 10.1 Bone marrow aspirate from a multiple myeloma showing clusters of plasma cells. × 1200, reduced to 71% on reproduction

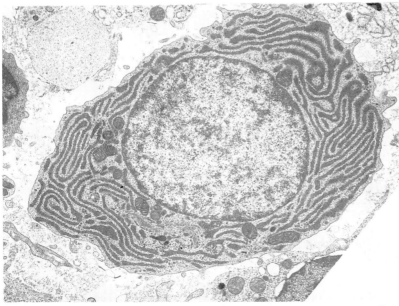

Figure 10.2 Electron micrograph of an immature plasma cell showing a moderately dilated endoplasmic reticulum (ER) covering the whole cytoplasm (× 16 000, reduced to 69% on reproduction). Because of their immaturity these cells were difficult to recognize as plasma cells by light microscopy examination

marrow specimens after chemotherapy may be difficult just in aspirates; a trephine biopsy is then essential to show residual foci of disease.

Immunostaining techniques can demonstrate whether plasma cells are monoclonal or not by showing heavy and light chain restriction. Rarely, it may be difficult to discriminate between multiple myeloma and benign monoclonal gammopathy, which is characterized by a slight excess of plasma cells (monoclonal in nature) but lacks bone lesions and has no immunoparesis (see below). In non-secretory myeloma, immunostaining can demonstrate monoclonality when plasma cells synthesize but do not excrete the Ig molecules. In the rare non-secretory cases without Ig synthesis such staining will be negative.

The diagnosis of the rare cases in which the plasma cells are very immature can be clarified by ultrastructural analysis which will show the typical pattern of concentric arrangement of the endoplasmic reticulum (ER) of the plasma cells (Figures 10.2 and 10.3). In non-secretory cases the cells usually show a markedly dilated ER (Figure 10.4). Electron microscopy is not, however, a technique routinely applied for diagnostic problems in myeloma but may be required in plasma cell leukaemia (see below).

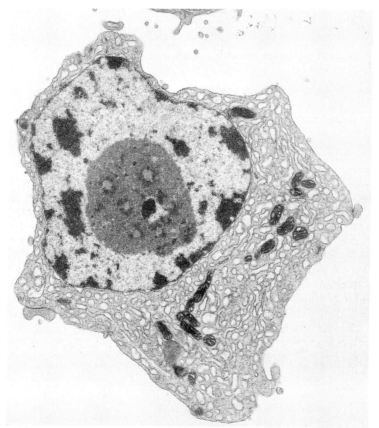

Figure 10.3 Plasmablast with a large nucleolus and short strands of dilated ER ($\times$ 14 000, reduced to 88% on reproduction). Sample obtained from the pleural effusion of an aggressive case of multiple myeloma whose karyotype is shown in Figure 10.6

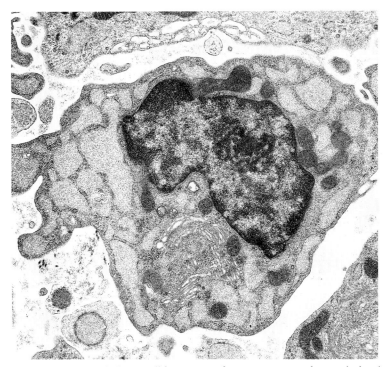

Figure 10.4 Abnormal plasma cell from a case of non-secretory myelomatosis showing a prominent Golgi apparatus and a very dilated ER containing Ig molecules; this was demonstrated by light microscopy immunofluorescence with appropriate antibodies. × 16 500, reduced to 74% on reproduction

Imaging techniques
An extensive radiographic survey should always be performed at diagnosis and this may demonstrate typical lesions in the skull, spine, ribs etc. It is debatable whether bone scans are helpful in the diagnosis of bone marrow involvement in this disease. This is because there is no new bone formation in myeloma, also reflected in the normal serum alkaline phosphatase concentration, and thus bone scans may be negative. Together with their prognostic importance, osteolytic lesions represent a valuable parameter for the long-term follow-up of patients.

The value of new imaging techniques to detect vertebral lesions in myeloma has recently been evaluated[69]. While deviations in shape and height are probably more easily assessed by plain X-rays, osteolytic lesions in lower thoracic and lumbar spine are best seen by computed tomography (CT) and particularly by magnetic resonance imaging (MRI). The latter has been shown to be superior to radiology, CT scan and radionuclide bone scanning for detecting vertebral lesions[69].

Prognostic factors and staging

Several different parameters have been considered at various times with regard to prognosis. The value of some of them has been controversial, as for example the prognostic significance of the class of heavy and light chains. Despite this controversy, one study reviewing 133 cases of IgD myelomatosis[56] suggested that this rare form of myeloma has a poor prognosis, with a 60% mortality within the first year of diagnosis. Bence-Jones myeloma also appears to be associated with a poor prognosis.

There is general agreement that renal failure at presentation is one of the most unfavourable prognostic features[3, 24, 75, 76]. Several other parameters, either alone or in combination, have also been shown to have prognostic value. These include haemoglobin, serum calcium, albumin concentration, Bence-Jones proteinuria, bone lesions and Karnovsky's preformance status. A study with a maximum follow-up of 12 years, carried out by Buckman et al.[22] indicated that three important guides for prognosis are the haemoglobin level, the posthydration blood urea concentration and the performance status at presentation, independent of all other parameters. The prognostic value of this classification was demonstrated by the different 5-year survival for each group of patients (Table 10.2). In recent years, however, the determination of serum β_2-microglobulin (see below) has become the single most important factor in myelomatosis[14, 32, 69a].

Table 10.2 Features of prognostic value in myeloma from early MRC trials [22, 76]

Prognostic	Hb (g/dl)	Urea[a] (mmol/l)	Performance status	Percentage patients	5-year survival (%)
Good	>10	<8	Minimal symptoms	22	38.6
Poor	<7.5	>10	Restricted activity	22	2.7
Intermediate	Neither 'good' nor 'poor' prognosis features			56	12.5

[a] Posthydration concentration.

In 1975 Durie and Salmon[35] introduced a clinical staging system based on the majority of relevant prognostic factors recognized by different authors and which correlated well with the myeloma cell mass. The latter was based on an earlier observation that in IgG myeloma the tumour cell mass could be derived from quantifications of the M-component[102]. The staging system, illustrated in Table 10.3, is easily reproducible on clinical criteria only. Although the tumour mass is not routinely measured, the task can be easily performed with the aid of a programmable pocket computer[103]. The validity of this staging system has been confirmed by various retrospective and prospective studies which showed significant differences between patients in stages I, II and III[36, 104, 119]. These are summarized in Table 10.4.

The demonstration of different degrees of histological infiltration in the bone marrow biopsy specimens has also led to the suggestion of a three-stage prognostic classification[11]. On the other hand, Cavo et al.[28] showed that in stage I myeloma the degree of bone marrow infiltration assessed on aspirates correlated significantly with prognosis. Patients with less than 50% plasma cells had a significantly longer survival than patients with more than 50% plasma cells. In the latter group a good correlation was also observed between response to chemotherapy and survival.

There is now growing evidence that the pre-treatment levels of β_2-microglobulin have great prognostic significance[4, 32, 86, 105]. A strong correlation has been

Table 10.3 Durie and Salmon's staging system [35]

Stage	Criteria
I	All of the following: 1. Haemoglobin value > 10 g/dl 2. Serum calcium value normal (<2.65 μmol/l) 3. On roetgenogram, normal bone structure or solitary bone plasmacytoma only 4. Low M-component production rates: IgG value < 50 g/l IgA value < 30 g/l Urine light chain M-component on electrophoresis <4 g/24 hours
II	Fitting neither stage I nor stage III
III	One or more of the following: 1. Haemoglobin value <8.5 g/dl 2. Serum calcium value >2.65 μmol/l 3. Advanced lytic bone lesions 4. High M-component production rates: IgG value > 70 g/l IgA value > 50 g/l Urine light chain M-component on electrophoresis >12 g/24 hours

Subclassification:
A = Relatively normal renal function (serum creatinine value <170 μmol/l)
B = Abnormal renal function (serum creatinine value (>170 μmol/l)

A or B according to the absence or presence of renal impairment.
Reproduced with permission from Durie and Salmon [35].

Table 10.4 Survival according to Durie and Salmon's staging system in three series

Authors	No. of patients	Median survival in months		
		Stage I	Stage II	Stage III
Woodruff et al. [119]	237	64	32	6
Durie et al. [36]	150	61.2	54.5	22.4
Santoro et al. [104]	81	48	41	23

found between serum β_2-microglobulin and the total body myeloma cell mass and an inverse correlation with Karnovsky's performance status[105]. Overall survival is significantly better in patients with low β_2-microglobulin levels. The good correlation between β_2-microglobulin and survival has been shown both in patients with normal renal function and in those with stage III[105].

Analysis of data from the MRC fourth trial[32], which included 476 patients, concluded that β_2-microglobulin level, uncorrected for serum creatinine, is the most powerful prognostic variable in myeloma as it takes into consideration both diesase activity and renal function. Multivariate analysis showed that only haemoglobin could add some extra useful information to the β_2-microglobulin levels. The MRC study also showed that the β_2-microglobulin estimation during a stable plateau phase was important in predicting subsequent prognosis. A similar conclusion about the value of serum β_2-microglobulin was reached by Bataille et al. [14] who found it to be the most powerful single variable for prognosis. In this study the authors compared the Durie and Salmon staging (see Table 10.3) with the MRC criteria (see Table 10.2) and found both equally valuable. They also found the β_2-microglobulin levels a better indicator than the MRC criteria and the combination of β_2-microglobulin and albumin levels superior to the classic Durie and Salmon staging system [14].

Treatment

For symptomatic patients the need for treatment to relieve symptoms and control the disease is self-evident. There is instead no agreement on the requirement to treat immediately asymptomatic patients with minimal disease [62]. Kyle and Greipp [63] described a group of patients, defined as 'smouldering' myeloma, who remained stable without treatment for 5–16 years.

It is difficult to determine at the time of diagnosis the rate at which the disease will progress. There is, however, no risk in waiting to commence treatment and to assess the need for therapy on the basis of close follow-up. Myelomatosis is nevertheless a disease of poor prognosis and few clinically documented cures have been described. Advances in treatment have been rapid in the last few years with more intensive approaches but these have not yet been translated consistently into better survivals [9].

Chemotherapy

A major improvement in the management of myelomatosis was brought about in the 1950s by the use of the alkylating agent sarcolysin [16] and especially of its *laevo*-isomer melphalan which has become the drug of choice for this disease. Before the advent of alkylating agents the median survival time of patients was of the order of 7–11 months [53, 89]. Following the use of either cyclophosphamide or melphalan, the median survival has more than doubled [4, 9, 71, 74, 77]. Both agents have been employed in several different modalities either alone or in combination with prednisone. No significant differences have been reported on the efficacy of either melphalan or cyclophosphamide [74], on continuous vs intermittent therapy and on the addition of prednisone, although the latter does seem to prolong survival [1]. The median survival time with these agents is generally over 2 years from initiation of therapy. Until recently the standard treatment for newly diagnosed myelomatosis was intermittent courses of melphalan and prednisone. This combination has been used at dosages of melphalan of 0.25 mg/kg per day for 4 days every 3 weeks or of 10 mg/day for 7 days every 4 weeks, together with prednisone 50–100 mg/day.

Several attempts have been made to try to improve survival, particularly for stage III patients. Other cytotoxic drugs have been tested alone but the overall results have been either worse or similar to those obtained with melphalan or cyclophosphamide. In the last decade different combination chemotherapy regimens including vincristine, doxorubicin, bleomycin, BCNU (carmustine) etc. have been tried. Most of them have been shown to be effective. Convincing evidence for the value of vincristine and bleomycin in these combinations is, however, lacking. A British randomized trial showed unequivocally that the addition of vincristine to melphalan and prednisone was not beneficial [79]. Overall, the results have shown only limited improvement in the rate of remission and survival [6, 9].

One of the first reported regimens which appeared to be advantageous compared with conventional treatment was the five drug M2 protocol (vincristine, melphalan, cyclophosphamide, BCNU, prednisone)[27] of the Memorial Hospital of New York. This was confirmed by a report[91] describing a greater than 50% reduction in paraprotein in 78% of patients, most of whom were in stage III. Similar results were found by Salmon et al.[101] who demonstrated a 75% tumour mass regression using alternating combination chemotherapy (including vincristine, doxorubicin, alkylating agents and prednisone) compared with the standard melphalan and prednisone regimen. These improved responses were observed particularly in stage III patients.

The MRC fifth myelomatosis trial is one of the first to show conclusively, in a randomized fashion, the advantage of the four-drug combination ABCM (doxorubicin and BCNU, both intravenously at $30\,mg/m^2$ on week 1 and melphalan $6\,mg/m^2$ and cyclophosphamide $100\,mg/m^2$, both orally for 4 days, 3 weeks later) over single agent melphalan ($7\,mg/m^2$ for 4 days every 3 weeks). This effect was seen in patients younger than 65 years[69a].

The benefits of ABCM and of a potent regimen used first for relapsed patients, VAD[vincristine and doxorubicin (Adriamycin) in 4-day infusions and oral high dose dexamethasone] seem to stem from the use of an anthracycline as part of the treatment of myeloma. The combination VAD or VAMP (with high dose methylprednisolone) is successful in refractory patients[68] and has a high remission rate in previously untreated patients[102a], but may not improve overall survival[9]. Several groups, including that of Professor McElwain at The Royal Marsden Hospital, are evaluating VAMP to induce remission followed by high dose melphalan ($200\,mg/m^2$) and autologous bone marrow transplantation[47a]. A recent report from this group describes an overall response rate of 74% in 50 previously untreated patients; this includes 50% achieving complete remission defined by strict haematological and biochemical criteria[47a].

Encouraging results (a 27% complete remission rate) have been reported initially in patients treated with high dose melphalan ($100–140\,mg/m^2$) given intravenously[73, 105a] without bone marrow rescue. This regimen, which is associated with 4 weeks of severe leucopenia[105a], is currently being evaluated in a randomized trial (MRC sixth trial) which started in June 1986, in comparison with ABCM, with or without the addition of methylprednisolone. The use of these new intensive regimens requires supportive measures similar to those used for the treatment of acute leukaemia. The possibility of combining melphalan plus prednisone with α-interferon is also under investigation.

Maintenance treatment
Whatever cut-off parameter may be adopted, a considerable tumour burden remains when remission is achieved. For this reason, several attempts have been made to assess the role of maintenance chemotherapy. However, in no series has prolongation of treatment after completion of induction chemotherapy proved to be beneficial[5, 6].

With melphalan and prednisone, Paccagnella et al.[91], with the M2 protocol, showed that stopping treatment after 1 year in responding patients did not reduce the duration of remission. Data from the fourth MRC trial also suggest that patients allocated to interrupt treatment 6 months after the establishment of a plateau phase in their paraprotein concentration may fare no worse than those allocated to continue treatment[69a]. A new approach to maintenance treatment in myeloma derives from the recognized effect of α-interferon in this disease (see below).

Treatment of relapse

The optimal management of relapsed patients or of those resistant to alkylating agents is still uncertain. Partial responses, of the order of 25%, have been obtained using more intensive protocols, including BCNU, vincristine, doxorubicin etc.[30, 96] and with the M2 five-drug combination[27]. Merlini et al.[81] used a drug with both alkylating and antimetabolic properties, peptichemio, and showed that it was effective on melphalan- and cyclophosphamide-resistant patients and on patients with advanced disease. A different approach has been described by Brandes and Israels[18] who used a weekly combination of cyclophosphamide intravenously (once a week) and prednisone on alternate days (for the first 6–8 weeks) to treat patients with advanced plasma cell myeloma. This protocol, which can be substituted with cyclophosphamide orally $400\,mg/m^2$ given over 2 or 3 days, has been successful in the authors' own experience in controlling the disease in patients who appear to be refractory to melphalan and prednisone. One advantage of this weekly cyclophosphamide regimen is that it allows the use of higher doses of an alkylating agent without the myelotoxicity of melphalan. The authors have been able to use this protocol in numerous patients in whom melphalan could not be given often enough due to cytopenia.

Re-treatment with melphalan and prednisone or the M2 protocol has been shown to be effective in achieving a second remission in relapsed patients who stopped treatment after 1 year[4, 6, 91] with the duration of the second response being only slightly shorter than after the first treatment[91]. These data refer to good responders in whom the best policy at present may thus be to stop therapy until relapse. One problem in stopping therapy and re-treating upon relapse relates to the possibility of diagnosing relapse early enough. Frequent measurements of the M-component are essential for this purpose. One major argument for not giving continuous therapy is the need to reduce the incidence of secondary acute myeloid leukaemia. A point in favour of not stopping a beneficial treatment scheme is the observation that, sooner or later, all patients need to restart therapy.

As stated above, the VAD or VAMP regimens are currently the most effective salvage treatments for relapsed and/or refractory myeloma[9]. A variation of this, cyclo-VAMP or VCAD, has also been used successfully in melphalan refractory disease[9]. In a recent study, 50% of patients achieved a complete remission with VAD[68] with a median duration of response of 9 months. One-third of the remitters remained in stable remission without therapy for over 1 year. It should be noted that the complete remission rate with VAMP or VAD in newly diagnosed patients has been much lower in other series, e.g. 6%[47a] and 28%[102a], respectively.

At the present time there is no recognized cure rate for multiple myeloma. Only randomized controlled trials will clearly define the optimal approach at diagnosis and at relapse, particularly for patients in the poor or intermediate prognostic groups. The most significant progress is emerging from the use of more intensive regimens, α-interferon and autologous bone marrow transplantation.

Interferon

Great interest has surrounded the possible role of human interferon in the treament of haematological malignancies. Recent results suggest that human leucocyte interferon or recombinant α-interferon is capable of inducing tumour regression in a minority of myeloma cases[7, 9, 98]. This has been observed both in previously untreated patients and in non-responders with minimal side effects. The beneficial role of α-interferon is currently being assessed on larger series of patients as a maintenance therapy (after plateau phase) and/or in combination with different chemotherapy regimens to assess whether it exerts a synergistic effect, recognizing that the proportion of responses when used alone in previously treated patients is low and higher in untreated patients[98].

Radiation therapy
Treatment of local lesions plays an important part in the management of myeloma. Often radiotherapy is useful for the treatment of collapsed vertebrae and as a palliative approach for pain relief in other sites. Doses required vary from 1000 to 2000 cGy which can be given in fractionated doses of 250–400 cGy per session. Irradiation of the bone marrow (2000 cGy) has been attempted in previously treated patients with limited benefit and resulted in significant haematological toxicity[31]. Such treatment would be contraindicated if there is a possibility of performing an autologous bone marrow transplantation.

Plasmapheresis
This procedure may be useful in the rare cases of hyperviscosity syndrome[54]. Plasmapheresis has also been used with beneficial effects to prevent extensive renal damage due to light chain excretion[83].

Bone marrow transplantation
So far few patients have been transplated with bone marrow from their HLA identical sibling[44] or twin[41, 90]. Of the two identical twin transplantations, one patient was in partial remission and the other was in relapse. In both cases high-dose chemotherapy was given prior to rescue with the bone marrow cells. One patient relapsed 18 months later and the other, although in unmaintained remission 2 years after transplantation, still showed a serum paraprotein. These observations confirm the difficulty of obtaining a complete eradication of the malignant cells in multiple myeloma. A 28-year-old patient with Bence-Jones myeloma achieved remission with melphalan and prednisone and received an allogeneic bone marrow transplantation after conditioning with high-dose cyclophosphamide and total body irradiation (1000 cGy). The patient remained in complete clinical remission for over 23 months, but without complete normalization of the previously extensive osteolytic lesions. Three young myeloma patients (aged 34–43 years) underwent an allogeneic bone marrow transplantation in Italy[109a]. Whilst one died of acute graft vs host disease, the other two were in unmaintained complete remission at 4 and 20 months respectively.

   Allogeneic and syngeneic bone marrow transplantation, although effective, is not going to change radically the outlook for the majority of patients. More encouraging is the use of autologous bone marrow transplantation obtained after a good initial remission[9]. The use of VAMP followed by high-dose melphalan can induce 50% of complete remissions, some of them very prolonged as discussed above[47a].

Management of specific complications

Renal failure
Of the factors contributing towards the development of renal failure in this disease, two can be treated: (1) hypercalcaemia (see below) is certainly the most frequent

cause and (2) hyperuricaemia which should always be controlled or prevented by using allopurinol.

In an attempt to reduce complications due to renal failure and the high incidence of early deaths, vigorous hydration therapy should always be given at the time of commencing treatment, with a daily input of more than 3 litres. Data from the fourth MRC myelomatosis trial[78] show that renal failure in multiple myeloma may be controlled and also reversed by a policy of daily high fluid intake (>3 litres per 24 hours). Furthermore, the high mortality in patients presenting with renal failure improved markedly compared with previous studies in which the approach to liquid intake has been less stringent. In the presence of acute renal failure dialysis may be required; in rare cases this procedure may be of great value as these patients may still respond to treatment. The authors have treated a patient who required dialysis for over 2 years and who, after a good remission, managed to recover sufficient renal function not to require further dialysis.

Hypercalcaemia

It is important to keep the calcium levels under control throughout the course of the disease because hypercalcaemia represents a leading event towards renal failure. Active rehydration is essential and daily urinary excretion of more than 3 litres is a necessary and often urgent measure. This may not be possible with oral input only and intravenous adminstration of saline is often required to provide an adequate extracellular fluid expansion and increase glomerular filtration. Corticosteroids, either by mouth or intravenously, are also indicated in the management of hypercalcaemia and will provide additional effect. Mithramycin also inhibits bone resorption[109] and it has been used successfully but is considered of limited value because of the risk of severe bone marrow depression. Calcitonin has been used in patients resistant to more conventional treatment[21]. A new group of compounds, the diphosphonates[33], have been shown to act as potent inhibitors of osteoclastic bone resorption but there are limited data on their long-term use. New diphosphonates are currently being tested in the management of hypercalcaemia in multiple myeloma and other malignancies. One of these agents, disodium etidronate (given in 3-day courses intravenously by slow infusion), seems to be very effective. An oral agent, clodronate (dichloromethylene diphosphonate), is being tested by one of the MRC trials to see whether it has an effect in improving the osteolytic lesions when given together with the cytotoxic treatment for myeloma.

Infection

This represents one of the main complications in myeloma and the most common cause of death. Different mechanisms may concur in causing infections in this disease:

1. The reduced levels of normal serum Ig are a major predisposing factor towards the high incidence of infections, particularly by *Streptococcus pneumoniae*.
2. The granulocytopenia which follows treatment may lead to both Gram-positive or Gram-negative infections.
3. The well documented T-cell abnormalities (see below) may contribute to the progressive hypogammaglobulinaemia in these patients.

Special attention should be given to the early phases of treatment when infective complications are an important cause of death. In the fourth MRC trial 9% of all deaths in the first 100 days from entry were due to pyogenic infections. It is therefore essential that in the management of multiple myeloma physicians should be alert to the risk of infective complications as well as those of renal failure at any time throughout the course of the illness.

Monitoring treatment

Monitoring of the M-components is the single most valuable indicator of the progression of the disease and of the effectiveness of treatment; it also provides a good guide as to when treatment should be restarted. Blood values (haemoglobin, neutrophil and platelet count, renal function, calcium, uric acid) should also be monitored regularly. Bone lesions are not of great value as they often vary little even in responding patients. Changes in symptoms in individual patients are often useful to assess the efficacy of treatment or to indicate relapse. Changes in serum β_2-microglobulin concentrations have also been shown to be extremely useful to monitor progression during the plateau phase and to assess response to treatment. The decrease in the percentage of plasma cells in the bone marrow, although probably less reliable, is currently used in programmes which incorporate the use of intensive chemotherapy (e.g. high-dose melphalan) followed by autologous bone marrow grafting. In such cases, the aim is to reinject bone marrows with the minimum number of plasma cells. Most groups use 30% as the upper limit above which they do not consider it safe to reinfuse[47a].

Incidence of acute leukaemia

Acute leukaemia, usually myeloid (AML), is not an infrequent complication of multiple myeloma. Although the risk of developing acute leukaemia has greatly increased since the advent of alkylating agents as first choice in the management of the disease, nevertheless it should be noted that the association can occur without the use of these cytotoxic agents[85]. Recent retrospective studies indicate that the incidence of acute leukaemia is some 100- to 200-fold higher in myeloma patients than the expected incidence in the normal population, with an overall incidence ranging between 6% and 17% according to the series and duration of therapy[113]. Practically all types of acute myeloid leukaemia have been encountered and the timing of occurrence may vary from a few months to several years after the onset of multiple myeloma, often preceded by a myelodysplastic phase.

It has been suggested that the risk of acute leukaemia is much higher in multiple myeloma than in other conditions in which alkylating agents are currently employed. These observations lead to the suggestion that the high risk of acute leukaemia in multiple myeloma is in some way related to the primary disorder. The possibility cannot be exluded that haemopoietic precursor cells may be involved in multiple myeloma and may therefore explain the possibility of developing a second haematological malignancy. On the other hand, melphalan is the cytotoxic drug most commonly used in the management of multiple myeloma and it has been strongly suggested that it is more leukaemogenic than other alkylating agents used in this disease (e.g. cyclophosphamide) as shown by data accumulated from the MRC trials[22].

Immunoblastic transformation

The development of an immunoblastic (large cell) lymphoma in myelomatosis may be more common than is generally recognized. A report by Falini et al.[40]

describes such an event in 10 patients. The morphological change took place in extramedullary sites in 6 patients and within the bone marrow in 4 others. The authors provide evidence to suggest that the process represents a clonal evolution of the original B-cell tumour analogous to the development of Richter's syndrome in CLL (see Chapter 3).

Benign monoclonal gammopathy

In a proportion of apparently healthy individuals, which accounts for up to 3% of people over the age of 70[61], a monoclonal serum immunoglobulin can be found. These cases, who clearly differ from classic multiple myeloma, have been termed 'benign monoclonal gammopathies', 'monoclonal gammopathies of undetermined significance' or 'indolent myeloma'. Based on a study of 241 such patients reported by Kyle[60], 75% of them showed a monoclonal IgG proliferation, 10% had an IgA band and 15% an IgM band; 62% were of the κ light chain type, whilst 38% were λ. A monoclonal light chain in the urine was found in 10% of these patients. It is important to distinguish between these benign proliferations and the true malignancies of plasma cells because the former conditions have a good prognosis and generally do not require treatment. This distinction is particularly relevant in view of the different incidence of the two conditions, benign monoclonal gammopathy being about five- to six-fold more frequent than multiple myeloma[61]. The diagnostic criteria for benign monoclonal gammopathy are:

1. The presence of a serum M band of less than 2.5 g/l with no detectable light chain in the urine (although individual exceptions occur).
2. Less than 10% plasma cells in the bone marrow without bizarre forms.
3. Absence of osteolytic lesions.

The level of the polyclonal serum immunoglobulins, which is reduced in most cases of myeloma, is usually normal in these patients. However, a single report suggests that a proportion of patients with benign monoclonal gammopathy may also show a reduction of the uninvolved immunoglobulins. Exceptional cases of monoclonal light chain gammopathy have been described by Lindstrom and Dahlstrom[67] and by Kyle[61].

The differential diagnosis between benign monoclonal gammopathy and myelomatosis is not always easy on the basis of laboratory findings. A close clinical follow-up together with laboratory analysis are essential as benign monoclonal gammopathy generally shows no evidence of progression for over 5 years after diagnosis. Retrospective studies carried out on large series of patients with benign monoclonal gammopathy indicate that the best differential parameter between benign and malignant gammopathy is the sequential evaluation of the level of the paraprotein[25, 61]. In rare but well-documented cases, a progression to multiple myeloma can occur after a long period (5–10 years) of apparently stable benign monoclonal gammopathy. The bone marrow plasma cell labelling index has recently been suggested as being useful for the differential diagnosis between multiple myeloma and benign monoclonal gammopathy[49].

Solitary myeloma

In rare cases, a plasma cell tumour histologically indistinguishable from classic myelomatosis, but with no evidence of generalized bone involvement, may develop as a solitary lesion in a single bone site[117, 120]. This disorder has a mean age at presentation younger than in myeloma. The clinical course is also significantly more benign compared with myeloma, often showing no evidence of an 'M' band in the serum and generally with normal levels of the remaining immunoglobulins. Although surgery and/or radiotherapy are effective, the disease may recur locally or may proceed to overt myeloma over a period of several years. The prognosis is overall better than in myelomatosis[2].

Extramedullary plasmacytoma

This is a rare neoplasia which could arise in any soft tissue containing immunoglobulin-producing cells[57, 117]. The most frequent site is the upper respiratory tract including the oral cavity. Extramedullary plasmacytoma may affect other areas such as lower airways and the lungs, lymph nodes and spleen, skin and the subcutaneous tissues, digestive tract etc. Although generally solitary, this tumour may develop simultaneously in different sites[13, 117]. In many cases the disease may spread outside the site of presentation, most often to the bones, although other soft tissues may also be involved. CNS involvement has been described[117] and the authors have seen a patient with persistent refractory meningeal deposits. It is of interest that the bone lesions, unlike multiple myeloma, often do not affect the areas of active bone marrow.

Patients with extramedullary plasmacytoma generally fare better than those with overt multiple myeloma and show a better tolerance to treatment because of the bone marrow sparing by the tumour. In theory at least, these patients are better candidates for autologous bone marrow transplantation. Surgical removal and/or radiotherapy can generally control local disease. Good responses have also been achieved with chemotherapy, single alkylating agent or combinations, including patients with disseminated disease. The authors have observed a prolonged complete remission (so far over 4 years) to combination chemotherapy in a plasmacytoma arising from a mesenteric node. The diagnosis was established by immunohistochemistry showing light chain restriction.

Amyloidosis

The term 'amyloidosis' refers to the presence of an amorphous substance which involves different organs and tissues and has specific characteristics demonstrable at both light and electron microscopy. The metachromatic stains with methyl violet and crystal violet are typical of amyloid deposits. More specific for a correct diagnosis is the stain, under polarized light, with Congo red. A better insight into the structure of amyloid has been obtained with the advent of electron microscopy. This has revealed the fibrillar architecture of amyloid, with aggregates of fibrils with varying length and organization and a typical β-pleated sheet structure[46]. Amyloid fibrils are insoluble and resistant to proteolytic enzymes and can replace normal tissues, thus destroying the physiological structure of the sites involved.

Amyloidosis was initially associated with other diseases, particularly chronic infections, and thus classified as secondary. It is, however, well recognized now that a form of primary amyloidosis which is characterized by the deposition of amyloid fibrils in different tissues in the absence of other detectable disorders does exist. Amyloidosis is also a relatively frequent complication of all plasma cell diseases, particularly multiple myeloma, in which 5–15% of patients are affected.

Although it is common to consider separately the primary and the secondary forms of amyloidosis, it should be stressed that no real difference exists between the two forms with regard to staining properties and tissue distribution[29]. The nature of amyloid in both these forms is different. In secondary amyloidosis the material has been defined as A-component or amyloid of unknown origin (AUO), whilst in primary amyloidosis, including the one associated with multiple myeloma, the protein component is of immunoglobulin origin. Amino acid sequence studies have demonstrated the structural similarities between Bence-Jones proteins and amyloid fibrils[47]. The molecular weight of the fibrils indicates that amyloid deposits contain mostly fragments of monoclonal light chains, which appear to be represented by the variable portions of the light chain. Thus, the major protein component of primary amyloidosis is either an intact immunoglobulin light chain, or the amino terminal portion of the light chain or of both[10].

Clinical manifestations of primary amyloidosis
Together with general symptoms of fatigue and weight loss, and physical findings which include oedema, purpura, macroglossia etc., the clinical features are related to the organ distribution of the amyloid deposits. The most severe clinical manifestations result from renal and cardiac involvement, which often terminate in renal or congestive heart failure. Other frequent localizations include the gastrointestinal tract with a variety of symptoms, including diarrhoea, haemorrhage and malabsorption problems, the respiratory tract, the nervous system with peripheral neuropathies, the 'carpal tunnel syndrome' etc. Purpura, due to the damage of the skin vessels, occurs in several areas, most commonly in the face and neck.

Amyloidosis in myeloma
This association may be suspected on clinical grounds but needs laboratory confirmation. A variety of haematological and biochemical alterations, reflecting the different organs and tissues involved, may be present. However, in order to achieve a correct diagnosis appropriate staining procedures for amyloid must be performed on biopsy material. For this purpose a rectal biopsy is most frequently performed and is normally free of side effects and complications. According to the clinical picture, other sites may be biopsied. All material should be stained with Congo red and with the metachromatic stains. Electron microscopic studies may be necessary for a definitive diagnosis in doubtful cases. Prognosis for patients with primary and myeloma-associated amyloidosis is very poor, in the order of about 4 months[61] and so far all forms of treatment have been unsatisfactory.

Plasma cell leukaemia

Primary plasma cell leukaemia should be distinguished from a terminal event during the course of classic multiple myeloma, in which spill-over of plasma cells in the peripheral blood may occur. It is generally agreed that a diagnosis of plasma cell leukaemia can be made when more than 20% plasma cells are present in the peripheral blood or in the presence of an absolute number of plasma cells greater than $2 \times 10^9/l$[64, 92, 118]. WBC counts are most often between 10 and $50 \times 10^9/l$. Whilst the incidence of plasmacytosis associated with multiple myeloma is in the range of 1–2%[64], the incidence of plasma cell leukaemia is uncertain. Osanto et al. [88] reviewed 49 cases of plasma cell leukaemia published between 1965 and 1980 in which the criteria for a correct diagnosis were fulfilled.

Because the plasma cell may be morphologically small, the differential diagnosis from other lymphoid leukaemias may arise. In some patients the cells resemble blast cells and the differential diagnosis with an acute leukaemia (ALL or AML) should be considered. In this context marker studies and ultrastructural morphology may help the correct diagnosis. Plasma cells will show CyIg and reactivity with the monoclonal antibody OKT10 (CD38) and are often negative for HLA-DR and other B-cell antigens (CD19, CD21, CD24). These findings are no different from those seen in the plasma cells of myelomatosis[55]. There is no evidence that CD10, a marker associated with poor prognosis[9], is more frequent in plasma cell leukaemia. In fact, CD10 (tested with the monoclonal antibody J5) was negative in all the six cases tested by the authors[92].

Ten cases of plasma cell leukaemia have been studied by the authors in the last 5 years. The diagnosis in all of them was difficult by light microscopy. The cell morphology ranged from that of small lymphoid cells to that of poorly differentiated blasts. Ultrastructural analysis showed the characteristic concentric profiles of endoplasmic reticulum of plasma cells which are not seen in other cell types (Figure 10.5)[98]. Anaemia, renal failure and hypercalcaemia were findings in most cases. The WBC count ranged from 17 to 150 × 10⁹/l (median 58 × 10⁹/l). Bone lesions were demonstrated in half of them.

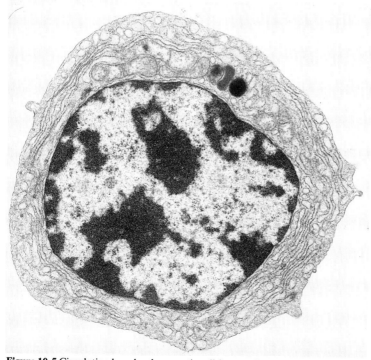

Figure 10.5 Circulating lymphoplasmacytic cell from a plasma cell leukaemia showing moderately abundant profiles of ER arranged in parallel arrays (× 16 000, reduced to 77% on reproduction). The membrane markers of these cells were intermediate between those of lymphoplasmacytic cells and plasma cells (SmIg+, FMC7+, HLA-DR−, OKT10+)

The prognosis for patients suffering from plasma cell leukaemia is generally poor. The therapeutic approach has not been uniform. Alkylating agents and corticosteroids alone or in combination have been used. Irrespective of the treatment, about two-thirds of the patients die within a few months of diagnosis. The median survival in the authors' series was less than 10 months. Nevertheless, a minority live for more than a year and in a few good responses have been observed. It is unquestionable that a very intensive approach is required to improve the response rate and survival of these patients. Regimens for myelomatosis, such as VAD or VAMP and high-dose melphalan, should be considered and/or new and more imaginative regimens.

Heavy chain disease

These represent B-cell disorders characterized by the proliferation of neoplastic cells which produce incomplete (or truncated) monoclonal heavy chains devoid of light chains. Diseases corresponding to the three main classes of human Ig have been described. The first case, reported in 1966 by Franklin et al. [43], was a patient with malignant lymphoma and high concentrations of the Fc portion of IgG (γ-chain) in serum and urine. Since then, several other reports have appeared in the literature, including cases with IgA (α-chain) and IgM (μ-chain) disease. Over 200 cases of heavy chain disease have now been reported. The most frequent of these is by far α-chain disease[106] and the rarest is μ-chain disease, first reported in 1970[42]. In all cases the abnormality can be demonstrated only with appropriate immunoelectrophoretic analysis of serum and urine which will demonstrate reactivity only with antisera against the specific heavy chain. The abnormal proteins are short chains which result from deletions of part or all of the variable region and one or two of the constant regions of the Ig heavy chain.

γ-Chain disease

This disease has been found in patients of all ages although it is rare under the age of 20 years. The clinical picture is frequently similar to that of Waldenströms's macroglobulinaemia[107] (see below). However, in about 20% of patients γ-chain disease is associated with an autoimmune disorder such as rheumatoid arthritis, lupus erythematosus, Sjögren's syndrome etc. The clinical features at presentation may be heterogeneous but lymphadenopathy and hepatosplenomegaly are the most common. Due to the frequent involvement of the nodes of Waldeyer's ring, both erythema and oedema of the palate are also frequent. Leucopenia also occurs in a high proportion of cases, and mild to moderate anaemia is a very frequent finding.

α-Chain disease

α-Chain disease, which often affects young patients from developing countries, involves mainly the anatomical sites of IgA production[107, 108]. In rare cases the disease can affect only the respiratory tract, whilst practically all cases display the digestive form of α-chain disease. The latter is characterized by a diffuse infiltration of lymphocytes and plasma cells of the small intestine and mesenteric lymph nodes. This gives rise to the clinical picture which is common to all patients: abdominal pain, diarrhoea, malabsorption, low serum albumin levels and steatorrhoea.

Lymphadenopathy and hepatosplenomegaly are often absent. The abnormal α-chain protein can be readily demonstrated in serum or urine of two-thirds of the patients. In cases with an otherwise compatible clinical picture and normal serum IgA, a careful search should be carried out on the jejunal fluid or at the intracellular level[99, 107].

Some degree of confusion on the similarities and differences between α-chain disease and Mediterranean lymphoma[39] has for a long time surrounded these two diseases. Initially, they were regarded as separate entities, mainly on the basis of the different morphology of the infiltrates. Later, however, it was shown that cases of α-chain disease may evolve towards a typical lymphoma with features of immunoblastic lymphoma, which was also shown to derive from the same clone as the original plasma cell dyscrasia[19, 99]. A WHO report described both diseases as corresponding to the same pathological entity[116]. However, the exact incidence of α-chain protein synthesis in Mediterranean lymphoma remains uncertain, because serum Ig analysis has not always been carried out in patients with this tumour.

μ-Chain disease

This disease presents almost invariably as a lymphoproliferative disorder, most often B-CLL and sometimes non-Hodgkin's lymphoma[20]. In most cases characteristic vacuolated plasma cells are found in the bone marrow. In B-CLL patients with significant hepatosplenomegaly and modest lymphadenopathy, serum Ig analysis should always be carried out. Clinically, patients show prominent hepatosplenomegaly and enlarged abdominal lymphadenopathy. Superficial lymph nodes are usually uninvolved.

Treatment

Chemotherapy with single or multiple agents has been employed against heavy chain disease. Altogether, patients with the different forms of heavy chain disease have an unfavourable prognosis. This is particularly evident in α-chain disease when patients develop a large cell immunoblastic lymphoma. On the other hand, some patients with α-chain disease and no evidence of lymphoma have achieved prolonged remissions with broad-spectrum antibiotics.

Waldenström's macroglobulinaemia

Waldenström's macroglobulinaemia is a chronic B-cell malignancy first described in 1944[114] and characterized by the abnormal production of monoclonal IgM. Along with the classic disease or primary macroglobulinaemia, which is a well-defined clinicopathological entity, a so-called secondary macroglobulinaemia can occur when increased levels of IgM are associated with other lymphoproliferative disorders, for instance B-CLL and B-PLL. It has been considered by many pathology groups that this disease is part of the spectrum of lymphoplasmacytic lymphoma (LPL) or immunocytoma. One group of patients with LPL and the presence of villous lymphocytes in the peripheral blood (splenic lymphoma with villous lymphocytes) has been discussed in Chapter 7. Although Waldenström's macroglobulinaemia occurs most often in the sixth and seventh decades of life, it has nevertheless been described also in young people. Males appear to be more affected than females. A more recent review of the disease was published by Waldenström in 1986[115].

Clinical and laboratory features

The clinical picture may present a wide range of manifestations. The most frequent complaints are fatigue, weakness and weight loss. Bleeding episodes often occur. Splenomegaly, hepatomegaly and lymphadenopathy are present in more than 50% of cases[58, 72, 114, 115]. In about 5–7% of patients central or peripheral neurological manifestations can be documented[58]. In contrast to myelomatosis, bone pain and bone lesions are uncommon. Similarly, both the incidence of renal disease and of amyloidosis are also much less frequent than in myeloma.

In the majority of patients, signs and symptoms related to hyperviscosity syndrome are present, namely visual disturbances, neurological complications and features of haemorrhagic diathesis, and these often suggest the diagnosis. Other symptoms of hyperviscosity, such as dizziness and headache, may occur and these are often accompanied by fundal changes, first in the form of dilated and tortuous veins and later as exudates and haemorrhages of the retina. The frequency of this syndrome is presumably related to the shape of the IgM molecules and to their high molecular weight and tendency to aggregate[15]. Symptoms related to the presence of cryoglobulins can also occur in a proportion of patients. Anaemia and a high erythrocyte sedimentation rate, classically over 100 mm, are seen in the majority of patients. Anaemia is often due to bone marrow infiltration by lymphoid cells, leading to inadequate red cell production, although haemolysis and blood loss may also be present. On the blood films rouleaux formation is often evident. The total leucocyte count is in general normal; in a proportion of cases lymphocytosis with intermediate features between lymphocytes and plasma cells may be present. Thrombocytopenia is seen in 30% of patients.

Diagnosis

The prerequisite for a correct diagnosis is the electrophoretic analysis of the serum. This shows a homogeneous high spike of mobility (M component) in the β or γ region. Immunoelectrophoresis is necessary in order establish the IgM origin of the monoclonal protein. Monoclonality is demonstrated by evidence of light chain restriction. In general the concentration of the IgM protein, a molecule with a sedimentation coefficient of 19 S, exceeds 20 g/1, although cases with lower values may be found. Often there is a concomitant decrease of IgG and IgA.

Bence-Jones proteinuria is found in approximately one-third of patients, although in some series a higher incidence has been reported[58]. The increase in serum viscosity can be measured using a viscosimeter tube assembly.

Bone marrow aspirates show hypercellularity with an infiltration by lymphocytes and plasmacytoid lymphocytes; a prominent component of mast cells is frequent. In many cases the aspirate is unsuccessful due to a marked increase in reticulin fibres. Bone marrow biopsies show hypercellularity with lymphoplasmacytic infiltration and fibrosis in practically all cases[12].

Management

The clinical course of Waldenström's macroglobulinaemia may vary considerably, and for some time treatment may not be necessary. Initiation of therapy is usually linked to clinico-laboratory findings and to the presence of symptoms related to hyperviscosity. Alkylating agents are the drugs of choice, chlorambucil being the most frequently used agent. Continuous[72] or intermittent courses of chlorambucil (6–10 mg daily for 2 weeks or 20 mg for 1 week) are generally given, sometimes in combination with pulses of prednisone. In many cases, repeated courses of chlorambucil are sufficient to keep the disease under control. Other alkylating agents, i.e. cyclophosphamide and melphalan, can be used with similar effect.

Good responders show a decrease in size of the spleen, liver and lymph nodes, and levels of IgM, an improvement in the symptoms related to hyperviscosity and an increase in the levels of haemoglobin. Treatment with alkylating agents may not be sufficient to control the hyperviscosity. In these cases regular plasmapheresis may be necessary, especially when a drastic decrease in the intravascular level of IgM is urgently required. It must be stressed that in general several plasmapheresis procedures are necessary and that the effects are only temporary. However, some patients have been maintained successfully with plasmapheresis alone for prolonged periods, particularly those resistant to chemotherapy.

In patients who respond well to alkylating agents the prognosis is relatively good. Median survivals of approximately 4 years have been reported[58]. A significant difference in prognosis between good and poor responders to alkylating agents has been noted[70]. In an attempt to improve survival, more aggressive treatment approaches are being attempted. For example, the five-drug combination M2 (vincristine, melphalan, cyclophosphamide, BCNU, prednisone) has also been employed in this disease, with some success[26]. A partial remission was achieved in 12 of 14 patients treated and a complete remission in the remaining 2. Furthermore, patients with symptomatic hyperviscosity did not require plasmapheresis. There is no reported evidence of the use of VAD or VAMP in Waldenström's macroglobulinaemia but these, or the combination CHOP (cyclophosphamide, hydroxydaunorubicin, oncovin and prednisone) are likely to be effective in patients primarily refractory to chlorambucil.

Special studies in plasma cell dyscrasias

In vitro cloning

The search for tests of drug sensitivity has been particularly active in multiple myeloma as overall prognosis has improved little in the last few years, despite the many therapeutic approaches and the various combinations of drugs used.

In 1977, Hamburger and Salmon[50] described an in vitro clonogenic assay which allowed the growth in soft agar of human myeloma cells. The possible applications and the theoretical potential of such a system, as in all tumour models, are easily foreseeable. This clonogenic system has been employed to predict the sensitivity of myeloma cells to different cytotoxic agents. Data from the same group who first described the assay suggest a good correlation between in vitro and in vivo drug sensitivity, particularly to indicate resistance to treatment[100]. In addition, the pattern of growth has been found to be of prognostic value[37]. However, this technique has not so far been widely applied.

A new double layer agar technique (agar/agar or agar/liquid) to consistently grow myeloma colonies has · recently been developed at The Royal Marsden Hospital[82]. Mononuclear cells from blood or bone marrow are cultured for 2–3 weeks, when colonies are formed. Two distinct types of myeloma cells grow in these cultures: large cells with plasmacytic features and smaller cells with lymphoid morphology. This technique apparently allows the colony growth from bone marrows with few plasma cells and can be used for drug sensitivity testing[82].

Cell kinetics

Cell kinetic techniques have been applied successfully to the study of myeloma cells. A good correlation has been established between the tritiated thymidine labelling index (LI) of myeloma cells and the clinical course of the disease with a better prognosis for patients with an LI of less than 1%[9, 17, 36]. Furthermore, a decline in LI can be documented when the patients are in remission, whilst the LI increases significantly at relapse. There appears to be a correlation between the percentage LI and myeloma colony growth, showing that the higher the LI the greater the chances of achieving in vitro growth[38]. It has been suggested that sensitivity in vitro to cytotoxic drugs and a low LI are associated with good prognosis, whilst a high LI and in vitro drug resistance correlate with a poor prognosis[38]. Another study[49] suggested that an LI greater than 0.4% is the best discriminating parameter between multiple myeloma, smouldering myeloma and benign monoclonal gammopathy. If this information is coupled with the percentage of bone marrow plasma cells, the discriminating accuracy of these measurements is even greater. In the same study it was also shown that patients initially diagnosed as smouldering myeloma or benign monoclonal gammopathy with an LI greater than 0.4% progressed to overt myeloma within 6 months. Thus, kinetic studies may prove to be a valuable diagnostic tool and an important therapeutic guide.

T-cell abnormalities in multiple myeloma

In recent years, as reported in the introductory chapter of this book, great interest has focused on the T-lymphocyte populations and on the possible role that abnormalities in the distribution and/or function of these subpopulations may play in the hypogammaglobulinaemia observed in several lymphoproliferative disorders.

Data based initially on Fcγ and Fcμ receptors and more recently on results with monoclonal antibodies have shown that in the majority of patients with multiple myeloma there is an increased proportion of Tγ and CD8+ cells (suppressor/cytotoxic phenotype) together with a reduced proportion of Tμ and CD4+ T-cells (helper/inducer phenotype)[65, 80, 87, 94]. These abnormalities are more pronounced in patients with advanced disease[65, 80]. Despite the increased proportion of CD8+ T-cells, the absolute number of these cells is normal or even reduced[65, 80].

Functional studies carried out on enriched myeloma T-cell lymphocytes are also indicative of a reduced helper capacity in a pokeweed mitogen (PWM) driven assay[65]. However, fractionation experiments suggest that these defects are probably due both to a reduced proportion of T-helper cells and to excessive suppressor activity by the Tγ CD8+ T-cell subset[65, 93]. Perri et al.[93] suggested that the increased suppressor activity may also be due to an enhanced sensitivity of B-cells in myeloma to T-cell suppression. Based on these observations, it is suggestive that the T-cell abnormalities observed within the T-cell subpopulations in multiple myeloma, paticularly in stage II–III patients, may contribute to the progressive hypogammaglobulinaemia and thus to the high incidence of infective complications.

These well-documented T-cell abnormalities in multiple myeloma may also be relevant to the understanding of the mechanism by which α-interferon exerts its anti-neoplastic effect in this disease: whether it acts directly on the pathological B-cell population or whether it may act as a biological modulator, possibly via the T-lymphocyte pathway.

Chromosome abnormalities

Several studies have described chromosome abnormalities in multiple myeloma and plasma cell leukaemia[34, 48, 66, 95, 110–112, 121]. The incidence of abnormal karyotypes in myeloma has been found to be between 20%[112] and 64%[95] (average 40%; Table 10.5). Patients with abnormal cytogenetic clones at diagnosis have a worse prognosis than those with a normal karyotype. A higher incidence of abnormalities has been reported in IgG3 myeloma[112] and in plasma cell leukaemia[34]. Hypodiploidy may be more common in Bence-Jones myeloma[48].

Table 10.5 Chromosome abnormalities in myelomatosis

Author	No. cases/ abnormal	Abnormalities	(No. cases)
Dewald et al. [34]	100/29	14q32	(11)
Gould et al. [48]	115/53	14q+	(9)
Liang et al. [66]	18/6	14q+	(5)
Philip et al. [95]	26/16	Trisomy 1q	(5)
		14q+	(2)
Ueshima et al. [110]	7/7	Trisomy 1q	(6)
		14q+	(3)
Van den Berghe [112]	26[b]/5	t(11;14)	(1)
Yamada et al. [121]	1/1	14q+	
Total	293/117 (40%)	14q+	(32)[a]

[a] Of the 32 cases with 14q abnormalities 11 (34%) had t(11;14) (q13;q32), 5 (15%) had t(8;14) (q24;q32) and 1 (3%) had t(14;18) (q32;q21). In one report the 4 cases with t(8;14) had IgA paraprotein [48].
[b] No growth in 7 additional cases; in another report [111] the authors described 4 cases with Ph chromosome, one with t(9;22), out of 70 studied (5.7%).

A marker 14q+, usually with breakpoint at 14q32, is the most frequent abnormality, having been observed in 21% of cases (Table 10.5); one-third of them had plasma cell leukaemia. The 14q+ marker results usually from the translocation t(11;14) which is also seen in other B-cell malignancies: B-CLL, B-PLL and some non-Hodgkin's lymphomas. The translocation t(8;14) characteristic of Burkitt's lymphoma has also been observed in cases of myeloma[48] and plasma cell leukaemia[121]. Other frequent abnormalities include trisomy 1q[34, 95, 110], trisomy 3, 5, 9 and 16[48], monosomy 13 and 16, abnormal chromosome 11 and, in

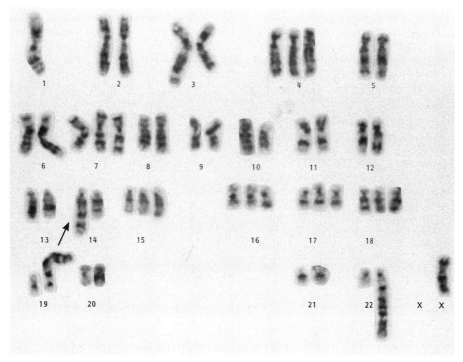

Figure 10.6 Karyotype of malignant cells from a case with advanced myelomatosis whose morphology was illustrated in Figure 10.3, showing complex chromosomal abnormalities. The arrow points to a marker 14q+ with a breakpoint at 14q32; the translocated material is p14–p27 from chromosome 3

one report[111], the Philadelphia (Ph) chromosome. The authors have seen a 14q+ marker (Figure 10.6) in all the metaphases obtained from the malignant pleural effusion of a patient with aggressive myeloma and poorly differentiated plasmablasts (see Figure 10.3). Chromosome abnormalities reported in Waldenström's macroglobulinaemia include trisomy 12 as in B-CLL[51].

The published data suggest that an abnormal karyotype is a feature of myelomas which are refractory to conventional therapy and have a shorter survival and that plasma cell leukaemia is almost always associated with 14q+. More prospective studies in newly diagnosed patients are necessary to assess more precisely the incidence and the nature of chromosome abnormalities seen in this disease. This information may be of value to consider whether patients with an abnormal karyotype should be treated differently from those with no abnormalities[34, 48]. A change in karyotype with the emergence of a new clone, e.g. monosomy 7, is associated with the development of myelodysplastic syndrome or acute myeloid leukaemia.

References

1. Ahre, A., Bjorkholm, M., Mellstedt, H. et al. (1983) Intermittent high dose melphalan/ prednisone vs continuous low dose melphalan treatment in multiple myeloma. *European Journal of Cancer and Clinical Oncology*, **19**, 499–506

2. Alexanian, R. (1980) Localized and indolent myeloma. *Blood*, **56**, 521–525
3. Alexanian, R., Balcerzak, S., Bonnet, J. D. et al. (1975) Prognostic factors in multiple myeloma. *Cancer*, **36**, 1192–1201
4. Alexanian, R., Bergsagel, D. E., Migliore, P. J., Vaughan, W. K. and Howe, C. D. (1968) Melphalan therapy for plasma cell myeloma. *Blood*, **31**, 1–10
5. Alexanian, R., Gehan, E., Haut, A., Saiki, J., Weick, J. for the Southwest Oncology Group (1978) Unmaintained remissions in multiple myeloma. *Blood*, **51**, 1005–1011
6. Alexanian, R., Salmon, S., Gutterman, J., Dixon, D., Bonnet, J. and Haut, A. (1981) Chemoimmunotherapy for multiple myeloma. *Cancer*, **47**, 1923–1929
7. Alexanian, R., Gutterman, J. and Levy, H. (1982) Interferon treatment for multiple myeloma. *Clinics in Haematology*, **11**, 211–220
8. Ameis, A., Ko, H. S. and Pruzanski, W. (1976) M components – a review of 1242 cases. *Canadian Medical Association Journal*, **114**, 889–895
9. Barlogie, B., Epstein, J., Selvanayagam, P. and Alexanian, R. (1989) Plasma cell myeloma – new biological insights and advances in therapy. *Blood*, **73**, 875–879
10. Barth, W. F., Willerson, J. T., Waldmann, T. A. and Decker, J. L. (1969) Primary amyloidosis. Clinical, immunochemical and immunoglobulin metabolism studies in fifteen patients. *American Journal of Medicine*, **47**, 259–273
11. Bartl, R., Frisch, B., Burkhardt, R. et al. (1982) Bone marrow histology in myeloma: its importance in diagnosis, prognosis, classification and staging. *British Journal of Haematology*, **51**, 361–375
12. Bartl, R., Frisch, B., Mahl, G. et al. (1983) Bone marrow histology in Waldenström's macroglobulinaemia. Clinical relevance of subtype recognition. *Scandinavian Journal of Haematology*, **31**, 359–375
13. Bataille, R. (1982) Localized plasmacytomas. *Clinics in Haematology*, **11**, 113–122
14. Bataille, R., Durie, B. G. M., Grenier, J. and Sany, J. (1986) Prognostic factors and staging in multiple myeloma: a reappraisal. *Journal of Clinical Oncology*, **4**, 80–87
15. Block, K. J. and Maki, D. G. (1973) Hyperviscosity syndromes associated with immunoglobulin abnormalities. *Seminars in Hematology*, **10**, 113–124
16. Blohkin, N., Larionov, L., Perevodchikova, N., Chebotareva, L. and Merkulova, N. (1958) Clinical experiences with sarcolysin in neoplastic diseases. *Annals of the New York Academy of Sciences*, **68**, 1128–1132
17. Boccadoro, M., Gavarotti, P., Fossati, G., Massaia, M., Pileri, A. and Durie, B. G. M. (1983) Kinetics of circulating B lymphocytes in human myeloma. *Blood*, **61**, 812–814
18. Brandes, L. H. and Israels, L. G. (1982) Treatment of advanced plasma cell myeloma with weekly cyclophosphamide and alternate-day prednisone. *Cancer Treatment Reports*, **66**, 1413–1415
19. Brouet, J. C., Mason, D. Y., Danon, F. et al. (1977) Alpha-chain disease: evidence for common clonal origin of intestinal immunoblastic lymphoma and plasmacytic proliferation. *Lancet*, i, 861
20. Brouet, J-C., Seligmann, M., Danon, F., Belpomme, D. and Fine, J. M. (1979) μ-Chain disease. Report of two new cases. *Archives of Internal Medicine*, **139**, 672–674
21. Brautbar, N. and Luboshitzky, R. (1977) Combined calcitonin and oral phosphate treatment for hypercalcemia in multiple myeloma. *Archives of Internal Medicine*, **7**, 914–916
22. Buckman, R., Cuzick, J. and Galton, D. A. G. (1982) Long-term survival in myelomatosis. A report to the MRC Working Party on Leukaemia in Adults. *British Journal of Haematology*, **52**, 589–599
23. Canale, D. D. Jr and Collins, R. D. (1974) Use of bone marrow particle sections in the diagnosis of multiple myeloma. *American Journal of Clinical Pathology*, **61**, 382–392
24. Carbone, P. P., Kellerhouse, L. E. and Gehan, E. A. (1967) Plasmacytic myeloma. A study of the relationship of survival to various clinical manifestations and anomalous protein type in 112 patients. *American Journal of Medicine*, **42**, 937–948
25. Carter, A. and Tatarsky, I. (1980) The physiopathological significance of benign monoclonal gammopathy: a study of 64 cases. *British Journal of Haematology*, **46**, 565–574
26. Case, D. C. Jr (1982) Combination chemotherapy (M-2) protocol (BCNU, Cyclophosphamide, Vincristine, Melphalan and Prednisone) for Waldenström's macroglobulinemia: preliminary report. *Blood*, **59**, 934–937

27. Case, D. C. Jr, Lee, B. J. III and Clarkson, B. D. (1977) Improved survival times in multiple myeloma treated with melphalan, prednisone, cyclophosphamide, vincristine and BCNU: M-2 protocol. *American Journal of Medicine*, **63**, 897–903

28. Cavo, M., Baccarani, M., Gobbi, M., Lipizer, A. and Tura, S. (1983) Prognostic value of bone marrow plasma cell infiltration in stage I multiple myeloma. *British Journal of Haematology*, **55**, 683–690

29. Cohen, A. S. and Shirahama, T. (1973) Electron microscopic analysis of isolated amyloid fibrils from patients with primary, secondary and myeloma-associated disease: A study utilizing shadowing and negative staining techniques. *Israel Journal of Medical Sciences*, **9**, 849–856

30. Cohen, H. J., Silberman, H. R., Larsen, W. E., Johnson, L., Bartolucci, A. A. and Durant, J. R. for the Southeastern Cancer Study Group (SECSG) (1979) Combination chemotherapy with intermittent 1-3-bis-(2-chloroethyl) 1-nitrosourea (BCNU), cyclophosphamide and prednisone for multiple myeloma. *Blood*, **54**, 824–836

31. Coleman, M., Saletan, S., Wolf, D., Nisce, L., Wasser, J., McIntyre, O. R. and Tulloh, M. (1982) Whole bone marrow irradiation for the treatment of multiple myeloma. *Cancer*, **49**, 1328–1333

32. Cuzick, J., Cooper, E. H. and MacLennan, I. C. M. (1985) The prognostic value of serum β2-microglobulin compared with other presentation features in myelomatosis. (A report to the Medical Research Council's Working Party on Leukaemia in Adults.) *British Journal of Cancer*, **52**, 1–6

33. Delamore, I. W. (1982) Hypercalcaemia and myeloma. *British Journal of Haematology*, **51**, 507–509

34. Dewald, G. W., Kyle, R. A., Hicks, G. A. and Greipp, P. R. (1985) The clinical significance of cytogenetic studies in 100 patients with multiple myeloma, plasma cell leukemia or amyloidosis. *Blood*, **66**, 380–390

35. Durie, B. G. M. and Salmon, S. E. (1975) A clinical staging system for multiple myeloma. Correlation of measured myeloma cell mass with presenting clinical features, response to treatment, and survival. *Cancer*, **36**, 842–854

36. Durie, B. G. M., Salmon, S. E. and Moon, T. E. (1980) Pretreatment tumor mass, cell kinetics and prognosis in multiple myeloma. *Blood*, **55**, 364–372

37. Durie, B. G. M., Salmon, S. E. and Mundy, G. R. (1981) Relation of osteoclast activating factor production to extent of bone disease in multiple myeloma. *British Journal of Haematology*, **47**, 21–30

38. Durie, B. G. M., Young, L. A. and Salmon, S. E. (1983) Human myeloma in vitro colony growth: interrelationships between drug sensitivity, cell kinetics and patient survival duration. *Blood*, **61**, 929–934

39. Eidelman, S., Parkins, R. A. and Rubin, C. E. (1966) Abdominal lymphoma presenting as malabsorption: a clinico-pathologic study of nine cases in Israel and a review of the literature. *Medicine*, **45**, 111–137

40. Falini, B., De Solas, I., Levine, A. M., Park, J. W., Lukes, R. J. and Taylor, C. R. (1982) Emergence of B-immunoblastic sarcoma in patients with multiple myeloma: a clinicopathologic study of 10 cases. *Blood*, **59**, 923–933

41. Fefer, A., Greenberg, P. D., Cheever, M. A. et al. (1982) Treatment of multiple myeloma (MM) with chemoradiotherapy and identical twin bone marrow transplantation (BMT). *Proceedings of the American Society of Clinical Oncology*, **1**, 188

42. Forte, F. A., Prelli, F., Yount, W. J., Jerry, L. M., Kochwa, S., Franklin, E. C. and Kunkel, H. G. (1970) Heavy chain disease of the μ (γM) type: report of the first case. *Blood*, **36**, 137–144

43. Franklin, E. C., Lowenstein, J., Bigelow, B. and Meltzer, M. (1964) Heavy chain disease: a new disorder of serum γ-globulins. Report of the first case. *American Journal of Medicine*, **37**, 332–350

44. Gallamini, A., Buffa, F., Bacigalupo, A. et al. (1987) Allogeneic bone marrow transplantation in multiple myeloma. *Acta Haematologica*, **77**, 111–114

45. Garrett, I. R., Durie, B. G. M., Nedwin, G. E. et al. (1987) Production of lymphotoxin, a bone-resorbing cytokine, by cultured human myeloma cells. *New England Journal of Medicine*, **317**, 526–532

46. Glenner, G. G. (1980) Amyloid deposits and amyloidosis. The B-fibrilloses. *New England Journal of Medicine*, **302**, 1283–1292

47. Glenner, G. G., Terry, W., Harada, M., Isersky, C. and Pape, D. (1971) Amyloid fibril proteins: proof of homology with immunoglobulin light chains by sequence analysis. *Science*, **172**, 1150–1151

47a. Gore, M. E., Selby, P. J., Viner, C. et al. (1989) Intensive treatment of multiple myeloma and criteria for complete remission. *Lancet*, **ii**, 779–882

48. Gould, J., Alexanian, R., Goodacre, A., Pathak, S., Hecht, B. and Barlogie, B. (1988) Plasma cell karyotype in multiple myeloma. *Blood*, **71**, 453–456

49. Greipp, P. R. and Kyle, R. A. (1983) Clinical, morphological and cell kinetic differences among multiple myeloma, monoclonal gammopathy of undetermined significance, and smoldering multiple myeloma. *Blood*, **62**, 166–171

50. Hamburger, A. W. and Salmon, S. E. (1977) Primary bioassay of human tumor stem cells. *Science*, **197**, 461–463

51. Han, T., Samadori, N., Takeuchi, J. et al. (1983) Clonal chromosome abnormalities in patients with Waldenström's and CLL-associated macroglobulinemia: significance of trisomy 12. *Blood*, **63**, 525–531

52. Hobbs, J. R. (1969) Immunochemical classes of myelomatosis. Including data from a therapeutic trial conducted by a Medical Research Council Working Party. *British Journal of Haematology*, **16**, 599–606

53. Holland, J. F., Hosley, H., Sharlau, C. et al. (1966) A controlled trial of urethane treatment in multiple myeloma. *Blood*, **27**, 328–342

54. Isbister, J. P., Biggs, J. C. and Penny, R. (1978) Experience with large volume plasmapheresis in malignant paraproteinaemia and immune disorders. *Australian and New Zealand Journal of Medicine*, **8**, 154–164

55. Jackson, N., Ling, N. R., Ball, J., Bromidge, E., Nathan, P. D. and Franklin, I. M. (1988) An analysis of myeloma plasma cell phenotype using antibodies defined at the IIIrd international workshop on human leukocyte differentiation antigens. *Clinical and Experimental Immunology*, **72**, 351–356

56. Jancelewicz, Z., Takatsuki, K., Sugai, S. and Pruzanski, W. (1975) IgD multiple myeloma. Review of 133 cases. *Archives of Internal Medicine*, **135**, 87–93

57. Kapadia, S. B., Desai, U. and Cheng, V. S. (1982) Extramedullary plasmacytoma of the head and neck. A clinicopathologic study of 20 cases. *Medicine*, **61**, 317–329

58. Krajny, M. and Pruzanski, W. (1976) Waldenström's macroglobulinaemia: review of 45 cases. *Canadian Medical Association Journal*, **114**, 899–905

59. Kyle, R. A. (1975) Multiple myeloma. Review of 869 cases. *Mayo Clinic Proceedings*, **50**, 29–40

60. Kyle, R. A. (1978) Monoclonal gammopathy of undetermined significance. Natural history in 241 cases. *American Journal of Medicine*, **64**, 814–826

61. Kyle, R. A. (1982) Monoclonal gammopathy of undetermined significance (MGUS): a review. *Clinics in Haematology*, **11**, 123–150

62. Kyle, R. A. (1987) Is there a correct time to begin treatment of multiple myeloma? *Haematologica*, **72**, 107–110

63. Kyle, R. A. and Griepp, P. R. (1980) Smoldering multiple myeloma. *New England Journal of Medicine*, **302**, 1347–1349

64. Kyle, R. A., Maldonado, J. E. and Bayrd, E. D. (1974) Plasma cell leukemia. Report on 17 cases. *Archives of Internal Medicine*, **133**, 813–818

65. Lauria, F., Foa, R., Cavo, M. et al. (1984) Membrane phenotype and functional behaviour of T lymphocytes in multiple myeloma: correlation with clinical stages of the disease. *Clinical and Experimental Immunology*, **56**, 653–658

66. Liang, W., Hopper, J. E. and Rowley, J. D. (1979) Karyotypic abnormalities and clinical aspects of patients with multiple myeloma and related paraproteinemic disorders. *Cancer*, **44**, 630–644

67. Lindstrom, F. D. and Dahlstrom, U. (1978) Multiple myeloma or benign monoclonal gammopathy? A study of differential diagnostic criteria in 44 cases. *Clinical Immunology and Immunopathology*, **10**, 168–174

68. Lokhorst, H. M., Meuwissen, O. J. A. Th., Bast, E. J. E. G. and Dekker, A. W. (1989) VAD chemotherapy for refractory multiple myeloma. *British Journal of Haematology*, **71**, 25–30

69. Ludwig, H., Fruhwald, F., Tscholakoff, D., Rasoul, S., Neuhold, A. and Fritz, E. (1987) Magnetic resonance imaging of the spine in multiple myeloma. *Lancet*, **ii**, 364–366

69a. MacLennan, I. C., Kelly, K., Crockson, R. A., Cooper, E. H., Cuzick, J. and Chapman, C. (1988) Results of the MRC myelomatosis trials for patients entered since 1980. *Hematological Oncology*, **6**, 145–158

70. Mackenzie, M. R. and Fudenberg, H. H. (1972) Macroglobulinemia: an analysis for forty patients. *Blood*, **39**, 874–889

71. McArthur, J. R., Athens, J. W., Wintrobe, M. M. and Cartwright, G. E. (1970) Melphalan and myeloma. Experience with a low-dose continuous regimen. *Annals of Internal Medicine*, **72**, 665–670

72. McCallister, B. D., Batrd, E. D., Harrison, E. G. Jr and McGuckin, W. F. (1967) Primary macroglobulinemia. Review with a report on thirty-one cases and notes on the value of continuous chlorambucil therapy. *American Journal of Medicine*, **43**, 394–434

73. McElwain, T. J. and Powles, R. L. (1983) High-dose intravenous melphalan for plasma-cell leukaemia and myeloma. *Lancet*, **ii**, 822–824

74. Medical Research Council (1971) Myelomatosis: comparison of melphalan and cyclophosphamide therapy. *British Medical Journal*, **1**, 640–641

75. Medical Research Council (1973) Report on the first myelomatosis trial. Part 1. Analysis of presenting features of prognostic importance. *British Journal of Haematology*, **24**, 123–139

76. Medical Research Council (1980) Prognostic features in the third MRC myelomatosis trial. *British Journal of Cancer*, **42**, 831–840

77. Medical Research Council (1980) Report on the second myelomatosis trial after five years of follow-up. *British Journal of Cancer*, **42**, 813–822

78. Medical Research Council (1984) Analysis and management of renal failure in fourth MRC myelomatosis trial. *British Medical Journal*, **288**, 1411–1416

79. Medical Research Council Working Party on Leukaemia in Adults (prepared by MacLennan, I. C. M. and Cusick, J.) (1985) Objective evaluation of the role of vincristine in induction and maintenance therapy for myelomatosis. *British Journal of Cancer*, **52**, 153–158

80. Mellstedt, H., Holm, G., Pettersson, D. et al. (1982) T cell in monoclonal gammapathies. *Scandinavian Journal of Haematology*, **29**, 57–64

81. Merlini, G., Gobbi, P. G., Riccardi, A., Riva, G., Sardi, C. and Perugini, S. (1982) Peptichemio induction therapy in myelomatosis. *Cancer Chemotherapy and Pharmacology*, **8**, 9–16

82. Millar, B. C., Bell, J. B. G., Lakhani, A., Ayliffe, M. J., Selby, P. J. and McElwain, T. J. (1988) A simple method for culturing myeloma cells from human bone marrow aspirates and peripheral blood in vitro. *British Journal of Haematology*, **69**, 197–203

83. Misiani, R., Remuzzi, G., Bertani, T. et al. (1979) Plasmapheresis in the treatment of acute renal failure in multiple myeloma. *American Journal of Medicine*, **66**, 684–688

84. Mundy, G. R., Raisz, L. G., Cooper, R. A., Schechter, G. R. and Salmon, S. E. (1974) Evidence for the secretion of an osteoclast stimulating factor in myeloma. *New England Journal of Medicine*, **291**, 1041–1046

85. Nordenson, N. G. (1966) Myelomatosis. A clinical review of 310 cases. *Acta Medica Scandinavica Supplementum*, **179** (445), 178–186

86. Norfolk, D., Child, J. A., Cooper, E. H., Kerruish, S. and Milford Ward, A. (1980) Serum β_2-microglobulin in myelomatosis: potential value in stratification and monitoring. *British Journal of Cancer*, **42**, 510–515

87. Oken, M. M. and Kay, N. E. (1981) T-cell subpopulations in multiple myeloma: correlation with clinical disease status. *British Journal of Haematology*, **49**, 629–634

88. Osanto, S., Muller, H. P., Schuit, H. R. E., Van Nieuwkoop, J. A. and Willemze, R. (1983) Primary plasma cell leukaemia. A case report and a review of the literature. *Acta Haematologica*, **70**, 122–129

89. Osgood, E. E. (1960) The survival time of patients with plasmocytic myeloma. *Cancer Chemotherapy Reports*, **9**, 1–10

90. Osserman, E. F., DiRe, L. B., DiRe, J., Sherman, W. H., Hersman, J. A. and Storb, R. (1982) Identical twin marrow transplantation in multiple myeloma. *Acta Haematologica*, **68**, 215–223

91. Paccagnella, A., Cartei, G., Fosser, V. et al. (1983) Treatment of multiple myeloma with M-2 protocol and without maintenance therapy. *European Journal of Cancer and Clinical Oncology*, **19**, 1345–1351

92. Parreira, A., Robinson, D. S. F., Melo, J. V. et al. (1985) Primary plasma cell leukaemia: immunological and ultrastructural studies in 6 cases. *Scandinavian Journal of Haematology*, **35**, 433–441

93. Perri, R. T., Oken, M. M. and Kay, N. E. (1982) Enhanced T cell suppression is directed toward sensitive circulating B cells in multiple myeloma. *Journal of Laboratory and Clinical Medicine*, **99**, 512–519

94. Pezzutto, A., Semenzato, G., Agostini, C., Raimondi, R. and Gasparotto, G. (1981) Subpopulations of T-lymphocytes in multiple myeloma. *Scandinavian Journal of Haematology*, **26**, 333–338

95. Philip, P., Drivsholm, A., Hansen, N. E., Jensen, M. K. and Killman, S-A. (1980) Chromosomes and survival in multiple myeloma. A banding study of 25 cases. *Cancer Genetics and Cytogenetics*, **2**, 243–257

96. Presant, C. A. and Klahr, C. (1978) Adriamycin, 1,3-bis(2-chloromethyl)-1-nitrosourea (BCNU, NSC 409962), cyclophosphamide plus prednisone (ABC-P) in melphalan-resistant multiple myeloma. *Cancer*, **42**, 1222–1227

97. Pruzansky, W. and Watt, J. G. (1972) Serum viscosity and hyperviscosity syndrome in IgG multiple myeloma. *Annals of Internal Medicine*, **77**, 853–860

98. Quesada, J. R., Alexanian, R., Hawkins, M., Barlogie, B., Borden, E., Itri, L. and Gutterman, J. U. (1986) Treatment of multiple myeloma with recombinant a-interferon. *Blood*, **67**, 275–278

99. Rambaud, J. C., Galian, A., Danon, F. G. et al. (1983) Alpha-chain disease without qualitative serum IgA abnormality. Report of two cases, including a 'nonsecretory' form. *Cancer*, **51**, 686–693

100. Salmon, S. E. (1982) In vitro cloning and chemosensitivity of human myeloma stem cells. *Clinics in Haematology*, **11**, 47–63

101. Salmon, S. E., Haut, A., Bonnet, J. D. et al. (1983) Alternating combination chemotherapy and levamisole improves survival in multiple myeloma: a Southwest Oncology Group Study. *Journal of Clinical Oncology*, **1**, 453–461

102. Salmon, S. E. and Smith, B. A. (1970) Immunoglobulin synthesis and total body tumor cell number in IgG multiple myeloma. *Journal of Clinical Investigation*, **49**, 1114–1121

102a. Samson, D., F Gaminara, E., Newland, A. et al. (1989) Infusion of vincristine and doxorubicin with oral dexamethasone as first-line therapy for multiple myeloma. *Lancet*, **ii**, 882–888

103. Salmon, S. E. and Wampler, S. B. (1977) Multiple myeloma: quantitative staging and assessment of response with a programmable pocket computer. *Blood*, **49**, 379–389

104. Santoro, A., Schieppati, G., Franchi, F., Valagussa, P. and Monfardini, S. (1983) Clinical staging and therapeutic results in multiple myeloma. *European Journal of Cancer and Clinical Oncology*, **19**, 1353–1359

105. Scarffe, J. H., Anderson, H., Palmer, M. K. and Crowther, D. (1983) Prognostic significance of pretreatment serum β2-microglobulin levels in multiple myeloma. *European Journal of Cancer and Clinical Oncology*, **19**, 1361–1364

105a. Selby, P. J., McElwain, T. J., Nandi, A. C. et al. (1987) Multiple myeloma treated with high dose intravenous melphalan. *British Journal of Haematology*, **66**, 55–62

106. Seligmann, M., Danon, F., Hurez, D., Mihaesco, E. and Preud'homme, J-L. (1968) Alpha-chain disease: a new immunoglobulin abnormality. *Science*, **162**, 1396–1397

107. Seligmann, M., Mihaesco, E., Preud'homme, J-L., Danon, F. and Brouet, J. C. (1979) Heavy chain diseases: current findings and concepts. *Immunology Reviews*, **48**, 145–167

108. Seligmann and Rambaud, J. C. (1969) IgA abnormalities in abdominal lymphoma (α-chain disease). *Israel Journal of Medical Sciences*, **5**, 151–157

109. Stamp, T. C. B., Child, J. A. and Walker, P. G. (1975) Treatment of osteolytic myelomatosis with mithramycin. *Lancet*, **i**, 719–722

109a. Tura, S., Cavo, M., Baccarani, M., Ricci, P. and Gobbi, M. (1986) Bone marrow transplantation in multiple myeloma. *Scandinavian Journal of Haematology*, **36**, 176–179

110. Ueshima, Y., Fukuhara, S., Nagai, K., Takatsuki, K. and Uchino, H. (1983) Cytogenetic studies and clinical aspects of patients with plasma cell leukemia and leukemic macroglobulinemia. *Cancer Research*, **43**, 905–912

111. Van Den Berge, H., Louwagie, A., Broeckaert-Van Orshoven, A. et al. (1979) Philadelphia chromosome in human multiple myeloma. *Journal of National Cancer Institute*, **63**, 11–16

112. Van Den Berghe, H., Vermaelen, K., Louwagie, A., Criel, A., Mecucci, C. and Vaerman, J. P. (1984) High incidence of chromosome abnormalities in IgG3 myeloma. *Cancer Genetics and Cytogenetics,* **11,** 381–387

113. Wahlin, A., Roos, G., Rudolphi, O. and Holm, J. (1982) Melphalan-related leukaemia in multiple myeloma. *Acta Medica Scandinavica,* **211,** 203–208

114. Waldenström, J. (1944) Incipient myelomatosis or 'essential' hyperglobulinaemia with fibrinogen-openia – a new syndrome? *Acta Medica Scandinavica,* **117,** 216–247

115. Waldenström, J. G. (1986) Macroglobulinaemia – a review. *Haematologica,* **71,** 437–440

116. WHO Meeting Report (1976) Alpha-chain disease and related small intestinal lymphoma. *Archives Françaises des Maladies de l'Appareil Digestif,* **65,** 591–607

117. Wiltshaw, E. (1976) The natural history of extramedullary plasmacytoma and its relation to solitary myeloma of bone and myelomatosis. *Medicine,* **55,** 217–238

118. Woodruff, R. K., Malpas, J. S., Paxton, A. M. and Lister, T. A. (1978) Plasma cell leukemia (PCL): a report on 15 patients. *Blood,* **52,** 839–845

119. Woodruff, R. K., Wadsworth, J., Malpas, J. S. and Tobias, J. S. (1979) Clinical staging in multiple myeloma. *British Journal of Haematology,* **42,** 199–205

120. Woodruff, R. K., Whittle, R. J. and Malpas, J. S. (1979) Solitary plasmocytoma I: Extramedullary soft tissue plasmocytoma. *Cancer,* **43,** 2340–2343

121. Yamada, K., Shionoya, S., Amano, M. and Imamura, Y. (1983) A Burkitt-type 8;14 translocation in a case of plasma cell leukemia. *Cancer Genetics and Cytogenetics,* **9,** 67–70

Index

Acid hydrolases, 38, 117, 119, 137, 144, 145, 147
Acid phosphatase, *see under* Cytochemistry
Acute leukaemia markers, 19
Acute lymphoblastic leukaemia, 32
  acid hydrolases, 38
  acid phosphatase, *see under* Cytochemistry
  adult-ALL, *see* Adult ALL
  ANAE, *see* Cytochemistry
  anaemia, 33
  antigen, 7, 8, 39, 42
  B-ALL, 34, 41, 48, 62, 63, 205, 206
  B- and T-markers, *see* Immunological classification
  biphenotypic, *see* Biphenotypic leukaemia
  blood counts, 33
  bone marrow, 33
  bone marrow transplantation, *see* Bone marrow transplantation
  Burkitt-type ALL, 34, 41, 48, 62, 63, 205, 206
  cell cycle, 36, 37, 45, 46, 53
  chromosomes, 58
    see also Chromosome abnormalities
  classification, immunological, *see* Immunological classification
  incidence of subtypes, 41, 64
  MIC classification, 60
  morphological, 33
  see also FAB classification
  clinical features, 32, 33
  see also under Anterior mediastinal mass
  CNS complications, 50, 52, 53, 55
  complete remission, 33
  common-ALL, *see* Common-ALL
  cytochemistry, *see* Cytochemistry
  epidemiology, 64, 65
  FAB types, *see under* FAB classification
  gene rearrangements, *see under* Gene rearrangements

Acute lymphoblastic leukaemia, (*cont.*)
  β-glucosaminidase, 38
  β-glucuronidase, 38
  granular ALL, 36
  hand-mirror variant, 36
  hypercalcaemia, immunological subtypes, *see* Immunological classification
  infections, *see under Infections*
  intravascular coagulation, 33
  isoenzymes, 39
  meningeal leukaemia, 53, 55
  monoclonal antibodies, *see* Monoclonal antibodies
  morphology, 33
    see also FAB classification
  myeloid antigens, 50
  non-T, non-B-ALL, 39
  null-ALL, 42, 48
  PAS reaction, 37
    see also Cytochemistry
  Ph-positive ALL, 60
    see also Philadelphia positive ALL
  pre-B-ALL, 16, 39, 41
  karyotype, 58, 60
  prognostic factors, 45
    see also Prognostic factors in ALL
  relapse, 54
    see also Relapse in ALL
  relation to NHL, 47
  scoring for ALL, 34
  special subtypes, 36, 47
  T-ALL, 40, 47
    see also T-lymphoblastic leukaemia
  TdT, 40
    see also Terminal transferase
  testicular relapse, 55, 56
  translocation t(4;11), 61, 62
  treatment, *see* Treatment of ALL
  WBC, 33, 46
Acute myeloid leukaemia, 18, 19, 49
  AML, MO, 50
  biphenotypic, 49
  chloroma in children, 65

Acute myeloid leukaemia, (*cont.*)
  cytochemistry, 18, 36
    see also Cytochemistry
  biphenotypic, 49
  gene rearrangements, 244, 246
  esterase, 18
  expression of CD7, 12
  Fc receptors, 19
  megakaryoblastic, 18
  monoblasts, 36
  myeloperoxidase, 18, 36
  non-specific binding of McAbs, 19
  phenotype, 19
  Sudan black B, 18
  TdT, 18
    see also Terminal transferase
Adenosine deaminase, 39
  ADA inhibitor, 39, 170, 267
  in treatment, *see* Deoxycoformycin
  deficiency, 267
  levels in ALL, 39
  levels in AML, 39
  levels in T-lymphoblasts, 267
Adult-ALL, 49
  danorubicin, 54
  differences with childhood ALL, 49
  induction therapy, 51
  meningeal leukaemia, 53
  morphology, 35
  prognosis, 49
  reinductions, 54
Adult T-cell leukaemia/lymphoma, 218
  acute ATLL, 218
  age of incidence, 219
  anaemia, 219, 221
  antibodies to HTLV-I, 227, 232, 233, 235
  anti-Tac, 15, 225, 227, 228
  association with HTLV-I, 231
    see also HTLV-I
  Black patients, 219
  blood counts, 221
  bone marrow, 219, 221, 222, 230
  Caribbean ATLL, 219, 233, 239
  Caribbean basin, 239
  Carribean immigrants to the UK, 239

Adult T-cell leukaemia/lymphoma, (cont.)
chest X-rays, 218
chromosome abnormalities, see Chromosome abnormalities
chronic ATLL, 219
clinical evolution, 119, 222
clinical features, 218, 219, 220
clinical forms, 219
clonality of viral integration, 218, 227, 243
CT scans, 218
cytochemistry, see Cytochemistry
diagnostic criteria, 227
diagnostic tests, 221, 277
differential diagnosis, 227
DNA analysis of provirus, 218, 228, 237, 243
epidemiology, 233, 234, 235, 238, 240
family studies, 234
function of ATLL cells, 226, 227
hepatomegaly, 219
histopathology, 228
HTLV-I, see under HTLV-I
hypercalcaemia, 218, 219, 225, 227, 230
IL-2 receptors, 15, 226, 231
in pathogenesis of ATLL, 227
see also Interleukin-2
incubation period, 240
laboratory findings, 219, 220, 221
long-term culture, 231
lymph node histology, 228, 229
lymphadenopathy, 218, 227
lymphocytosis, 221, 237
lymphoma-type ATLL, 219
lymphosarcoma-cell leukaemia, 222
markers, see phenotype
morphology, 221, 223, 224, 236
osteolytic lesions, 219, 230
pathogenesis of ATLL, 237, 243
peripheral T-cell lymphoma, 228, 229
phenotype, 17, 18, 119, 225, 277
low density CD3, 225
relation to function, 224, 227
subset analysis, 226
terminal transferase, 225
presenting features, 219, 220
prognosis, 240, 241
racial factors, 240
serology, 228, 235, 238
see also HTLV-I
skin lesions, 218, 219, 230
smouldering ATLL, 218, 237
south west of Japan, 233, 239
splenomegaly, 219
stages of HTLV-I infection, 235
Strongyloides, 236, 237
thrombocytopenia, 221
treatment, 240, 241
ultrastructure, 230, 231, 232, 236
WBC, 220, 221
Amyloidosis, 173, 293, 294
Anterior mediastinal mass, 32
in ALL, 33, 46

Anterior mediastinal mass, (cont.)
prognostic factor, 46
in T-ALL, 47
thymic tumour, 47
In T-LbLy, 47
Aplastic anaemia, 24
role of T-cells, 24

B-cell chronic lymphocytic leukaemia, 73
age, 83, 84
alkylating agents, 96
anaemia, 76
of advanced CLL, 76
haemolytic, 76, 88
prognosis, 84
red cell aplasia, see Red cell aplasia
secondary, 76, 94
in staging, 86, 89
see also Immune haemolytic anaemia
animal model, 74
association with Hodgkin's disease, 94
association with myeloma, 90
association with other malignancies, 94
autoimmune phenomena, 88, 89
blood counts, 76
bone marrow, 77, 84, 99
causes of death, 84
CD5 antigen, 15, 17, 80
cell volume, 81, 174, 204
chest X-ray, 75
chromosome abnormalities, see under Chromosome abnormalities
class II antigen, 8
clinical findings, 75, 85
CLL/PL, 84, 90, 132
clonality, 78
complications, 86
Coombs' test, 88
corticosteroids, 97, 98
crystalline inclusions, 76
CyIg, 80, 81, 92
diagnosis, 75
electron microscopy, 82, 83
epithelial cancers, 94
Evans' syndrome, 88
familial CLL, 74
FMC7, 8, 9, 17, 80, 81, 90
gene rearrangements, 79, 140, 244
see also under Gene rearrangements
haemophagocytic syndrome, 88
HLA-linkage, 74
hypercalcaemia, 78, 89
hypersplenism, 95
hypogammaglobulinaemia, 86
IL-2 receptors, 80, 102
imaging, 75
immunity, 86, 88
immunoblastic lymphoma, 77
incidence, 73
indications for treatment, 94
infections, 86

B-cell chronic lymphocytic leukaemia, (cont.)
karotype, 104
laboratory tests, 75, 78
lymph node biopsy, 78
lymphocyte count, 76, 84
lymphocyte doubling time, 83, 84
markers, see phenotype
maturation, 81, 176
'M' bands, 78, 92, 133
M:F ratio, 74, 204
morphology, 76, 84
M-rosettes, 5, 17, 79, 90
nephrotic syndrome, 89
osetolytic lesions, 89, 173
phenotype, 5, 8, 15, 16, 17, 79, 80
changes with maturation, 81
differences from NHL, 187
McAbs, 80
see also Monoclonal antibodies
membrane CD22, 7, 80
platelet counts, 76
presenting symptoms, 75
prognostic factors, see Prognostic factors in CLL
progressive disease, 94
prolymphocytes, 76
increase in, 90, 91
prognostic value, 92
ultrastructure, 82
prolymphocytoid transformation, 76, 90
CLL/PL, 90, 92
morphology, 90, 91
phenotype, 80, 90, 92
prognosis, 84, 92
response to treatment, 92
survival, 92
ultrastructure, 82
radiation, 98
red cell aplasia, 24, 89
response to treatment, 85, 92, 95
see also Treatment of B-CLL
prognostic value, see Prognostic factors in B-CLL
Richter's syndrome, 17, 75, 78, 92, 93
second neoplasms, 94
serum Ig, 78
sex, 83, 84
skin cancer, 94
SmIg, 17, 78, 80, 81
splenectomy, 86, 99, 100
splenic form, 75
splenic sequestration, 99
staging systems, 85
Binet, 84, 86, 87
International, 75, 76, 85, 87
Rai, 75, 76, 84, 85, 87
survival, 85, 87, 92
T-cell function, 21, 100, 101, 102
T-cell imbalance, 101, 102
thrombocytopenia, 76
immune, 88, 89, 97, 99
pathogenesis, 76
prognosis, 84
staging, 86, 89
T-lymphocytes, 76, 80, 101, 102

B-cell chronic lymphocytic
    leukaemia, (cont.)
    transformation, 90
        acute leukaemia, 90, 93
        immunoblastic, 90, 92
        plasmacytoma, 90
        prolymphocytoid, 90
    treatment, see under Treatment
        of B-CLL
    tumour necrosis factor, 106
    urticarial reactions, 88
B-cell differentiation, 9, 16, 21
    anti-HC2, 176
    in B-CLL, 81
    pathway, 40
    T-cell help, 21, 24
Benign monoclonal gammopathy,
    292, 300
Biphenotypic leukaemias, 49
    chromosome abnormalities, 40
    clinical significance, 50
    co-expression of markers, 50
    cytochemistry, 37, 50
    phenotypic switch, 49
    prognostic significance, 50
    translocation t(4;11), 50, 61
    translocation t(9;22), 50
    treatment, 50
B-lymphocytes, 5, 6
    acid hydrolases, 145
    antigens, 6, 7, 10, 15
    cell lines, 25
    colonies, 25
    function, 20
    pre-B-cells, 39
Bone marrow, 33, 77
    in ALL, 33
    in B-CLL, 77, 84, 99
    in Burkitt's lymphoma, 48
    in HCL, 158
    myelofibrosis, 33
    in PLL, 141
    in T-ALL, 47
    in T-LbLy, 47
    T-markers, 14
    transplantation, see Bone
        marrow transplantation
Bone marrow transplantation, 57
    in ALL, 57
    in ALL-L3 type, 207, 211
    allogeneic, 49, 57
    in AML, 57
    with antibody purging, 212
    autologous, 58, 212
    in B-ALL, 49
    in CGL, 57
    in complete remission, 57, 58, 212
    in HCL, 170
    in high-grade NHL, 212
    in myeloma, 287, 289
    non-T-ALL, 57
    T-ALL, 57
Burkitt's lymphoma, 34, 47, 48, 62,
    205
    ALL, L3 type, 34, 205, 206, 207
    B-ALL, Burkitt type, 48, 62
        abdominal masses, 48, 205,
            206
        karyotype, 62

Burkitt's lymphoma, (cont.)
    B-ALL, Burkitt type, (cont.)
        nerve involvement, 62
        phenotype, 41, 206
        presentation, 48
        survival, 63
    bilateral hypoaesthesia, 62
    bone marrow involvement, 34,
        48, 205, 207
    bone marrow transplantation, 49
    C3b receptors, 205
    chromosome changes, 34, 48, 59,
        60, 62, 63, 205, 207, 212,
        213, 214
        abnormal no. 1, 62
        breakpoints, 63, 213
        correlation with phenotype, 207
        correspondence with light
            chains, 63
        errors during Ig gene
            rearrangement, 207, 213,
            214
        t(2;8), 60, 62, 63, 207, 213
        t(8;14), 59, 60, 62, 207, 212,
            213, 214
        t(8;22), 60, 62, 63, 207, 213
    clinical course, 207
    clinical features, 48, 62, 205
    c-myc gene, 63, 64, 213, 214
    CNS leukaemia, 206
    CNS prophylaxis, 211
    cytotoxic T-lymphocytes, 206
    endemic form, 48, 62, 205, 206
    epidemiology, 64
    Epstein–Barr virus, 205, 206
    histological classification, 205
    immune response, 206
    jaw tumour, 48, 205
    lactic dehydrogenase, 207
    lymph node histology, 205
    lymph node imprint, 34, 205
    malaria, 206
    metabolic abnormalities, 48
    molecular basis, 63
    morphology, 205
    non-endemic form, 48, 205, 206,
        207
    pathogenesis, 206
    phenotype, 205, 206
    presentation as B-ALL, 48
    prognosis, 207
    similarities to B-ALL, 48
    treatment, 207, 211
    tumour lysis syndrome, 48
    types of, 205
    variant translocations, 62, 213
    WBC, 48

Cell cycle, 20, 45
    in ALL, 36, 37, 45, 46, 53
    ploidy of Sézary cells, 269
    T-lymphocytes, 20
Cell kinetics in ALL, 36, 37, 45, 46,
    53
Cell markers, see immunological
    markers and monoclonal
    antibodies
Cell volume estimations, 81, 204
    in B-CLL, 81, 174, 204

Cell volume estimations, (cont.)
    in CLL/PL, 81, 84
    in follicular lymphoma, 185
    in HCL, 82, 174, 175, 186, 204
    in HCL-variant, 174, 175, 204
    immunoblasts, 82, 185, 186
    in NHL, 185
    in PLL, 82, 174, 186, 204
    in Sézary syndrome, 257
    in SLVL, 185, 204
Centrocytic lymphoma, see
    Intermediate lymphoma
Chromosome abnormalities, 59
    in ALL, 46, 58, 59
        correlation with phenotype,
            58, 60
        prognostic value, 46, 59
    in ATLL, 242
        breakpoints in no. 14, 242
        clinical progression, 243
        trisomies, 153, 242, 243, 270
    in B-ALL, 48
    in B-cell lines, 25, 206, 207
    in B-CLL, 104
        analysis by McAbs, 106
        common abnormalities, 104
        marker 14q+, 105
        normal metaphases, 106
        prognostic value, 85, 105
        translocation t(11;14), 214,
            301
        trisomy 12, 105, 106, 214, 215
    in biphenotypic leukaemias, 50
    in B-PLL, 60, 151, 152, 214, 301
    in Burkitt lymphoma, 25, 48,
        206, 212
    in Burkitt-type ALL, 62, 214
        abnormal chromosome 1, 62
        variant translocations, 62, 207,
            213
        see also under Burkitt's
            lymphoma
    in CGL blast crisis, 61
    in CTCL, 269, 270
    errors during gene
        rearrangement, 150, 207, 214
    in follicular lymphoma, see
        Follicular lymphoma
    frequency in ALL, 59
    in HCL, 177
    hyperdiploidy in ALL, 59
    hypotetraploid in Sézary cells,
        269
    in intermediate lymphoma, 213,
        214
    inversion 14, 126, 152, 242
    involvement of oncogenes, 213,
        214
        see also Oncogenes
    juxtaposition of Ig genes and
        oncogenes, 213, 214
        see also Oncogenes
    in large cell NHL, 212, 213
    in lymphocytic NHL, 213, 214
    in myeloma, 301, 302
    in NHLs, 212, 213, 214, 215, 301
    Ph-positive ALL, 60, 61, 63
    in plasma cell leukaemia, 301
    prognostic value in ALL, 45, 59

Chromosome abnormalities, (*cont.*)
  prolymphocytic leukaemia, 150
  pseudodiploidy in ALL, 59
  in T-ALL, 58, 60, 152
  in T-CLL, 126
  in T-PLL, 126, 152, 153
  translocations in ALL, 58, 59
    survival, 59
    t(1;19), 58, 60
    t(4;11), 59, 61, 62
    t(8;14), 48, 59
      see also under Burkitt's
        lymphoma
    t(9;22), 59
      see also Philadelphia
        positive ALL
    t(11;14), 58, 60, 152
  trisomy 12, 105, 213, 214, 215,
    302
  in Waldenström's
    macroglobulinaemia, 302
Chronic lymphocytic leukaemia,
  see B-cell CLL and T-cell CLL
Class II MHC antigens, *see under*
  Monoclonal antibodies and
  HLA-DR
CNS complications in ALL, 50, 52,
  53, 55
Common-ALL, 16, 39, 42
  cALL antigen, 7, 8, 39, 42
  cALL gene, 42
  epidemiology, 64
  gene rearrangements, 43
  karyotype, 58
  monoclonal antibody, 7, 16, 39
  neutral endopeptidase, 42
  phenotype, 41, 42
  phorbol ester effect, 42
  polyclonal antiserum, 39
  in thymic cells, 43
Common leucocyte antigen, 14
Complement receptors, 8
  C3b, 205
  C3d, 8
  CR2, 8
Cutaneous T-cell lymphomas, 253
  blood chemistry, 255
  blood counts, 254
  blood films, 262
  bone marrow, 255
  causes of death, 263
  cell markers, *see phenotype*
  chest X-rays, 255
  chromosome abnormalities, 269,
    270
  clinical features, 253
  colonies, 21
  cytochemistry, 119, 258
    see also Cytochemistry
  delayed hypersensitivity, 268
  dermatopathic
    lymphadenopathy, 262
  diagnosis, 256
  differences with ATLL, 219
  differential diagnosis, 261
  evolution, 119
  gene rearrangement, *see under*
    T-cell receptor gene
  hepatomegaly, 253, 264

Cutaneous T-cell lymphomas, (*cont.*)
  histopathology, 259
    epidermotropism, 259
    lymph nodes, 260
    skin, 259
  HTLV-I serology, 228
  IL-2 receptor, 15
  immunocytochemistry, 261
  incidence, 253
  infections, 263
  laboratory findings, 253
  lymph nodes, 253, 264
  lymphomatoid papulosis, 262
  'M' bands, 255
  mycosis fungoides, *see* Mycosis
    fungoides
  natural history, 262
  nature of the Sézary cell, *see*
    Sézary syndrome
  phenotype, 15, 17, 18, 119, 260,
    261, 269
  prognosis, 262, 263, 264
  serum Igs, 255
  Sézary syndrome, *see* Sézary
    syndrome
  skin lesions, 255, 263
  staging systems, 263
  T-cell activation, 269
  TCR rearrangement, 262
  T-lymphocyte function, 268, 269
  treatment, 264
    alkylating agents, 266
    anti-thymocyte globulin, 268
    bleomycin, 266
    carmustine, 265
    chemotherapy, 266
    CHOP, COP, HOP, 266, 267
    combined approach, 267
    cytosine arabinoside, 265
    DCF, *see under*
      Deoxycoformycin
    doxorubicin, 266
    electron beam therapy, 266
    extracorporeal
      photoactivation, 265
    folinic acid, 266
    leucapheresis, 267
    mechloretamine, 265
    methotrexate, 266
    methoxsalen, 265
    8-methoxysporalen, 265
    monoclonal antibodies, 268
    photochemotherapy, 265
    phototherapy, 265
    radiotherapy, 266
    retinoic acid, 267
    topical, 265
    ultraviolet light, 265
    ultrastructural analysis, 257,
      258, 259, 264, 269
Cytochemistry, 36, 144
  acid hydrolases, 38, 117, 119,
    137, 145, 147
  acid phosphatase, 37, 38, 145
    ALL, 37
    ATLL, 119, 144
    B-cells, 145
    B-CLL, 144
    B-PLL, 144, 146

Cytochemistry, (*cont.*)
  acid phosphatase, (*cont.*)
    fetal thymocytes, 37
    HCL, 144, 145, 160
    isoenzyme, 5, 145, 160
    lymphoplasmacytic
      lymphoma, 144
    myeloma, 144
    plasma cells, 145
    pre-T-ALL, 37, 38, 145, 147
    prognostic factor, 38
    Sézary cells, 119, 144
    SLVL, 144, 147
    T-ALL, 37, 48, 144
    tartrate resistant, 144, 147,
      160, 204
    T-cell leukaemias, 119, 144, 147
    T-cell lymphomas, 147
    T-cells, 145
    T-CLL, 117, 119, 144
    T-LbLy, 37, 48, 144
    T-PLL, 119, 144, 145, 146
    ultrastructure, 37
  ANAE, 36, 38, 145
    ALL, 38, 39
    AML, 36
    ATLL, 144
    B-CLL, 144
    B-lineage ALL, 145
    B-PLL, 144
    CD4+ cells, 145
    CD8+ cells, 145
    dot-like pattern, 145
    gall bodiess, 137, 145
    HCL, 144, 161
    large granular lymphocytes,
      145
    lymphoplasmacytic
      lymphoma, 144
    monocytes, 145
    myeloma, 144, 145
    NaF sensitive, 36, 145
    plasma cells, 145
    Sézary cells, 144, 258, 269
    SLVL, 144
    T-ALL, 144
    T-CLL, 117, 144
    T-LbLy, 144
    Tγ-lymphocytes, 145
    T-lymphocytes, 145, 269
    T-PLL, 119, 144, 145
  B-cell leukaemias, 144
  biphenotypic leukaemias, 49
  β-glucosaminidase, 38, 117, 144,
    147
    B-cell disorders, 144, 147
    T-cell disorders, 117, 144, 147
  β-glucuronidase, 38, 147, 258
    B-cell disorders, 144
    T-cell disorders, 146
  DAP I and II, 144
  DAP IV, 117, 144, 146, 147
  hexosaminidase, 39
  isoenzymes, 39
  myeloperoxidase, 36, 48, 49
  non-specific esterase, *see* ANAE
  PAS reaction, 37
  Sudan black, 13, 36, 50
  T-cell leukaemias, 144

Deoxycoformycin, 99, 241
in ATLL, 241
in B-CLL, 99
in B-PLL, 149, 150
in CTCL, 267
in HCL, 170, 171
infections, 171, 267
nephrotoxicity, 170
in Sézary syndrome, 267
side effects, 171, 267
in T-ALL, 170
in T-cell leukaemia, 241
correlation with phenotype,
123, 150, 241, 267
in T-CLL, 123
toxicity, 171
in T-PLL, 150
Dipeptidylaminopeptidase IV
(DAP IV), 117, 144, 146, 147

Epidemiology of ALL, 64
ALL in Africa, 64
ALL in Gaza Strip, 64
ALL in Western countries, 64
Burkitt's in Africa, 65, 205
socioeconomic factors, 65
Epstein–Barr virus, 8, 25, 152, 206
antibody titres, 206
B-cell lines, 25, 152, 205, 206
B-PLL cell lines, 152
differences in Burkitt's
lymphoma types, 205
EBV nuclear antigen, 205, 206
effect on B-CLL, 81
isolation, 206
as mitogen, 151
receptor, 8, 25
relation to Burkitt's lymphoma,
205, 206
relation to malaria, 206

FAB classification, 33
ALL, 33
L1, 33, 35, 36
L2, 33, 35, 36
L3, 34, 48
AML, 18, 19
aneuploidy, 45
cell kinetics, 36, 45
see also Cell kinetics in ALL
cell size, 34, 35
convoluted nucleus, 35, 48, 49
nucleo-/cytoplasmic ratio, 33, 35
prognostic value, 35, 36, 46
scoring for ALL, 34
Follicular lymphoma, 190
anaemia, 194
bcl-2 gene, 214
blastic phase, 193
bone marrow histology, 186, 193
cell volume, 185
chromosome abnormality, 213
classification, 190
clinical features, 190, 193
clinical history, 190
course of the disease, 194
CT scan, 193
detection of minimal residual
disease, 214

Follicular lymphoma, (cont.)
electron microscopy, 191, 192,
193
epidemiology, 191
hepatomegaly, 194
leukaemic phase, 189
correlation with del 13q32, 214
correlation with histology, 190
evolution, 194
evolution to pre B-ALL, 214
incidence, 189
old designations, 190
presentation as ALL, 214
prognostic significance, 194
terminal event, 193
treatment, 211
lymph node histology, 190
patterns of growth, 190
predominant cell type, 190
lymphadenopathy, 193, 194
lymphocytosis resembling CLL,
190, 191
morphology of circulating cells,
191, 192, 193
phenotype, 8, 9, 17, 187
difference from B-CLL, 187,
194
expression of CD25 and
CD10, 188
of leukaemic phase cells, 194,
214
SmIg, 188, 194
TdT, 214
prognosis, 195
prognostic groups, 181
sex predominance, 190
splenic form, 194, 211
splenomegaly, 194
subtypes, 190
thromboycytopenia, 194
transformation, 190, 195
translocation t(14;18), 213, 214
treatment, 194
CHOP/COP/chlorambucil,
194, 211
delay policy, 195
response, 190
single agent vs combination,
195, 211
splenectomy, 211
survival, 190, 195
WBC, 191, 194

Gene rearrangements, 40, 43, 243,
244
in All, 43
in chronic leukaemias, 44, 79
Ig genes, 40, 43, 44
see also under
Immunoglobulin genes
in lymphoid leukaemias, 43, 79
in translocations, 64, 207
in NHLs, 188
in NK cells, 128
sensitivity, 188
significance, 188
T-cell receptor, see under T-cell
receptor gene
unexpected, 246

Haemophagocytic syndrome, 57,
88
Hairy cell leukaemia, 156
age incidence, 156
amyloidosis, 173
anaemia, 156
incidence, 157
isotope studies, 163
pathogenesis, 157, 163
prognostic factor, 165
anti-hairy cell McAbs, 9, 176
B-ly7, 10, 163
CD25, see anti-Tac
HC1, 7, 163, 176
HC2, 6, 7, 8, 9, 163, 164, 174,
176, 204
LeuM5, 10, 163, 164, 174, 204
PCA-1, 10
anti-Tac, 15, 81, 163, 164, 174,
176, 204
associations, 171
atypical forms, 173
autoimmune phenomena, 88
B-cell nature, see under
phenotype and nature of
hairy cells
blood counts, 157
bone marrow, 158
aspirate, 158
biopsy, 158, 167
dry tap, 158
function, 163
normal haemopoiesis, 159
pattern of infiltration, 159
prediction of response to
splenectomy, 159, 167
reticulin, 158
bone marrow form of HCL, 165,
166
cell volume, 81, 162, 174, 175
see also Cell volume
estimations
chromosome abnormalities, 177
clinical features, 156, 157
complications, 177
cutaneous involvement, 173
cytochemistry, see
Cytochemistry
cytopenia, 156, 172
diagnosis, 157
differential diagnosis, 161, 164
with B-CLL, 164
with B-PLL, 164
with follicular lymphoma, 159
with myelofibrosis, 164
with SLVL, 164, 199
with Waldenström's
macroglobulinaemia, 164
electron microscopy, 161, 162
Fc receptors, 163, 177
FMC7, see Monoclonal
antibodies
gene rearrangement, 176
granulocytopenia, 172
see under Neutropenia
hairy cells, 157, 158, 159
in blood films, 157
difference from villous
lymphocytes, 157

Hairy cell leukaemia, (cont.)
  hairy cells, (cont.)
    in HCL-variant, 158, 159, 173, 174
    normal counterparts, 157, 176
    origin, 174
    relation to plasma cells, 173
    relation to prognosis, 165
  HCL-variant, 10, 15, 158, 173
    blood counts, 173
    cell volume, 174, 175
    clinical features, 173
    disease course, 178
    membrane IgG, 173
    M:F ratio, 204
    morphology, 173
    phenotype, 9, 10, 15, 174
    relation to B-PLL, 142, 158, 174
    splenomegaly, 173
    treatment, 174
    ultrastructure, 174
    WBC, 173
  hepatomegaly, 156
  bone marrow, 159
  incidence, 157
  liver, 160
  lymph node, 160
  spleen, 142, 160, 199, 202
  IL-2 receptor, see under anti-Tac
  infections, 156, 171, 172
    α-interferon, 168, 169
  isoenzyme 5, 160
  laboratory findings, 156, 157
  leucocytosis, 157
  leucopenia, 157
  lymphadenopathy, 156, 173
  markers, see phenotype
  'M' bands, 173
  M:F ratio, 204
  monocytopenia, 157, 172
  morphology, 157
    see also hairy cells
  nature of hairy cells, 9, 10, 156, 175
    B-cell features, 173, 175, 176
    monocyte origin, 162, 175
  neutropenia, 156, 165, 172
  non-specific esterases, 161
  osteolytic lesions, 164, 173
  phase contrast, 156
  phenotype, 9, 15, 17, 162, 175, 176
    common to B-cell disorders, 163, 176, 204
    differences from B-CLL, 163, 187
    differences from NHL, 187
    high affinity Fc receptors, 163
    McAbs, 176
    mouse rosettes, 163, 176
    SmIg, 163, 175, 204
    technique, 163
    unique features, 163
  prognostic features, 165, 167
  relation to B-CLL, 81
  RFB1, 16, 163
  spleen function, 163
  spleen histology, 160, 163, 165, 199, 202

Hairy cell leukaemia, (cont.)
  splenectomy, 160, 165, 166, 167, 172
  splenic form, 163, 165
  splenic pooling, 163
  splenomegaly, 156, 157, 163, 165
  staging, 165
  survival, 165
  systemic vasculitis, 172
  T-cell function, 103, 177
  T-cell HCL, 177
  thrombocytopenia, 156, 157
  TRAP activity, 160, 204
    see under Cytochemistry
  treatment, 166
    anthracyclines, 167
    before DCF, 171
    bone marrow transplant, 170
    chemotherapy, 167
    chlorambucil, 167, 168
    cyclophosphamide, 167
    deoxycoformycin, 170, 71
    α-interferon, 168
      see under Interferon
    lithium carbonate, 170
    mononuclear cells, 170
    splenectomy, 166
    splenic irradiation, 170
  WBC, 157
Hairy cell variant, see under Hairy cell leukaemia
Hand-mirror ALL, 36
Heavy chain disease, see under Plasma cell neoplasias
Helper/inducer cells, see under T-lymphocytes
Hodgkin's disease, 16
  confusion with Richter's syndrome, 92, 94
  Ki-1 antigen, 16
  Reed–Sternberg cells, 92
HTLV-I, 231
  antibodies, 233, 238
    in ATLL, 232, 235
    in family members, 234
    in healthy donors, 235, 236
    in T-cell leukaemias, 141, 235
  in Africa, 240
  in ATLL, 231, 237, 238
  cell lines, 232
  in the Caribbean basin, 233, 239
  in Chile, 238
  clonal integration, 218, 228, 233, 236
  in Cuba, 240
  DNA sequences, 237
  HIV, 233, 237
  HTLV-II, 177, 233, 237
  isolation, 232
  in Japan, 239
  mode of transmission, 233, 234
  proviral DNA, 218, 228, 231, 236
  retrovirus in primates, 234
  reverse transcriptase, 231, 237
  risk of ATLL, 236
  RNA tumour viruses, 231
  role in T-cell growth, 231
  serological assays, 238
  stages of HTLV-I infection, 235

HTLV-I, (cont.)
  STLV-I, 235
  tat gene, 227
  tropical spastic paraparesis, 233, 238
Hyperviscosity syndrome, 279, 298

Immune haemolytic anaemia, 76, 88
  in B-CLL, 76, 88, 89
  Evans' syndrome, 88
  idiopathic, 88
  splenectomy, 99
  treatment, 89, 97
Immune thrombocytopenic purpura, 88
  in B-CLL, 88, 89
  Evans' syndrome, 88
  splenectomy, 99
  T-cell abnormalities, 88
  treatment, 89, 97, 99
Immunoglobulin genes, 16, 43
  as clonal markers, 246
  for detection of minimal disease, 247
  errors during rearrangement, 207
  heavy chain gene, 44
  light chain gene, 44
  order of light chain rearrangement, 207
  rearrangements, 44, 242
    in AML, 246
    in B-CLL, 44, 79
    in B-PLL, 44
    in cALL, 44
    in HCL, 44, 176, 247
    in large cell NHL, 208
    in lymphoid leukaemia, 44, 246
    in null-ALL, 44
    in T-ALL, 44, 246
    in T-CLL, 44
    in T-PLL, 44
  relation to chromosome translocations, 207
Immunoglobulins, 5, 41
  as B-markers, see Immunological markers
  gene rearrangement, see under Immunoglobulin genes
  serum Igs in B-CLL, 78
Immunogold method, 10, 236
  B-lymphocytes, 10
  CD4+ cells, 236, 269
  hairy cell counterparts, 176
  in HTLV-I infection, 237
  large granular lymphocytes, 116
  Tac+ lymphocytes, 237
  T-lymphocytes, 102
Immunological classification, 16, 39
  ALL, 16, 39, 40, 41
  AML, 18, 19
  B-ALL, 39, 48
    see also Burkitt's lymphoma
  B-cell nature of HCL, 175, 176
  B-CLL, 79
    see also under B-cell CLL
  biphenotypic leukaemia, 49

Immunological classification,
    (cont.)
  B-PLL, 90
  chronic B-cell leukaemia, 17, 90,
      163, 174, 187, 204
  chronic T-cell leukaemia, 119
  CLL/PL, 90
  common-ALL, 16, 39, 41, 42
    see also Common-ALL
  early B-lineage, 42
  gene rearrangements, 43
    see also Gene rearrangements
  immature T-cell leukaemias, 17,
      18, 117
  lymphoid leukaemias, 16, 39
    B-cell, 16, 17
    T-cell, 17, 18, 117
  mature T-cell leukaemias, 18
  MIC classification, 60
  NHL in leukaemic phase, 187
  non-T-ALL, 12, 16, 43
  non-T, non-B-ALL, 39
  null-ALL, 42
  pre-B-ALL, 16, 39, 41
  pre-T-ALL, 17, 18, 41
  prognosis, 46
  T-ALL, 17, 18, 39, 40, 48
  T-CLL, 117
  terminal transferase, 39
    see also Terminal transferase
  T-PLL, 140, 141
Immunological markers, 1
  acute leukaemia, 18, 19, 39, 49
  in ALL, 40
  anti-hairy cell McAbs, 9, 163,
      174, 176, 204
  anti-plasma cell McAbs, 10
  anti-Tac, 14, 163, 204, 225
  B-lineage, 40, 42, 140
  B-malignancies, 16, 17
  B-markers, 5, 6, 7, 8, 17, 39, 79,
      204
    CyIg, 5, 21, 80
    Cyμ, 39, 42
    monoclonals, 6, 204
    see also Monoclonal
      antibodies
  class II antigens, 14
  E-rosettes, 3, 6, 11, 17, 23, 39,
      80, 226
    in ALL, 39, 40
    in B-CLL, 80
    see also under B-cell CLL
    in Sézary syndrome, 260
  FACS analyser, 4, 82
  Fc receptors, 3, 13, 80, 101
    in B-CLL, 80
    in cytotoxic cells, 23
    in hairy cells, 163, 177
    in T-CLL, 117
  Fc rosettes, 3, 23, 80
  immunofluorescence, 5, 80
  immunoglobulins, see
      Immunoglobulins
  immunoperoxidase, 3, 80
  methodology, 3, 19
  monoclonal antibodies see
      Monoclonal antibodies
  M-rosettes, 3, 5, 17

Immunological markers, (cont.)
  M-rosettes, (cont.)
    in B-CLL, 79, 90
    in HCL, 163, 176
  myeloid antigens, 18, 19
    in ALL, 50
    in AML, MO, 5
    in biphenotypic leukaemia, 49
  rosettes, 3
  SmIg, 5, 8, 17, 79, 163, 204
  TdT, see under Terminal
      transferase
  T-lineage, 40
  T-malignancies, 17, 18, 41, 117
  T-markers, 5, 10, 12, 14, 17, 18,
      39
    antigens, 39, 140
    monoclonals, see Monoclonal
      antibodies
Infections, 56, 86
  in ALL, 56, 57
  in CLL, 86, 88, 100
  in CTCL, 263
  in HCL, 171, 172
Interferon, 100, 168
  in B-CLL, 100
  in B-PLL, 150
  in HCL, 168, 169, 171
  γ-interferon, 24, 102
  mechanism of action, 168
  in myeloma, 288
  receptors, 169
  release by normal T-cells, 125
  side effects, 169
Interleukin-1, 20
  in myeloma, 278
  in T-cell colonies, 4
Interleukin-2, 14, 20, 102
  antibodies, 14
  gene, 23
  in leukaemia, 15, 80, 118, 261,
      269
  in long-term cultures, 231
  purified IL-2, 23
  receptor, 14, 80, 179, 269
  recombinant IL-2, 23
  release by T-CLL cells, 125
  release by T-lymphocytes, 125
  role in T-cell clones, 23
  role in T-cell growth, 23, 231
  source, 23, 24
  in T-cell colonies, 21
Intermediate lymphoma, 195
  age of incidence, 197
  alternative designations, 195
  anaemia, 197
  bone marrow histology, 196
  chromosome abnormalities, 213,
      214
  clinical course, 198
  clinical features, 197
  constitutional symptoms, 197
  leukaemic phase, 195, 196, 198
  lymph node histology, 195, 196
  lymphocytosis, 196
  M:F ratio, 197
  morphology of circulating cells,
      195, 196
  phenotype, 187, 188, 197

Intermediate lymphoma, (cont.)
  prognosis, 198
  spleen histology, 196
  stage of NHL, 197
  survival, 198
  thrombocytopenia, 197
  treatment responses, 198, 211
  WBC, 196, 197, 198

Killer cells, 13, 22, 23, 24, 102, 103

Large cell NHL in leukaemic
    phase, see under non-
      Hodgkin's lymphoma
Large granular lymphocytes, 115
  cytochemistry, 145
  cytotoxicity, 23
  function, 23, 126
  markers, 13
  in T-CLL, 115
    see also T-cell chronic
      lymphocytic leukaemia
  ultrastructure, 102, 116
    PTAs, 116, 117
Large granular lymphocytic
    leukaemia, see T-cell chronic
      lymphocytic leukaemia
Leukaemic phase of non-Hodgkin's
    lymphoma, see under non-
      Hodgkin's lymphoma
Lymph node biopsy, 78, 92
  in ATLL, 228, 229
  in B-PLL, 142
  in B-CLL, 78
  in NHLs, see under non-
      Hodgkin's lymphoma
  in Richter's syndrome, 92
Lymphoblastoid B-cell lines, 25,
    206
  B-CLL cell lines, 25
  B-PLL cell lines, 25, 152
  Burkitt cell lines, 25, 206, 207
  HCL lines, 25, 177
  immortalization by EBV, 152
  normal B-cells, 25
Lymphocyte function tests, 19
  antibody-dependent, see
      cytotoxic assays
  B-cell lines, 25, 152
  B-colonies, 20, 25
  colony growth, 20, 21, 23, 103
  cytotoxic assays, 22
    in B-cell leukaemia, 104
    killer cells, 22
    natural killer, 22, 268
    in T-CLL, 23, 124
  helper function, 21
    assay, 21
    CD4+ subsets, 22
    in leukaemia, 22, 102, 103,
        104, 124, 141, 268
    PWM driven, 21
  phytohaemagglutinin, 20, 24
  release of soluble factors, 125
  soluble factors, 24, 241
  suppressor function, 21, 124
    assay, 21
    cells, 21

Lymphocyte function assays,
    (cont.)
  suppressor function, (cont.)
    in leukaemia, 22, 24, 104, 124,
      268
    myeloid colonies, 125, 126
  T-cell clones, 23, 24
  T-cell colonies, 20, 23
    in CTCL, 268
    in leukaemia, 21, 101, 103, 104
    in T-CLL, 125
  T-cell growth, 23
  T-cell lines, 23, 24
  T-cell related, 20
  TPA, 23
  transformation, 20
Lymphocyte transformation, 20
Lymphocytes, see under B- and
    T-lymphocytes
Lymphoplasmacytic lymphoma,
    16, 17, 198, 199, 202, 297

Mantle zone NHL, 195
Mitogens, 15
  B-cell mitogens, 81, 85
  concanavalin A, 21
  effect on B-CLL, 176
  Epstein–Barr virus, see under
    Epstein–Barr virus
  lipopolysaccharide, 81
  phytohaemagglutinin, 20, 21, 24,
    101, 103, 104
    decreased response in T-CLL,
      124, 125, 126
    in HTLV-I+ individuals, 235
    in Sézary syndrome, 268
  pokeweed mitogen, 81, 101, 103,
    176, 268
  polyclonal B-cell activators, 104,
    177
  T-cell mitogens, 15, 20
    antigen changes, 15, 16
    response in CTCL, 268
    source of IL-2, 23, 102
  TPA, 106
Mixed acute leukaemia, see under
    Biphenotypic leukaemia
Monoclonal antibodies, 1, 6, 7, 10,
    11, 40
  in ALL, 19, 40
    see also Immunological
      classification
  in AML, 18, 19
  against B and T antigens, 15
  B-cell antigens, 6, 7, 40
  in B-CLL, 80, 204
  BE1, BE2, 11, 14, 18, 261
  in biphenotypic leukaemia, 49
  B-ly7, 7, 10, 163
  BU11, 140, 143, 204
  CD1a, 11, 12, 18, 40, 117, 118,
    260
  CD2, 6, 11, 13, 18, 40, 117, 260
  CD3, 11, 12, 13, 14, 18, 40, 41,
    117, 118, 123, 225, 226, 243,
    260
  CD4, 11, 13, 14, 18, 21, 22, 23,
    40, 101, 103, 145, 147, 226,
    236, 243, 260, 268

Monoclonal antibodies, (cont.)
  CD5, 11, 13, 15, 17, 18, 40, 80,
    118, 163
  CD7, 11, 12, 13, 18, 19, 40, 118,
    140, 228, 260
  CD8, 11, 13, 14, 18, 21, 22, 23,
    24, 40, 101, 103, 118, 123,
    147, 243, 260, 268
  CD9, 6, 7, 8, 10
  CD10, 7, 8, 16, 17, 39, 40, 41
  CD11b, 11, 13, 22, 23, 116, 117,
    118
  CD11c, 10, 81, 163, 174, 204
  CD13, 19
  CD16, 11, 13, 23, 102, 116
  CD19, 6, 7, 16, 17, 19, 40, 80
  CD20, 6, 7, 17, 40, 80, 81, 163
  CD21, 8, 17, 80, 81, 163
  CD22, 7, 9, 163
    cytoplasmic, 16, 40, 42
  CD23, 7, 80
  CD24, 6, 7, 16, 40, 80
  CD25, 11, 14, 15, 17, 18, 20, 118,
    174, 261
    in ATLL, 225, 228
    in B-CLL, 80, 81, 204
    in HCL, 81, 163, 176, 204
  CD29, 11, 13, 14, 226
  CD33, 18, 19
  CD34, 18, 19
  CD38, 7, 10, 15, 16, 17, 188, 203,
    269
  CD45O, 11, 13, 14, 21
  CD45R, 11, 13, 14, 21, 226
  CD57, 11, 13, 23, 102, 103, 117,
    118
  CD70, 16
  clusters of differentiation, 7, 11
  in CSF, 55
  FMC7, 6, 7, 8, 9, 17, 80, 81, 90,
    140, 163, 176, 188, 203, 204
  HC1, 7, 9, 163
  HC2, 6, 7, 9, 17, 163, 174, 176,
    203, 204
  HLA-DR, 7, 8, 17, 118, 163
  Leu8, 11, 14, 268
  myeloid antigens, 18, 19
    in null-ALL, 42
  PCA-1, PC-1, 6, 7, 10, 18
  R1-3, 6, 7, 10
  SN1, SN2, 14
  T17, 11, 12, 18, 118
  in T-ALL, 17, 18, 19, 39, 40, 41,
    48
  T-cell antigens, 10, 11, 18, 19,
    37, 40
  T-cell leukaemias, 12, 13, 14, 17,
    18, 19, 40, 41, 117
    in T-CLL, 117
  Y29/55, 7
Mycosis fungoides, 253
  blood involvement, 264
  clinical findings, 254
  laboratory findings, 254
  lymphadenopathy, 253
  skin lesions, 219, 230, 255, 262
  stages, 254
  treatment, 264
  visceral involvement, 264

Myeloid antigens, 43
  in ALL, 49
  in biphenotypic leukaemia, 50
  in null-ALL, 43
  significance, 50
Myelomatosis, 277
  age, 277
  amyloidosis, 173, 293, 294
  anaemia, 278, 279
  Bence Jones proteinuria, 278,
    280, 284
  blood counts, 278, 279
  bone lesions, 278, 283
  bone marrow, 280, 281, 284
  cell kinetics, 300
  chromosome abnormalities, 301,
    302
  circulating plasma cells, 294
  clinical features, 278
  complications, 289
  cord compression, 280
  CT scan, 283
  cultures/colonies, 299
  diagnosis, 280, 282
  differential diagnosis, 280, 282
  electron microscopy, 281, 282,
    283, 295
  fractures, 278
  granulocytopenia, 279, 290
  hypercalcaemia, 278, 279, 290
  hypercalciuria, 279
  hyperviscosity syndrome, 279
  hyperuricaemia, 279, 289
  hypogammaglobulinaemia, 279,
    280, 290
  imaging techniques, 283
  immunoelectrophoresis, 280
  immunoparesis, 280
  immunostaining, 282
  incidence, 277
  incidence of acute leukaemia,
    291
  infections, 279, 290
  labelling index, 45, 46
  leucopenia, 279
  magnetic resonance, 283
  M-component, 277, 278, 280, 284
  β_2-microglobulin, 284, 285
  monitoring therapy, 291
  myeloma kidney, 279
  non-secretory myeloma, 278,
    280, 282, 283
  osteoclast activating factor, 278
  osteolytic lesions, 278, 283
  paraprotein, 277, 278, 280, 284
  phenotype, 16, 17
  plasma cell leukaemia, 294
  plasmacytoma, extramedullary,
    see under Plasma cell
      neoplasias
  prognostic factors, 278, 279, 283,
    284, 285
  renal failure, 279, 284, 289, 290
  renal function, 279
  secondary acute leukaemia, 291,
    302
  serum alkaline phosphatase, 283
  serum creatinine, 285
  smouldering myeloma, 286, 300

Myelomatosis, (cont.)
  solitary myeloma, 292, 293
  staging of myeloma, 283, 284, 285, 286
  survival, 284, 285, 286
  T-cell function, 103, 104, 290, 300
  tests for drug sensitivity, 299, 300
  thrombocytopenia, 279
  transformation, 291, 292
  treatment, 286
    ABCM protocol, 287
    alkylating agents, 286
    autologous BMT, 287
    BCNU, 286, 287, 288
    BMT, allogeneic, syngeneic, 289
    calcitonin, 290
    chemotherpay, 286
    combinations, 286, 287
    cyclophosphamide, 286, 288
    diphosphonates, 290
    doxorubicin, 286, 287, 288
    high dose melphalan, 287, 296
    hydration therapy, 290
    interferon, 288
    M2 protocol, 287
    maintenance, 287
    melphalan, 286, 287, 288
    monitoring, 288, 291
    plasmapheresis, 289
    plateau phase, 287
    prednisone, 286, 287, 290
    radiation, 289
    relapses, 288
    remission rate, 287, 288
    response criteria, 287
    sarcolysin, 286
    trials, 286, 287
    VAD, 286, 287, 296
    VAMP, 287, 288, 296
    vincristine, 286, 287, 288
    weekly cyclophosphamide, 288
  X-rays, 283

Natural killer cells, 13, 22, 23, 102, 128
Non-Hodgkin's lymphoma, 182
  bone marrow histology, 186, 187, 193, 196
  bone 'spill-over', 186, 196
  B-lymphoblastic, 183
  cell volume, 185
  centrocytic, 195
  chromosome abnormalities, 212, 213, 214, 215, 301
  classification, 182
    Kiel, 183
    place of ATLL, 184, 190, 229
    Rappaport, 182
    working formulation, 183, 190, 229
  clinical course, 211
  diagnosis, 189
  differential diagnosis, 185, 187, 188
  DNA analysis, 188
    see also under Gene rearrangements

Non-Hodgkin's lymphoma, (cont.)
  follicular lymphoma, 190
    see also under Follicular lymphoma
  high-grade NHL, 189
  histology, 186
  imaging, 15, 193
  immunoblastic, 229
  immunocytochemistry, 187
  immunocytoma, see under Lymphoplasmacytic lymphoma and Splenic lymphoma with villous lymphocytes
  intermediate or mantle zone, 195
    see under Intermediate lymphoma
  laboratory investigations, 184, 185
  large cell NHL, 207
    B and T types, 208, 229
    bone marrow involvement, 207
    complete remissions, 208, 209, 212
    leukaemic phase, 207
    morphology, 207, 208, 209
    phenotype, 188, 208
    prognosis, 190, 208
    treatment, 212
  leukaemia/lymphoma syndromes, 184, 190, 199
  leukaemic phase, 182, 183
    definition, 189
    diagnosis, 189
    of follicular lymphoma, 190
      see under Follicular lymphoma
    incidence, 189
    of intermediate lymphoma, 196
    of large cell lymphoma, 207
    prognostic significance, 189, 194, 210
  lymphoplasmacytic lymphoma, 198, 199
    clinicopathological syndromes, 198
    diagnostic criteria, 198
    incidence, 198
    'M' bands, 198
    phenotype, 16, 17
    spleen histology, 202
    Waldenström's, see Waldenström's macroglobulinaemia
    with IgG or IgA paraprotein, 199
  low-grade NHL, 189, 190, 198
  membrane markers, 17, 187, 188, 197
  morphology, 185
  phenotype, 17, 187, 188, 197
  prognosis, 189, 211
  prognostic factors, 190
  SLVL, see Splenic lymphoma with villous lymphocytes
  spleen histology, 186, 202
  T-immunoblastic, 184, 208, 211

Non-Hodgkin's lymphoma, (cont.)
  treatment, 209, 211, 212
  WBC, 190

Oncogenes, 63
  bcl-1, 214
  bcl-2, 213, 214
  c-abl, 61, 63, 64
  c-myc, 63, 64, 213, 214
  c-is in CGL, 64

Parallel tubular arrays, 116, 117
PAS reaction, 37
Philadelphia-positive ALL, 60, 61, 63
Phorbol esters, 42
  in ALL, 42
  in B-CLL, 81
  in T-cell growth, 23
  TPA as mitogen in B-CLL, 106
Plasma cell leukaemia, 294
  anaemia, 295
  chromosomes, 301
  diagnostic criteria, 294, 295
  differential diagnosis, 295
  hypercalcaemia, 295
  incidence, 294
  median survival, 296
  plasma cell numbers, 294, 295
  phenotype, 16, 17, 295
  prognosis, 296
  renal failure, 295
  treatment, 296
  ultrastructure, 295
Plasma cell neoplasias, 277
  amyloidosis, 293
  anti-plasma cell McAbs, 10
  B-cell antigens, 10
  benign monoclonal gammopathy, 292, 300
  cell kinetics, 300
  α-chain disease, 296, 297
  γ-chain disease, 296
  μ-chain disease, 297
  chromosome abnormalities, 301
  classification, 277
  extramedullary plasmacytoma, 293
  heavy chain disease, 296, 297
  in vitro cloning, 299
  myelomatosis, 277
  phenotype, 16, 17
  plasma cell leukaemia, see under Plasma cell leukaemia
  solitary myeloma, 292, 293
  special studies, 299
  T-cell abnormalities, 103, 104, 290, 300
  Waldenström's macroglobulinaemia, 297
Prognostic factors in ALL, 45, 46, 47, 51, 59
Prognostic factors in B-CLL, 82
  age, 83, 84
  anaemia, 83, 84
  bone marrow histology, 83, 84
  doubling time, 83, 84
  haemoglobin, 84
  hepatosplenomegaly, 83

Prognostic factors in B-CLL,
    (cont.)
  karyotype, 83, 85
  light chains, 85
  lymphadenopathy, 83
  lymphocyte count, 83, 84
  multivariate analysis, 82, 86
  prolymphocyte count, 83, 84, 92
  response to mitogens, 85
  response to treatment, 83, 85
  sex, 83, 84
  splenomegaly, 83
  staging, 83, 85, 87
    Binet, 84, 86, 87
    International, 85, 87
    Rai, 84, 85, 87
  thrombocytopenia, 83, 84
  tumour mass, 84
Prolymphocytic leukaemia, 132
  age, 133
  anaemia, 133
  ascites, 133
  biochemistry, 133
  bone marrow biopsy, 141
  B-PLL, 90, 133, 135, 142
  cell volume, 82, 174, 186, 204
  chromosomes, 150
    B-PLL, 60, 151
    T-PLL, 152
  clinical course, 119, 147
  clinical features, 132
  cytochemistry, 119, 144
    see also Cytochemistry
  diagnosis, 133
  differences between B- and T-
    PLL, 133
  differences from CLL/PL, 134
  differential diagnosis, 134, 140,
    142
    with ATLL, 143
    with B-CLL, 142
    with CLL/PL, 142
    with HCL-V, 142, 143
    with NHL, 143
    score for borderline cases, 142
    with Sézary cell leukaemia, 143
    with Sézary syndrome, 143
    with SLVL, 143, 204
    with T-CLL, 144
  electron microscopy, 82, 83, 135,
    137, 138
  functional assays, 141, 227
  gene rearrangements, 140, 244,
    245
  histopathology, 141
  HTLV-I status, 141, 143
  immunoblasts, 134
  incidence between B- and T-
    disorders, 132
  inclusions in B-PLL cells, see
    electron microsocpy
  laboratory findings, 132, 133
  lymph node histology, 142
  lymphadenopathy, 133
  'M' bands, 133
  markers, see phenotype
  M:F ratio, 133, 204
  morphology, 119, 133, 134, 135,
    136

Prolymphocytic leukaemia, (cont.)
  natural history, 148
  percentage prolymphocytes, 90,
    134
  phenotype, 7, 140
    B-PLL, 7, 8, 9, 17, 80, 140, 176
    BU11 McAb, 140, 143, 204
    co-expression of CD4 and
      CD8, 140
    differences from B-CLL, 140
    membrane Igs, 140, 204
    origin of T-prolymphocytes,
      141
    relation to HCL, 140, 174, 176
    T-PLL, 12, 15, 17, 18, 119, 140
  pleural effusions, 133
  presenting symptoms, 133
  prognosis, 147
  Rai staging for B-PLL, 148
  relation to B-CLL, 90, 92
  relation to HCL-variant, 142,
    158, 174
  relative incidence, 153
  serum Igs, 133
  skin lesions, 133
  spleen histology, 142
  splenectomy, 148, 149
  splenomegaly, 132, 133
  survival, 133, 148, 150
  thrombocytopenia, 133
  T-lymphocyte function, 102, 141
  T-PLL, 18, 113, 135, 143
    Caribbean born, 228
    helper function, 227
    other designations, 137
    small cell type, 136, 137, 143
    T-colonies, 21
  treatment, 147, 148
    B-PLL, 148
    chlorambucil, 150
    CHOP, 149, 150
    deoxycoformycin, 149, 150
    α-interferon, 150
    intrathecal methotrexate, 150
    leucapheresis, 149
    prednisolone, 150
    splenectomy, 148, 149
    splenic irradiation, 148
    'thymic' irradiation, 150
    T-PLL, 150
  variant forms of T-PLL, 119
  WBC, 133
Prolymphocytoid transformation,
  90

Rai staging, 75, 76, 84, 85, 87
Red cell aplasia, 24
  in B-CLL, 24, 89
  in T-CLL, 114, 126
Relapse in ALL, 54
  bone marrow, 53, 54
  CNS, 50, 52, 53, 55
  eye, 54
  iris, 54
  meningeal, 50, 52, 53, 55
  optic nerve, 54
  ovaries, 54
  prophylactic irradiation, 56
  testicular, 55, 56

Relapse in ALL, (cont.)
  testicular biopsy, 56
  time of relapse, 54
Richter's syndrome, 90, 92, 93

Serum immunoglobulins, 78
  in B-CLL, 78
  in B-PLL, 133
  in myeloma, 279, 280
Sézary cell leukaemia, 228, 261
Sézary cells, see under Sézary
    syndrome
Sézary syndrome, 218, 232, 253
  bone marrow sparing, 255
  cell markers, 260
  cell volume, 257
  clinical findings, 254
  cytochemistry, 119, 144, 147,
    258, 269
  electron microscopy, 137, 257
  helper function, 227, 268
  hepatomegaly, 253, 264
  karyotype, 269, 270
    see also Chromosome
      abnormalities
  laboratory findings, 254
  lymph node histology, 260
  lymphadenopathy, 253, 264
  Lutzner cells, 256
  morphology, see Sézary cells
  phenotype, 14, 260, 269
  Sézary cell leukaemia, 261
    HTLV-I status, 228
    phenotype, 261
  Sézary cells, 221, 222, 256, 264
    analogy with hairy cells, 269
    in ATLL, 230
    in cord blood, 269
    differences from ATLL, 222,
      268
    DNA content, 269
    function, 268
    large, 256, 262, 263, 269
    normal counterpart, 269
    in normals, 236, 269
    ploidy, 269
    in prognosis, 263
    response to PHA, 269
    small, 256, 269
    T-cell nature, 269
  skin histology, 259, 260
  skin lesions, 219, 230, 256
  splenomegaly, 253
  treatment, see under Cutaneous
    T-cell lymphoma
Splenectomy, 99, 166
  in B-CLL, 86, 99, 100
  in B-PLL, 149
  in HCL, 166
  in SLVL, 202, 204, 211
  in T-CLL, 123
Splenic lymphoma with villous
    lymphocytes, 199
  age, 202, 204
  anaemia, 202
  bone marrow, 202
  cell volume, 186, 204
  clinical course, 204, 211
  clinical features, 202, 203

Splenic lymphoma with villous
    lymphocytes, (cont.)
cytochemistry, 144, 147, 200
cytopenia, 204
diagnosis, 199, 202
differential diagnosis, 199, 200,
    202, 203, 204
laboratory findings, 202, 203
light chains in urine, 203
lymph node histology, 202
lymphocytosis, 202
'M' band, 199, 202, 203, 204
marker studies, 187, 203, 204
membrane Ig, 204
monocytopenia, 202
morphology, 199, 200, 203, 204
neutropenia, 202
phenotype, 187, 203, 204
prognosis, 204
relation to immunocytoma, 184
relation to lymphoplasmacytic
    NHL, 184, 199
sex predominance, 202
spleen histology, 197, 199, 202,
    204
splenectomy, 202, 204
splenomegalic B-cell disorders,
    204
splenomegaly, 202, 204
tartrate-resistant acid
    phosphatase, 200, 204
thrombocytopenia, 202
treatment, 202, 204, 211
types of villous projections, 200
ultrastructure, 200, 201
WBC, 202, 204

T-cell activation, 13, 14, 15, 16, 20,
    24
T-cell chronic lymphocytic
    leukaemia, 113
age distribution, 114
alternative names, 113, 119, 127
anaemia, 114
animal model, 113
blood counts, 114
bone marrow, 114, 116
cell markers, see phenotype
chromosome abnormalities, 126
clinical course, 119, 120, 121
clinical features, 113, 114
clonal nature, 127
cytochemistry, 117, 119
cytopenias, 114, 121
cytotoxic function, 123
diagnostic criteria, 115
differential diagnosis, 115, 118,
    119, 120
functional studies, 123, 124, 125
hypergammaglobulinaemia, 115
hypogammaglobulinaemia, 115,
    124, 126
incidence within CLL, 113
infections, 120
'knobby' type of CLL, 137
laboratory findings, 113
management, 121
morphology, 115, 119
myeloid colonies, 125

T-cell chronic lymphocytic
    leukaemia, (cont.)
natural history, 120
nature of T-cell proliferation,
    127
pathogenesis of anaemia, 24, 125
pathogenesis of neutropenia, 24,
    125, 126
phenotype, 17, 18, 117, 118, 119,
    124, 125
prognosis, 120, 121
red cell hypoplasia, 114, 126
relation to rheumatoid arthritis,
    115, 145
spontaneous regression, 127
survival, 121
TCR rearrangements, 127, 128
    see also T-cell receptor gene
thrombocytopenia, 114
T-lymphocytosis, 113, 117, 123
transformation, 121
treatment, 120, 121, 123
ultrastructure, 115, 116, 117
WBC, 114, 119, 123
T-cell colonies, see under
    Lymphocyte function assays
T-cell function, see under T-
    lymphocytes
T-cell lines, 23, 24
T-cell lymphocytosis, 113, 117, 123
T-cell receptor gene, 13, 14, 40, 45,
    243
in B-CLL, 79
in CD3− T-CLL, 128
CD3 complex, 12, 243, 244
chronic T-cell leukaemias, 127,
    128, 245
as clonal marker, 246
for detection of minimal disease,
    247
genes, 13, 243
    α-chain, 243
    β-chain, 13, 127, 128, 243, 244
    δ-chain, 128, 243
    γ-chain, 13, 127, 128, 243, 244
germ-line, 128, 244
in NK cells, 128
rearrangements, 244
    in AML, 246
    in B-CLL, 246
    in B-lineage ALL, 246
    in CTCL, 262
    in HCL, 246
    in leukaemia, 244
    in lymphomatoid papulosis,
        262
    in relapse, 246
    in T-ALL, 244
    in T-CLL, 127, 128
    in TdT+ AML, 246
relation to T-phenotype, 243
T-CLL/T-cell lymphocytosis,
    127, 245
types of TCR, 243
unexpected rearrangements, 246
Terminal transferase, 39
in ALL, 18, 19, 39, 40, 41
in AML, 12, 18, 19, 39, 49
in biphenotypic leukaemia, 49, 50

Terminal transferase, (cont.)
in CSF fluid, 55
lymphoid precursor cells, 40
in pre-T-ALL, 41
role in gene rearrangement, 246
in T-ALL, 41, 188
in T-cell leukaemias, 12, 17, 18,
    19, 188
TdT positive AML, 49
in T-lymphoblastic lymphoma,
    188
T-lymphoblastic leukaemia, 47
age incidence, 48
blood counts, 48
cell markers, see under
    phenotype
cytochemistry, 37, 48, 144, 147
epidemiology, 64, 65
facial palsy, 55
hepatosplenomegaly, 48
incidence, 41, 64
karyotype, 58, 60
lymphadenopathy, 48
mediastinal mass, 32, 47
morphology, 34, 48
    see also FAB classification
phenotype, 11, 12, 15, 17, 18, 19,
    39, 40, 41, 48
    clinical relevance, 41
    early and late phenotype, 41
    differences from T-LbLy, 48,
        184
presenting features, 48
pre-T-ALL, 17, 18, 39
prognosis, 46, 48
relation to T-LbLy, 47, 48, 184
T-lymphoblastic lymphoma, 47
acid phosphatase, 38, 48, 144
age of incidence, 48
cell markers, see under
    phenotype
cytochemistry, 48, 144
mediastinal mass, 47
phenotype, 11, 17, 18, 39, 48,
    184
pleural effusions, 48
prognosis, 48
relation to T-ALL, 47, 48, 184,
    211
treatment, 211
T-lymphocytes, 10, 12, 100
abnormalities in B-cell
    leukaemia, 104, 206
antigens, 10, 11, 14, 15, 39, 41
in B-cell leukaemias, 100
    B-PLL, 102, 104
    Burkitt's lymphoma, 206
    CLL, 101, 102, 104
    HCL, 103, 104
    myelomatosis, 103, 104
colonies, 20, 21, 23, 29
    in B-CLL, 101
    in HCL, 103
    in T-CLL, 125
cytochemistry, 144, 145
cytotoxic, 12, 13, 22, 23, 103
functional assays, 19
    see also Lymphocyte function
        assays

T-lymphocytes, (cont.)
  helper/inducer, 12, 13, 14
    helper function, 21, 102
    response to PHA, 20
  inhibition of haemopoiesis, 24,
    125, 126
  interaction with other cells, 24
  killer cells, 13, 22, 23, 24, 102,
    103
  large granular, see under Large
    granular lymphocytes
  natural killer cells, 13, 22, 23,
    102, 103, 128
  post-thymic, 13
  receptor, see under T-cell
    receptor gene
  resting, 15
  role in aplastic anaemia, 24
  subsets, 12, 13, 14, 21
  suppressor, 12, 13, 14, 20
    function, 21, 124
    of Ig synthesis, 124, 126
  T-cell clones, 23
  Tγ-cells, 3, 13, 23, 24, 101, 116,
    117
  Tμ-cells, 3, 101, 117
  transformation, 20, 21
  sensitivity to steroids, 24
Thymic phenotype, 11, 12, 40, 48
  acid phosphatase, 37
  cortical thymocytes, 12
  differences betwen T-ALL and
    T-LbLy, 48
  post-thymic cells, 13, 17, 113
Treatment of ALL, 50
  Ara-C, 50, 52
  BFM studies, 52, 54
  bone marrow transplantation,
    57, 58, 211
    see also Bone marrow
      transplantation
  CALGB studies, 51
  CNS prophylaxis, 50, 51, 52
  consolidation, 51
  cranial irradiation, 52

Treatment of ALL, (cont.)
  cyclophosphamide, 52, 57
  daunorubicin, 51
  dexamethasone, 52
  doxorubicin, 51, 52
  etoposide, 52
  folinic acid, 52
  induction, 51
  landmarks, 50
  L-asparaginase, 50, 51
  Leucovorin, 52
  maintenance, 51, 53, 54
  meningeal leukaemia, 52, 53
  6-mercaptopurine, 52, 53, 54
  methotrexate, 52, 53, 54
  mitozantrone, 50
  prednisolone, 51
  prednisone, 51
  reinductions, 50, 54
  teniposide, 50
  total body irradiation, 57
  total therapy, 50
  UKALL trials, 51, 52, 53, 56
  vincristine, 51, 52
Treatment of B-CLL, 94
  alkylating agents, 96
  α-interferon, 100
  carmustine, 96
  chemotherapy, 96
  chlorambucil, 96, 97
  CHOP, 96
  complete response, 95
  COP, 96
  corticosteroids, 97, 98
  deoxycoformycin, 99
  fludarabine, 99
  hydroxydaunorubicin, 96
  improvement, 95
  indications, 94
  M2 protocol, 96
  melphalan, 96
  MRC CLL Trial, 96, 97
  oncovin, 96
  partial response, 95
  prednisolone, 96

Treatment of B-CLL, (cont.)
  radiation, 98
  splenectomy, 86, 96, 99, 100
Tumour necrosis factor, 106
  in CLL, 106
  effect of anti-TNF antibodies,
    106
  levels in cell proliferation, 106
  in myeloma, 278

Waldenström's
  macroglobulinaemia, 198, 297
  age of incidence, 297
  anaemia, 298
  Bence Jones proteinuria, 298
  blood films, 298
  bone marrow, 298
  bone pain/lesions, 298
  chromosomes, 302
  clincial course, 298
  clinical features, 298
  cryoglobulins, 298
  diagnosis, 298
  differential diagnosis, 199
  hepatomegaly, 298
  hyperviscosity syndrome, 279,
    298
  laboratory findings, 298
  lymphadenopathy, 298
  lymphocytosis, 298
  'M' band, 198, 199, 297, 298
  management, 298
  osteolytic lesions, 173, 298
  phenotype, 17
  prognosis, 299
  relation to lymphoplasmacytic
    lymphoma, 198, 297
  serum Igs, 298
  serum viscosity, 298
  survival, 299
  symptoms, 298
  thrombocytopenia, 298
  treatment, 299